Teen Health Series

D1502170

Multiple Sclerosis
SOURCEBOOK

Health Reference Series

First Edition

Multiple Sclerosis
SOURCEBOOK

*Basic Consumer Health Information about Multiple
Sclerosis (MS) and Its Effects on Mobility, Vision, Bladder
Function, Speech, Swallowing, and Cognition, Including
Facts about Risk Factors, Causes, Diagnostic Procedures,
Pain Management, Drug Treatments, and Physical and
Occupational Therapies*

*Along with Guidelines for Nutrition and Exercise, Tips
on Choosing Assistive Equipment, Information about
Disability, Work, Financial, and Legal Issues, a Glossary
of Related Terms, and a Directory of Additional Resources*

Edited by
Joyce Brennfleck Shannon

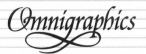

Omnigraphics

P.O. Box 31-1640, Detroit, MI 48231-1640

Bibliographic Note

Because this page cannot legibly accommodate all the copyright notices, the Bibliographic Note portion of the Preface constitutes an extension of the copyright notice.

Edited by Joyce Brennfleck Shannon

Health Reference Series

Karen Bellenir, *Managing Editor*
David A. Cooke, M.D., *Medical Consultant*
Elizabeth Collins, *Research and Permissions Coordinator*
Cherry Stockdale, *Permissions Assistant*
EdIndex, Services for Publishers, *Indexers*

* * *

Omnigraphics, Inc.

Matthew P. Barbour, *Senior Vice President*
Kay Gill, *Vice President—Directories*
Kevin M. Hayes, *Operations Manager*

* * *

Peter E. Ruffner, *Publisher*

Copyright © 2007 Omnigraphics, Inc.

ISBN 978-0-7808-0998-7

Library of Congress Cataloging-in-Publication Data

Multiple sclerosis sourcebook : basic consumer health information about multiple sclerosis (MS) and its effects on mobility, vision, bladder function, speech, swallowing, and cognition, including facts about risk factors, causes, diagnostic procedures, pain management, drug treatments, and physical and occupational therapies; along with guidelines for nutrition and exercise, tips on choosing assistive equipment, information about disability, work, financial, and legal issues, a glossary of related terms, and a directory of additional resources / edited by Joyce Brennfleck Shannon. -- 1st ed.
   p. cm. -- (Health references series)
   Summary: "Provides basic consumer health information about symptoms, diagnosis, treatment, and management of multiple sclerosis. Includes index, glossary of related terms, and other resources"--Provided by publisher.
   Includes bibliographical references and index.
   ISBN 978-0-7808-0998-7 (hardcover : alk. paper) 1. Multiple sclerosis--Popular works. I. Shannon, Joyce Brennfleck.
   RC377.M8638 2007
   616.8'34--dc22

                                                              2007037548

Table of Contents

Visit www.healthreferenceseries.com to view *A Contents Guide to the Health Reference Series*, a listing of more than 13,000 topics and the volumes in which they are covered.

Part II: Symptoms of Multiple Sclerosis

Part III: Diagnostic Tests, Treatments, and Therapies for Multiple Sclerosis

Part V: Multiple Sclerosis and Work, Financial, and Legal Issues

Part VI: Additional Help and Information

Preface

About This Book

With approximately 10,000 new cases diagnosed each year in the United States, multiple sclerosis is the most common neurological disorder that strikes young adults. The risk is double for Caucasian women; however, men, children, and other racial groups also contract multiple sclerosis. It is a difficult, unpredictable autoimmune disease that affects the central nervous system. Symptoms may include pain, sudden weakness, or difficulties with vision, speech, or mobility. Many people with multiple sclerosis experience problems such as fatigue, a limp, or difficulties with bladder control, and about 15% need to use a wheelchair full-time. Currently, there is no cure, but several therapies can relieve the symptoms and, in some cases, delay disease progression.

Multiple Sclerosis Sourcebook, First Edition provides information about risk factors, causes, and types of multiple sclerosis and its effects on mobility, vision, bladder function, speech, swallowing, and cognition. Treatments and rehabilitation therapies are described, guidelines for nutrition and exercise are discussed, and tips on choosing assistive equipment are provided. Information about issues related to disability resources, workplace concerns, and financial planning is also included, along with a glossary and directory of resources.

How to Use This Book

This book is divided into parts and chapters. Parts focus on broad areas of interest. Chapters are devoted to single topics within a part.

Part I: Multiple Sclerosis: Causes, Risk Factors, and Disease Course presents information about autoimmune disease and the cellular, genetic, nerve, and myelin processes involved with MS. It includes facts about how toxic agents, nutrition, or infection may trigger MS and describes other demyelinating disorders and diseases that mimic MS. Individual chapters explain the progression of MS and how MS impacts specific segments of the population.

Part II: Symptoms of Multiple Sclerosis describes the types of physical concerns that develop in people with MS, including movement problems, tremors, pain, fatigue, speech, swallowing, and vision problems. Information is also included about complications that impact breathing, bladder control, cognition, and mental health. A separate chapter addresses pregnancy-related concerns for women with MS.

Part III: Diagnostic Tests, Treatments, and Therapies for Multiple Sclerosis describes various ways MS is diagnosed, managed, and monitored, including benign treatment, drug treatments, pain management, and management of involuntary movement and tremor. Physical, occupational, and counseling therapies are explained, and information is presented about complementary and alternative medical treatments, plasmapheresis, cooling therapy, and clinical studies of MS.

Part IV: Living with Multiple Sclerosis offers guidelines for discussing MS with family, friends, and employers. It includes information about nutrition and exercise and offers techniques for managing fatigue and stress. Individual chapters provide tips for developing a support group, offer tools for caregivers of individuals with MS, describe home accessibility guidelines, and discuss equipment that promotes self-care, mobility, and independence.

Part V: Multiple Sclerosis and Work, Financial, and Legal Issues describes how individuals with MS can navigate workplace challenges and prepare for the future. Financial planning needs, disability benefits, home care, assisted living, and skilled nursing health care options are described and written advance directives are explained.

Part VI: Additional Help and Information includes a glossary of related terms and a directory of resources.

Bibliographic Note

This volume contains documents and excerpts from publications issued by the following U.S. government agencies: Administration on

Aging; Centers for Medicare and Medicaid Services (CMS); National Institute of Diabetes and Digestive and Kidney Diseases (NIDDK); National Institute of Neurological Disorders and Stroke (NINDS); National Institute on Aging (NIA); National Institute on Disability and Rehabilitation Research (NIDRR); National Institutes of Health (NIH) Clinical Center; National Women's Health Information Center (NWHIC); Social Security Administration (SSA); U.S. Food and Drug Administration (FDA); U.S. Department of Health and Human Services (HHS); and the U.S. Department of Labor (DOL).

In addition, this volume contains copyrighted documents from the following individuals and organizations: Accelerated Cure Project for Multiple Sclerosis; A.D.A.M., Inc.; American Hospital Association; Pamela Cazzolli, RN; Cleveland Clinic; Consortium of Multiple Sclerosis Centers; Frederick W. Foley, Ph.D.; Rosalind Joffe; Jennie Q. Lou, MD; Multiple Sclerosis Association of America; Multiple Sclerosis Association of King County; Multiple Sclerosis Foundation; Multiple Sclerosis International Federation; National Academies Press; National Center on Physical Activity and Disability; National Multiple Sclerosis Society; and WoltersKluwer Health.

Acknowledgements

In addition to the listed organizations, agencies, and individuals who have contributed to this *Sourcebook*, special thanks go to managing editor Karen Bellenir, research and permissions coordinator Liz Collins, and document engineer Bruce Bellenir for their help and support.

About the Health Reference Series

The *Health Reference Series* is designed to provide basic medical information for patients, families, caregivers, and the general public. Each volume takes a particular topic and provides comprehensive coverage. This is especially important for people who may be dealing with a newly diagnosed disease or a chronic disorder in themselves or in a family member. People looking for preventive guidance, information about disease warning signs, medical statistics, and risk factors for health problems will also find answers to their questions in the *Health Reference Series*. The *Series*, however, is not intended to serve as a tool for diagnosing illness, in prescribing treatments, or as a substitute for the physician/patient relationship. All people concerned about medical symptoms or the possibility of disease are encouraged to seek professional care from an appropriate health care provider.

A Note about Spelling and Style

Health Reference Series editors use *Stedman's Medical Dictionary* as an authority for questions related to the spelling of medical terms and the *Chicago Manual of Style* for questions related to grammatical structures, punctuation, and other editorial concerns. Consistent adherence is not always possible, however, because the individual volumes within the *Series* include many documents from a wide variety of different producers and copyright holders, and the editor's primary goal is to present material from each source as accurately as is possible following the terms specified by each document's producer. This sometimes means that information in different chapters or sections may follow other guidelines and alternate spelling authorities. For example, occasionally a copyright holder may require that eponymous terms be shown in possessive forms (Crohn's disease *vs.* Crohn disease) or that British spelling norms be retained (leukaemia *vs.* leukemia).

Locating Information within the Health Reference Series

The *Health Reference Series* contains a wealth of information about a wide variety of medical topics. Ensuring easy access to all the fact sheets, research reports, in-depth discussions, and other material contained within the individual books of the *Series* remains one of our highest priorities. As the *Series* continues to grow in size and scope, however, locating the precise information needed by a reader may become more challenging.

A *Contents Guide to the Health Reference Series* was developed to direct readers to the specific volumes that address their concerns. It presents an extensive list of diseases, treatments, and other topics of general interest compiled from the Tables of Contents and major index headings. To access *A Contents Guide to the Health Reference Series*, visit www.healthreferenceseries.com.

Medical Consultant

Medical consultation services are provided to the *Health Reference Series* editors by David A. Cooke, M.D. Dr. Cooke is a graduate of Brandeis University, and he received his M.D. degree from the University of Michigan. He completed residency training at the University of Wisconsin Hospital and Clinics. He is board-certified in Internal Medicine. Dr. Cooke currently works as part of the University of Michigan Health System and practices in Brighton, MI. In his free time, he enjoys writing, science fiction, and spending time with his family.

Our Advisory Board

We would like to thank the following board members for providing guidance to the development of this *Series*:

- Dr. Lynda Baker, Associate Professor of Library and Information Science, Wayne State University, Detroit, MI

- Nancy Bulgarelli, William Beaumont Hospital Library, Royal Oak, MI

- Karen Imarisio, Bloomfield Township Public Library, Bloomfield Township, MI

- Karen Morgan, Mardigian Library, University of Michigan-Dearborn, Dearborn, MI

- Rosemary Orlando, St. Clair Shores Public Library, St. Clair Shores, MI

Health Reference Series *Update Policy*

The inaugural book in the *Health Reference Series* was the first edition of *Cancer Sourcebook* published in 1989. Since then, the *Series* has been enthusiastically received by librarians and in the medical community. In order to maintain the standard of providing high-quality health information for the layperson the editorial staff at Omnigraphics felt it was necessary to implement a policy of updating volumes when warranted.

Medical researchers have been making tremendous strides, and it is the purpose of the *Health Reference Series* to stay current with the most recent advances. Each decision to update a volume is made on an individual basis. Some of the considerations include how much new information is available and the feedback we receive from people who use the books. If there is a topic you would like to see added to the update list, or an area of medical concern you feel has not been adequately addressed, please write to:

Editor
Health Reference Series
Omnigraphics, Inc.
P.O. Box 31-1640
Detroit, MI 48231-1640
E-mail: editorial@omnigraphics.com

Part One

Multiple Sclerosis: Causes, Risk Factors, and Disease Course

Chapter 1

Multiple Sclerosis (MS) Overview

Although multiple sclerosis (MS) was first diagnosed in 1849, the earliest known description of a person with possible MS dates from fourteenth century Holland. An unpredictable disease of the central nervous system, MS can range from relatively benign to somewhat disabling to devastating as communication between the brain and other parts of the body is disrupted.

The vast majority of patients are mildly affected, but in the worst cases, MS can render a person unable to write, speak, or walk. A physician can diagnose MS in some patients soon after the onset of the illness. In others, however, physicians may not be able to readily identify the cause of the symptoms, leading to years of uncertainty and multiple diagnoses punctuated by baffling symptoms that mysteriously wax and wane. Once a diagnosis is made with confidence, patients must consider a profusion of information—and misinformation—associated with this complex disease.

What is multiple sclerosis?

During an MS attack, inflammation occurs in areas of the white matter of the central nervous system in random patches called plaques. This process is followed by destruction of myelin, the fatty covering that insulates nerve cell fibers in the brain and spinal cord. Myelin

Excerpted from "Multiple Sclerosis: Hope Through Research," National Institute of Neurological Disorders and Stroke (NINDS), NIH Publication No. 96-75, updated April 16, 2007.

facilitates the smooth, high-speed transmission of electrochemical messages between the brain, the spinal cord, and the rest of the body; when it is damaged, neurological transmission of messages may be slowed or blocked completely, leading to diminished or lost function. The name "multiple sclerosis" signifies both the number (multiple) and condition (sclerosis, from the Greek term for scarring or hardening) of the demyelinated areas in the central nervous system.

How many people have MS?

No one knows exactly how many people have MS. It is believed that, currently, there are approximately 250,000 to 350,000 people in the United States with MS diagnosed by a physician. This estimate suggests that approximately 200 new cases are diagnosed each week.

Who gets MS?

Most people experience their first symptoms of MS between the ages of 20 and 40, but a diagnosis is often delayed. This is due to both the transitory nature of the disease and the lack of a specific diagnostic test—specific symptoms and changes in the brain must develop before the diagnosis is confirmed.

Although scientists have documented cases of MS in young children and elderly adults, symptoms rarely begin before age 15 or after age 60. Whites are more than twice as likely as other races to develop MS. In general, women are affected at almost twice the rate of men; however, among patients who develop the symptoms of MS at a later age, the gender ratio is more balanced.

MS is five times more prevalent in temperate climates—such as those found in the northern United States, Canada, and Europe—than in tropical regions. Furthermore, the age of 15 seems to be significant in terms of risk for developing the disease. Some studies indicate that a person moving from a high-risk (temperate) to a low-risk (tropical) area before the age of 15 tends to adopt the risk (in this case, low) of the new area and vice versa. Other studies suggest that people moving after age 15 maintain the risk of the area where they grew up.

These findings indicate a strong role for an environmental factor in the cause of MS. It is possible that, at the time of or immediately following puberty, patients acquire an infection with a long latency period. Or, conversely, people in some areas may come in contact with an unknown protective agent during the time before puberty. Other studies suggest that the unknown geographic or climatic element may

4

actually be simply a matter of genetic predilection and reflect racial and ethnic susceptibility factors.

Periodically, scientists receive reports of MS clusters. The most famous of these MS "epidemics" took place in the Faeroe Islands north of Scotland in the years following the arrival of British troops during World War II. Despite intense study of this and other clusters, no direct environmental factor has been identified. Nor has any definitive evidence been found to link daily stress to MS attacks, although there is evidence that the risk of worsening is greater after acute viral illnesses.

How much does MS cost America?

MS is a lifelong chronic disease diagnosed primarily in young adults who have a virtually normal life expectancy. Consequently, the economic, social, and medical costs associated with the disease are significant. Estimates place the annual cost of MS in the United States in the billions of dollars.

What causes MS?

Scientists have learned a great deal about MS in recent years; still, its cause remains elusive. Many investigators believe MS to be an autoimmune disease—one in which the body, through its immune system, launches a defensive attack against its own tissues. In the case of MS, it is the nerve-insulating myelin that comes under assault. Such assaults may be linked to an unknown environmental trigger, perhaps a virus.

The Immune System

To understand what is happening when a person has MS, it is first necessary to know a little about how the healthy immune system works. The immune system—a complex network of specialized cells and organs—defends the body against attacks by "foreign" invaders such as bacteria, viruses, fungi, and parasites. It does this by seeking out and destroying the interlopers as they enter the body. Substances capable of triggering an immune response are called antigens.

The immune system displays both enormous diversity and extraordinary specificity. It can recognize millions of distinctive foreign molecules and produce its own molecules and cells to match up with and counteract each of them. In order to have room for enough cells to match the millions of possible foreign invaders, the immune system stores just a few cells for each specific antigen. When an antigen appears, those few specifically matched cells are stimulated to multiply into a full-scale army. Later, to prevent this army from over-expanding, powerful mechanisms to suppress the immune response come into play.

T cells, so named because they are processed in the thymus, appear to play a particularly important role in MS. They travel widely and continuously throughout the body patrolling for foreign invaders. In order to recognize and respond to each specific antigen, each T cell's surface carries special receptor molecules for particular antigens.

T cells contribute to the body's defenses in two major ways. Regulatory T cells help orchestrate the elaborate immune system. For instance, they assist other cells to make antibodies, proteins programmed to match one specific antigen much as a key matches a lock. Antibodies typically interact with circulating antigens, such as bacteria, but are unable to penetrate living cells. Chief among the regulatory T cells are those known as helper (or inducer) cells. Helper T cells are essential for activating the body's defenses against foreign substances. Yet another subset of regulatory T cells acts to turn off, or suppress, various immune system cells when their job is done.

Killer T cells, on the other hand, directly attack diseased or damaged body cells by binding to them and bombarding them with lethal chemicals called cytokines. Since T cells can attack cells directly, they must be able to discriminate between "self" cells (those of the body) and "nonself" cells (foreign invaders). To enable the immune system to distinguish the self, each body cell carries identifying molecules on its surface. T cells likely to react against the self are usually eliminated before leaving the thymus; the remaining T cells recognize the molecular markers and coexist peaceably with body tissues in a state of self-tolerance.

In autoimmune diseases such as MS, the détente between the immune system and the body is disrupted when the immune system seems to wrongly identify self as nonself and declares war on the part of the body (myelin) it no longer recognizes. Through intensive research efforts, scientists are unraveling the complex secrets of the malfunctioning immune system of patients with MS.

Components of myelin such as myelin basic protein have been the focus of much research because, when injected into laboratory animals, they can precipitate experimental allergic encephalomyelitis (EAE), a chronic relapsing brain and spinal cord disease that resembles MS. The injected myelin probably stimulates the immune system to produce anti-myelin T cells that attack the animal's own myelin.

Investigators are also looking for abnormalities or malfunctions in the blood/brain barrier, a protective membrane that controls the passage of substances from the blood into the central nervous system. It is possible that, in MS, components of the immune system get through the barrier and cause nervous system damage.

Scientists have studied a number of infectious agents (such as viruses) that have been suspected of causing MS, but have been unable to implicate any one particular agent. Viral infections are usually accompanied by inflammation and the production of gamma interferon, a naturally occurring body chemical that has been shown to worsen the clinical course of MS. It is possible that the immune response to viral infections may themselves precipitate an MS attack. There seems to be little doubt that something in the environment is involved in triggering MS.

Genetics

In addition, increasing scientific evidence suggests that genetics may play a role in determining a person's susceptibility to MS. Some populations, such as Gypsies, Eskimos, and Bantus, never get MS. Native Indians of North and South America, the Japanese, and other Asian peoples have very low incidence rates. It is unclear whether this is due mostly to genetic or environmental factors. In the population at large, the chance of developing MS is less than a tenth of one percent. However, if one person in a family has MS, that person's first-degree relatives—parents, children, and siblings—have a one to three percent chance of getting the disease.

For identical twins, the likelihood that the second twin may develop MS if the first twin does is about 30 percent; for fraternal twins (who do not inherit identical gene pools), the likelihood is closer to that for non-twin siblings, or about 4 percent. The fact that the rate for identical twins both developing MS is significantly less than 100 percent suggests that the disease is not entirely genetically controlled. Some (but definitely not all) of this effect may be due to shared exposure to something in the environment, or to the fact that some people with MS lesions remain essentially asymptomatic throughout their lives.

Further indications that more than one gene is involved in MS susceptibility come from studies of families in which more than one member has MS. Several research teams found that people with MS inherit certain regions on individual genes more frequently than people without MS. Of particular interest are the human leukocyte antigens

(HLA) or major histocompatibility complex region on chromosome 6. HLA are genetically determined proteins that influence the immune system.

The HLA patterns of MS patients tend to be different from those of people without the disease. Investigations in northern Europe and America have detected three HLA that are more prevalent in people with MS than in the general population. Studies of American MS patients have shown that people with MS also tend to exhibit these HLA in combination—that is, they have more than one of the three HLA—more frequently than the rest of the population. Furthermore, there is evidence that different combinations of the HLA may correspond to variations in disease severity and progression.

Studies of families with multiple cases of MS and research comparing genetic regions of humans to those of mice with experimental allergic encephalitis (EAE) suggest that another area related to MS susceptibility may be located on chromosome 5. Other regions on chromosomes 2, 3, 7, 11, 17, 19, and X have also been identified as possibly containing genes involved in the development of MS.

These studies strengthen the theory that MS is the result of a number of factors rather than a single gene or other agent. Development of MS is likely to be influenced by the interactions of a number of genes, each of which (individually) has only a modest effect. Additional studies are needed to specifically pinpoint which genes are involved, determine their function, and learn how each gene's interactions with other genes and with the environment make an individual susceptible to MS. In addition to leading to better ways to diagnose MS, such studies should yield clues to the underlying causes of MS and, eventually, to better treatments or a way to prevent the disease.

What is the course of MS?

Each case of MS displays one of several patterns of presentation and subsequent course. Most commonly, MS first manifests itself as a series of attacks followed by complete or partial remissions as symptoms mysteriously lessen, only to return later after a period of stability. This is called relapsing-remitting (RR) MS. Primary-progressive (PP) MS is characterized by a gradual clinical decline with no distinct remissions, although there may be temporary plateaus or minor relief from symptoms. Secondary-progressive (SP) MS begins with a relapsing-remitting course followed by a later primary-progressive course. Rarely, patients may have a progressive-relapsing (PR) course in which the disease takes a progressive path punctuated by acute attacks. PP, SP, and PR are sometimes lumped together and called chronic progressive MS.

In addition, twenty percent of the MS population has a benign form of the disease in which symptoms show little or no progression after the initial attack; these patients remain fully functional. A few patients experience malignant MS, defined as a swift and relentless decline resulting in significant disability or even death shortly after disease onset. However, MS is very rarely fatal and most people with MS have a fairly normal life expectancy.

Studies throughout the world are causing investigators to redefine the natural course of the disease. These studies use a technique called magnetic resonance imaging (MRI) to visualize the evolution of MS lesions in the white matter of the brain. Bright spots on a T2 MRI scan indicate the presence of lesions, but do not provide information about when they developed.

Because investigators speculate that the breakdown of the blood/ brain barrier is the first step in the development of MS lesions, it is important to distinguish new lesions from old. To do this, physicians give patients injections of gadolinium, a chemical contrast agent that normally does not cross the blood/brain barrier, before performing a scan. On this type of scan, called T1, the appearance of bright areas indicates periods of recent disease activity (when gadolinium is able to cross the barrier). The ability to estimate the age of lesions through MRI has allowed investigators to show that, in some patients, lesions occur frequently throughout the course of the disease even when no symptoms are present.

Can life events affect the course of MS?

While there is no good evidence that daily stress or trauma affects the course of MS, there is data on the influence of pregnancy. Since MS generally strikes during childbearing years, a common concern among women with the disease is whether or not to have a baby. Studies on the subject have shown that MS has no adverse effects on the course of pregnancy, labor, or delivery; in fact, symptoms often stabilize or remit during pregnancy. This temporary improvement is thought to relate to changes in a woman's immune system that allow her body to carry a baby. Because every fetus has genetic material from the father as well as the mother, the mother's body should identify the growing fetus as foreign tissue and try to reject it in much the same way the body seeks to reject a transplanted organ. To prevent

9

this from happening, a natural process takes place to suppress the mother's immune system in the uterus during pregnancy.

However, women with MS who are considering pregnancy need to be aware that certain drugs used to treat MS should be avoided during pregnancy and while breast feeding. These drugs can cause birth defects and can be passed to the fetus via blood and to an infant via breast milk. Among them are prednisone, corticotropin, azathioprine, cyclophosphamide, diazepam, phenytoin, carbamazepine, and baclofen.

Unfortunately, between 20 and 40 percent of women with MS do have a relapse in the three months following delivery. However, there is no evidence that pregnancy and childbirth affect the overall course of the disease one way or the other. Also, while MS is not in itself a reason to avoid pregnancy and poses no significant risks to the fetus, physical limitations can make child care more difficult. It is therefore important that MS patients planning families discuss these issues with both their partner and physician.

Diagnosis

There is no single test that unequivocally detects MS. When faced with a patient whose symptoms, neurological exam results, and medical history suggest MS, physicians use a variety of tools to rule out other possible disorders and perform a series of laboratory tests which, if positive, confirm the diagnosis.

Magnetic Resonance Imaging (MRI)

Imaging technologies such as MRI can help locate central nervous system lesions resulting from myelin loss. MRI is painless, noninvasive, and does not expose the body to radiation. It is often used in conjunction with the contrast agent gadolinium, which helps distinguish new plaques from old. However, since these lesions can also occur in several other neurological disorders, they are not absolute evidence of MS.

Several new MRI techniques may help quantify and characterize MS lesions that are too subtle to be detected using conventional MRI scans. While standard MRI provides an anatomical picture of lesions, magnetic resonance spectroscopy (MRS) yields information about the brain's biochemistry; specifically, it can measure the brain chemical N-acetyl aspartate. Decreased levels of this chemical can indicate nerve damage.

- **Magnetization transfer imaging (MTI)** is able to detect white matter abnormalities before lesions can be seen on standard MRI scans by calculating the amount of "free" water in tissues. Demyelinated tissues and damaged nerves show increased levels of "free" (versus "bound") water particles.

- **Diffusion-tensor magnetic resonance imaging (DT-MRI or DTI)** measures the random motion of water molecules. Individual water molecules are constantly in motion, colliding with each other at extremely high speeds. This causes them to spread out, or diffuse. DT-MRI maps this diffusion to produce intricate, three-dimensional images indicating the size and location of demyelinated areas of the brain. Changes in this process can then be measured and correlated with disease progression.

- **Functional MRI (fMRI)** uses radio waves and a strong magnetic field to measure the correlation between physical changes in the brain (such as blood flow) and mental functioning during the performance of cognitive tasks.

In addition to helping scientists and physicians better understand how MS develops—an important first step in devising new treatments—these approaches offer earlier diagnosis and enhance efforts to monitor disease progression and the effects of treatment.

Other Tests That Diagnose MS

Other tests that may be used to diagnosis MS include visual evoked potential (VEP) tests and studies of cerebrospinal fluid (the colorless liquid that circulates through the brain and spinal cord). VEP tests measure the speed of the brain's response to visual stimuli. VEP can sometimes detect lesions that the scanners miss and is particularly useful when abnormalities seen on MRI do not meet the specific criteria for MS. Auditory and sensory evoked potentials have also been used in the past, but are no longer believed to contribute significantly to the diagnosis of MS. Like imaging technologies, VEP is helpful but not conclusive because it cannot identify the cause of lesions.

Examination of cerebrospinal fluid can show cellular and chemical abnormalities often associated with MS. These abnormalities include increased numbers of white blood cells and higher-than-average amounts of protein, especially myelin basic protein and an antibody called immunoglobulin G. Physicians can use several different laboratory techniques to separate and graph the various proteins in MS patients' cerebrospinal fluid. This process often identifies the presence of a characteristic pattern called oligoclonal bands.

While it can still be difficult for the physician to differentiate between an MS attack and symptoms that can follow a viral infection or even an immunization, our growing understanding of disease mechanisms and the expanded use of MRI is enabling physicians to diagnose MS with far more confidence than ever before. Today, most patients who undergo a diagnostic evaluation for MS will be classified as either having MS or not having MS, although there are still cases where a person may have the clinical symptoms of MS but not meet all the criteria to confirm a diagnosis of MS. In these cases, a diagnosis of "possible MS" is used.

A number of other diseases may produce symptoms similar to those seen in MS. Other conditions with an intermittent course and MS-like lesions of the brain's white matter include polyarteritis, lupus erythematosus, syringomyelia, tropical spastic paraparesis, some cancers, and certain tumors that compress the brainstem or spinal cord. Progressive multifocal leukoencephalopathy can mimic the acute stage of an MS attack. Physicians will also need to rule out stroke, neurosyphilis, spinocerebellar ataxias, pernicious anemia, diabetes, Sjögren disease, and vitamin B_{12} deficiency. Acute transverse myelitis may signal the first attack of MS, or it may indicate other problems such as infection with the Epstein-Barr or herpes simplex B viruses. Recent reports suggest that the neurological problems associated with Lyme disease may present a clinical picture much like MS.

Investigators are continuing their search for a definitive test for MS. Until one is developed, however, evidence of both multiple attacks and central nervous system lesions must be found before a diagnosis of MS is given.

MS Treatment

There is as yet no cure for MS. Many patients do well with no therapy at all, especially since many medications have serious side effects and some carry significant risks. Naturally occurring or spontaneous remissions make it difficult to determine therapeutic effects of experimental treatments; however, the emerging evidence that MRIs can chart the development of lesions is already helping scientists evaluate new therapies.

In the past, the principal medications physicians used to treat MS were steroids possessing anti-inflammatory properties; these include adrenocorticotropic hormone (better known as ACTH), prednisone, prednisolone, methylprednisolone, betamethasone, and dexamethasone. Studies suggest that intravenous methylprednisolone may be superior to the more traditional intravenous ACTH for patients experiencing acute relapses; no strong evidence exists to support the use of these drugs to treat progressive forms of MS. Also, there is some indication that steroids may be more appropriate for people with movement, rather than sensory, symptoms.

While steroids do not affect the course of MS over time, they can reduce the duration and severity of attacks in some patients. The mechanism behind this effect is not known; one study suggests the medications work by restoring the effectiveness of the blood/brain barrier. Because steroids can produce numerous adverse side effects (acne, weight gain, seizures, psychosis), they are not recommended for long-term use.

One of the most promising MS research areas involves naturally occurring antiviral proteins known as interferons. Three forms of beta interferon (Avonex, Betaseron, and Rebif) have now been approved by the Food and Drug Administration for treatment of relapsing-remitting MS. Beta interferon has been shown to reduce the number of exacerbations and may slow the progression of physical disability. When attacks do occur, they tend to be shorter and less severe. In addition, MRI scans suggest that beta interferon can decrease myelin destruction.

Investigators speculate that the effects of beta interferon may be due to the drug's ability to correct an MS-related deficiency of certain white blood cells that suppress the immune system and/or its ability to inhibit gamma interferon, a substance believed to be involved in MS attacks. Alpha interferon is also being studied as a possible treatment for MS. Common side effects of interferons include fever, chills, sweating, muscle aches, fatigue, depression, and injection site reactions.

Scientists continue their extensive efforts to create new and better therapies for MS. Goals of therapy are threefold: to improve recovery from attacks, to prevent or lessen the number of relapses, and to halt disease progression.

Immunotherapy

As evidence of immune system involvement in the development of MS has grown, trials of various new treatments to alter or suppress immune response are being conducted. Most of these therapies are, at this time, still considered experimental.

Results of recent clinical trials have shown that immunosuppressive agents and techniques can positively (if temporarily) affect the course of MS; however, toxic side effects often preclude their widespread use. In addition, generalized immunosuppression leaves the patient open to a variety of viral, bacterial, and fungal infections.

Over the years, MS investigators have studied a number of immunosuppressant treatments. One such treatment, Novantrone (mitoxantrone), was approved by the Food and Drug Administration (FDA) for the treatment of advanced or chronic MS. Other therapies being studied are cyclosporine (Sandimmune), cyclophosphamide (Cytoxan), methotrexate, azathioprine (Imuran), and total lymphoid irradiation (a process whereby the MS patient's lymph nodes are irradiated with x-rays in small doses over a few weeks to destroy lymphoid tissue, which is actively involved in tissue destruction in autoimmune diseases). Inconclusive and/or contradictory results of these trials, combined with the therapies' potentially dangerous side effects, dictate that further research is necessary to determine what, if any, role they should play in the management of MS. Studies are also being conducted with the immune system modulating drug cladribine (Leustatin).

Another potential treatment for MS is monoclonal antibodies, which are identical, laboratory-produced antibodies that are highly specific for a single antigen. They are injected into the patient in the hope that they will alter the patient's immune response. One monoclonal antibody, natalizumab (Tysabri), was shown in clinical trials to significantly reduce the frequency of attacks in people with relapsing forms of MS and was approved for marketing by the FDA in 2004. However, in 2005 the drug's manufacturer voluntarily suspended marketing of the drug after several reports of significant adverse events. In 2006, the FDA again approved sale of the drug for MS but under strict treatment guidelines involving infusion centers where patients can be monitored by specially trained physicians.

Another experimental treatment for MS is plasma exchange, or plasmapheresis. Plasmapheresis is a procedure in which blood is removed from the patient and the blood plasma is separated from other blood substances that may contain antibodies and other immunologically active products. These other blood substances are discarded and the plasma is then transfused back into the patient. Because its worth as a treatment for MS has not yet been proven, this experimental treatment remains at the stage of clinical testing.

Bone marrow transplantation (a procedure in which bone marrow from a healthy donor is infused into patients who have undergone drug or radiation therapy to suppress their immune system so they will not reject the donated marrow) and injections of venom from honey bees are also being studied. Each of these therapies carries the risk of potentially severe side effects.

Therapy to Improve Nerve Impulse Conduction

Because the transmission of electrochemical messages between the brain and body is disrupted in MS, medications to improve the conduction of nerve impulses are being investigated. Since demyelinated nerves show abnormalities of potassium activity, scientists are studying drugs that block the channels through which potassium moves, thereby restoring conduction of the nerve impulse. In several small experimental trials, derivatives of a drug called aminopyridine temporarily improved vision, coordination, and strength when given to MS patients who suffered from both visual symptoms and heightened sensitivity to temperature. Possible side effects of these therapies include paresthesias (tingling sensations), dizziness, and seizures.

Therapies Targeting an Antigen

Trials of a synthetic form of myelin basic protein, called copolymer I (Copaxone), were successful, leading the FDA to approve the agent for the treatment of relapsing-remitting MS. Copolymer I, unlike so many drugs tested for the treatment of MS, has few side effects, and studies indicate that the agent can reduce the relapse rate by almost one-third. In addition, patients given copolymer I are more likely to show neurologic improvement than those given a placebo.

Investigators are also looking at the possibility of developing an MS vaccine. Myelin-attacking T cells were removed, inactivated, and injected back into animals with experimental allergic encephalomyelitis (EAE). This procedure results in destruction of the immune system cells that were attacking myelin basic protein. In a couple of small trials scientists have tested a similar vaccine in humans. The product was well-tolerated and had no side effects, but the studies were too small to establish efficacy. Patients with progressive forms of MS did not appear to benefit, although relapsing-remitting patients showed some neurologic improvement and had fewer relapses and reduced numbers of lesions in one study. Unfortunately, the benefits did not last beyond two years.

A similar approach, known as peptide therapy, is based on evidence that the body can mount an immune response against the T cells that destroy myelin, but this response is not strong enough to overcome the disease. To induce this response, the investigator scans the myelin-attacking T cells for the myelin-recognizing receptors on the cells' surface. A fragment, or peptide, of those receptors is then injected into the body. The immune system identifies the injected peptide as a foreign invader and launches an attack on any myelin-destroying T cells that carry the peptide. The injection of portions of T cell receptors may heighten the immune system reaction against the errant T cells much the same way a booster shot heightens immunity to tetanus. Or, peptide therapy may jam the errant cells' receptors, preventing the cells from attacking myelin.

Despite these promising early results, there are some major obstacles to developing vaccine and peptide therapies. Individual patients' T cells vary so much that it may not be possible to develop a standard vaccine or peptide therapy beneficial to all, or even most, MS patients. At this time, each treatment involves extracting cells from each individual patient, purifying the cells, and then growing them in culture before inactivating and chemically altering them. This makes the production of quantities sufficient for therapy extremely time consuming, labor intensive, and expensive. Further studies are necessary to determine whether universal inoculations can be developed to induce suppression of MS patients' overactive immune systems.

Protein antigen feeding is similar to peptide therapy, but is a potentially simpler means to the same end. Whenever we eat, the digestive system breaks each food or substance into its primary "non-antigenic" building blocks, thereby averting a potentially harmful immune attack. So, strange as it may seem, antigens that trigger an immune response when they are injected can encourage immune system tolerance when taken orally. Furthermore, this reaction is directed solely at the specific antigen being fed; wholesale immunosuppression, which can leave the body open to a variety of infections, does not occur. Studies have shown that when rodents with EAE are fed myelin protein antigens, they experience fewer relapses. Data from a small, preliminary trial of antigen feeding in humans found limited suggestion of improvement, but the results were not statistically significant. A multi-center trial is being conducted to determine whether protein antigen feeding is effective.

Cytokines

As our growing insight into the workings of the immune system gives us new knowledge about the function of cytokines, the powerful chemicals produced by T cells, the possibility of using them to manipulate the immune system becomes more attractive. Scientists are studying a variety of substances that may block harmful cytokines, such as those involved in inflammation, or that encourage the production of protective cytokines.

A drug that has been tested as a depression treatment, rolipram, has been shown to reduce levels of several destructive cytokines in animal models of MS. Its potential as a therapy for MS is not known at this time, but side effects seem modest. Protein antigen feeding may release transforming growth factor beta (TGF), a protective cytokine that inhibits or regulates the activity of certain immune cells. Preliminary tests indicate that it may reduce the number of immune cells commonly found in MS patients' spinal fluid. Side effects include anemia and altered kidney function.

Interleukin 4 (IL-4) is able to diminish demyelination and improve the clinical course of mice with EAE, apparently by influencing developing T cells to become protective rather than harmful. This also appears to be true of a group of chemicals called retinoids. When fed to rodents with EAE, retinoids increase levels of TGF and IL-4, which encourage protective T cells, while decreasing numbers of harmful T cells. This results in improvement of the animals' clinical symptoms.

Remyelination

Some studies focus on strategies to reverse the damage to myelin and oligodendrocytes (the cells that make and maintain myelin in the central nervous system), both of which are destroyed during MS attacks. Scientists now know that oligodendrocytes may proliferate and form new myelin after an attack. Therefore, there is a great deal of interest in agents that may stimulate this reaction. To learn more about the process, investigators are looking at how drugs used in MS trials affect remyelination. Studies of animal models indicate that monoclonal antibodies and two immunosuppressant drugs, cyclophosphamide and azathioprine, may accelerate remyelination, while steroids may inhibit it. The ability of intravenous immunoglobulin (IVIg) to restore visual acuity and/or muscle strength is also being investigated.

Diet

Over the years, many people have tried to implicate diet as a cause of, or treatment for, MS. Some physicians have advocated a diet low in saturated fats; others have suggested increasing the patient's intake of linoleic acid, a polyunsaturated fat, via supplements of sunflower seed, safflower, or evening primrose oils. Other proposed dietary remedies include megavitamin therapy, including increased intake of vitamins B_{12} or C; various liquid diets; and sucrose-, tobacco-, or gluten-free diets. To date, clinical studies have not been able to confirm benefits from dietary changes. In the absence of any evidence that diet therapy is effective, patients are best advised to eat a balanced, wholesome diet.

Unproven Therapies

MS is a disease with a natural tendency to remit spontaneously, and for which there is no universally effective treatment and no known cause. These factors open the door for an array of unsubstantiated claims of cures. At one time or another, many ineffective and even potentially dangerous therapies have been promoted as treatments for MS. A partial list of these therapies includes: injections of snake venom, electrical stimulation of the spinal cord's dorsal column, removal of the thymus gland, breathing pressurized (hyperbaric) oxygen in a special chamber, injections of beef heart and hog pancreas extracts, intravenous or oral calcium orotate (calcium ethanol phosphate [EAP]), hysterectomy, removal of dental fillings containing silver or mercury amalgams, and surgical implantation of pig brain into the patient's abdomen. None of these treatments is an effective therapy for MS or any of its symptoms.

What recent advances have been made in MS research?

Many advances, on several fronts, have been made in the war against MS. Each advance interacts with the others, adding greater depth and meaning to each new discovery. Four areas, in particular, stand out.

1. Over the last decade, our knowledge about how the immune system works has grown at an amazing rate. Major gains have been made in recognizing and defining the role of this system in the development of MS lesions, giving scientists the ability to devise ways to alter the immune response. Such work is expected to yield a variety of new potential therapies that may ameliorate MS without harmful side effects.

2. New tools such as MRI have redefined the natural history of MS and are proving invaluable in monitoring disease activity.

Scientists are now able to visualize and follow the development of MS lesions in the brain and spinal cord using MRI; this ability is a tremendous aid in the assessment of new therapies and can speed the process of evaluating new treatments.

3. Other tools have been developed that make the painstaking work of teasing out the disease's genetic secrets possible. Such studies have strengthened scientists' conviction that MS is a disease with many genetic components, none of which is dominant. Immune system-related genetic factors that predispose an individual to the development of MS have been identified, and may lead to new ways to treat or prevent the disease.

4. A treatment that may actually slow the course of the disease has been found and a growing number of therapies are now available that effectively treat some MS symptoms.

In addition, there are a number of treatments under investigation that may curtail attacks or improve function of demyelinated nerve fibers. Over a dozen clinical trials testing potential therapies are under way, and additional new treatments are being devised and tested in animal models.

What research remains to be done?

The role of genetic risk factors, and how they can be modified, must be more clearly defined. Environmental triggers, such as viruses or toxins, need to be investigated further. The specific cellular and sub-cellular targets of immune attack in the brain and spinal cord, and the subsets of T cells involved in that attack, need to be identified. Knowledge of these aspects of the disease will enable scientists to develop new methods for halting—or reversing and repairing—the destruction of myelin that causes the symptoms of MS.

How can I help research?

The NINDS contributes to the support of the Human Brain and Spinal Fluid Resource Center in Los Angeles. This bank supplies investigators around the world with tissue from patients with neurological and other disorders. Tissue from individuals with MS is needed to enable scientists to study this disorder more intensely. Prospective donors may contact:

Human Brain and Spinal Fluid Resource Center
W. LA Healthcare Cntr., Bldg. 212, Rm. 16
11301 Wilshire Blvd. (127A)
Los Angeles, CA 90073
Phone: 310-268-3536
Fax: 310-268-4768
24-hour pager: 310-636-5199
Website: http://www.loni.ucla.edu/uclabrainbank
E-mail: RMNbbank@ucla.edu

Additional Information

American Autoimmune Related Diseases Association
22100 Gratiot Ave., Eastpointe
East Detroit, MI 48021-2227
Toll-Free: 800-598-4668
Phone: 586-776-3900
Fax: 586-776-3903
Website: http://www.aarda.org
E-mail: aarda@aarda.org

Brain Resources and Information Network (BRAIN)
P.O. Box 5801
Bethesda, MD 20824
Toll-Free: 800-352-9424
Website: http://www.ninds.nih.gov
E-mail: braininfo@ninds.nih.gov

Multiple Sclerosis Association of America
706 Haddonfield Road
Cherry Hill, NJ 08002
Toll-Free: 800-532-7667
Phone: 856-488-4500
Fax: 856-661-9797
Website: http://www.msassociation.org
E-mail: msaa@msaa.com

Multiple Sclerosis Foundation
6350 North Andrews Avenue
Ft. Lauderdale, FL 33309-2130
Toll-Free: 888-MSFOCUS (673-6287)
Phone: 954-776-6805

Fax: 954-351-0630
Website: http://www.msfocus.org
E-mail: support@msfocus.org

National Multiple Sclerosis Society
733 Third Ave., 6th Fl.
New York, NY 10017-3288
Toll-Free: 800-344-4867 (FIGHTMS)
Phone: 212-986-3240
Fax: 212-986-7981
Website: http://www.nationalmssociety.org
E-mail: nat@nmss.org

Chapter 2

Autoimmune Disease

Autoimmune Diseases: Overview

What are autoimmune diseases?

Our bodies have an immune system that protects us from disease and infection. But if you have an autoimmune disease, your immune system attacks itself by mistake, and you can get sick. Autoimmune diseases can affect connective tissue in your body (the tissue which binds together body tissues and organs). Autoimmune disease can affect many parts of your body, like your nerves, muscles, endocrine system (system that directs your body's hormones and other chemicals), and digestive system.

Who is at risk for getting autoimmune diseases?

Most autoimmune diseases occur in women, and most often during their childbearing years. Some of these diseases also affect African American, American Indian, and Latina women more than white women. These diseases tend to run in families, so your genes, along with the way your immune system responds to certain triggers or things in the environment, affect your chances of getting one of these

This chapter includes: "Autoimmune Diseases: Overview," National Women's Health Information Center, January 2005; and, "Chemical Messenger Inactivates Cellular 'Police' in Multiple Sclerosis," by Michelle D. Jones-London, Ph.D., National Institute of Neurological Disorders and Stroke (NINDS), October 2005.

diseases. If you think you may have an autoimmune disease, ask your family members if they have had symptoms like yours. The good news is that if you have an autoimmune disease, there are things you can do to feel better.

What are the most common symptoms of autoimmune diseases?

There are more than 80 types of autoimmune diseases. Learning the symptoms of some of the more common autoimmune diseases can help you recognize the signs if you get one. But some autoimmune diseases share similar symptoms. This makes it hard for doctors to find out if you really have one of these diseases, and which one it might be. This can make your trip to doctors long and stressful. But if you are having symptoms that bother you, you need to persist to make sure you get relief. Following are descriptions of some common autoimmune diseases.

Hashimoto thyroiditis (underactive thyroid) symptoms may include:

- tiredness
- depression
- sensitivity to cold
- weight gain
- muscle weakness and cramps
- dry hair
- tough skin
- constipation
- sometimes there are no symptoms

Testing for Hashimoto thyroiditis is done with a blood test for thyroid stimulating hormone (TSH).

Grave disease (overactive thyroid) symptoms may include:

- insomnia (not able to sleep)
- irritability
- weight loss without dieting

- heat sensitivity
- sweating
- fine brittle hair
- weakness in your muscles
- light menstrual periods
- bulging eyes
- shaky hands
- sometimes there are no symptoms

A blood test for thyroid stimulating hormone (TSH) is used to test for Grave disease.

Lupus symptoms may include:

- swelling and damage to the joints, skin, kidneys, heart, lungs, blood vessels, and brain
- butterfly rash across the nose and cheeks
- rashes on other parts of the body
- painful and swollen joints
- sensitivity to the sun

Tests to find lupus include body lab tests such as the antinuclear antibody (ANA) test, blood tests, and urine tests.

Multiple sclerosis (MS) symptoms may include:

- weakness and trouble with coordination, balance, speaking, and walking
- paralysis
- tremors
- numbness and tingling feeling in arms, legs, hands, and feet

Tests for multiple sclerosis may include:

- exam of your body
- exam of your brain, spinal cord, and nerves (neurological exam)

- x-ray tests (magnetic resonance imaging [MRI] and magnetic resonance spectroscopy [MRS])
- other tests on the brain and spinal cord fluid to look for things linked to these diseases

Rheumatoid arthritis symptoms may include:

- inflammation begins in the tissue lining your joints and then spreads to the whole joint (hand joints are the most common site, but it can affect most joints in the body)
- muscle pain
- deformed joints
- weakness
- fatigue
- loss of appetite
- weight loss
- becoming confined to bed in severe cases

Blood tests may show that you have anemia (when your body does not have enough red blood cells) and an antibody called rheumatoid factor (RF). Some people with RF never get this disease, and others with the disease never have RF.

Are chronic fatigue syndrome and fibromyalgia autoimmune diseases?

Chronic fatigue syndrome (CFS) and fibromyalgia (FM) are not autoimmune diseases, but they often have symptoms—like being tired all the time and pain—that may seem like other autoimmune diseases.

- CFS can cause you to be very tired, have trouble concentrating, feel weak, and have muscle pain. Symptoms of CFS come and go. The cause of CFS is not known.
- FM is a disorder with symptoms of widespread muscle pain, fatigue (feeling tired and having low energy), and multiple tender points. Tender points are located in the neck, spine, shoulders, hips, and knees and are painful when pressure is applied to them. FM mainly occurs in women of childbearing age, but children, the elderly, and men are sometimes diagnosed with FM. The cause is not known.

What are flare ups?

Symptoms of autoimmune diseases can come and go, ranging in how bad they are, or all go away for a while (called remission). Flare-ups, or the sudden and severe onset of symptoms, can also happen. It is best to work closely and often with your doctor and other members of your health care team to manage your illness. If you have a flare-up, it is best to first call your doctor. Don't try a cure you heard about from a friend or relative.

Are there medicines to treat autoimmune diseases?

You can take medicines to help your symptoms, which your doctor(s) will talk with you about. The type of medicine you take depends on which disease you have and what your symptoms are. Some people can take over-the-counter drugs, like aspirin and ibuprofen for pain. Others with more severe symptoms may have to take certain kinds of prescription drugs that can help with pain, swelling, depression, anxiety, sleep problems, fatigue, or rashes. You also might be able to take medicine to help slow the progress of your disease. New treatments for autoimmune diseases are being studied all the time.

How can I manage my life now that I have an autoimmune disease?

Although there is no cure for autoimmune disease, you can treat your symptoms and learn to manage your disease, so you can enjoy life. People with autoimmune disease lead full, active lives. Your life goals should not have to change. It is important, though, to see a doctor who specializes in these types of diseases.

What are some things I can do to feel better?

If you are living with an autoimmune disease, there are things you can do each day to feel better.

- **Eat a healthy diet.** Keep your immune system as healthy as can be. The list of nutrients that you need for a healthy immune system is long. But do not try to overload on vitamins because that could be worse for your health. Try to get all you need from food, rather than from vitamin pills. Eat balanced meals with foods from all of the food groups. Include yummy fruits and vegetables and whole grains. Also eat calcium-rich foods, such as fat-free or low-fat milk and yogurt. Avoid fatty foods.

27

- **Get regular exercise** (but be careful not to overdo it). Thirty minutes most days of the week is best, but talk with your doctor about what types of exercise you can do. A gradual and gentle exercise program often works well for people with long-lasting muscle and joint pain. Some types of yoga or tai chi exercises may be helpful.

- **Get enough rest.** Rest allows your body tissues and joints the time they need to repair. Sleeping is a great way you can help both your body and mind. If you do not get enough sleep, your stress level and your symptoms could get worse. You also cannot fight off sickness as well when you sleep poorly. With enough sleep, you can tackle your problems better and lower your risk for illness. Try to get at least seven hours of sleep every night.

- **Reduce stress and try to manage pain.** You also might be able to lessen your pain or muscle spasms and deal with other aspects of living with your disease if you try meditation or self-hypnosis. You can learn to do these through self-help books, tapes, or with the help of an instructor. You also can use imagery (use the power of your thoughts to destroy your pain) or distract your focus on your pain by doing a hobby or something else you enjoy.

What kinds of doctors will I need to treat my autoimmune disease?

Juggling your health care needs among different doctors and other types of health care providers can be hard. But visiting other types of health care workers, along with your main doctor, may be helpful in managing some symptoms of your autoimmune disease. If you are visiting many types of health care workers, make sure you have a supportive main doctor to help you. Often, your family doctor may help you coordinate care. Following are some other kinds of health care workers that may be useful.

- **Nephrologist:** A doctor who will look at how well your kidneys are working. Kidneys are organs that clean the blood and produce urine.

- **Rheumatologist:** A doctor who specializes in arthritis and other diseases.

- **Endocrinologist:** A doctor who specializes in diseases which affect your glands (organs in your body that make hormones).

Glands help control the body's reproduction, energy levels, weight, food and waste production, and growth and development.

- **Physical therapist:** A health care worker who can help you with stiffness, weakness, restricted body movement, and with finding out the proper level of exercise for your body.

- **Occupational therapist:** A health care worker who can help you find devices or make changes in your home or workplace to make life easier for you. They also can teach you ways to do all you have to despite your pain and other health problems.

- **Speech therapist:** A health care worker who can be helpful for people with MS who have speech problems.

- **Vocational therapist:** A health care worker who offers job training for people who cannot do their current jobs because of their illness or other health problems. You can find this type of person through both public and private agencies.

- **Counselor for emotional support:** A health care worker who is specially trained to help you to find ways to cope with your illness. You can work through your feelings of anger, fear, denial, and frustration.

- **Support groups:** Some people find that talking with others who have the same health problem is helpful in finding new ways to cope with it.

- **Chiropractor:** A type of doctor who might be helpful in relieving some of your symptoms, such as muscle spasms and backaches. But you should only see this type of doctor along with your regular autoimmune disease doctor, not in place of him or her.

Chemical Messenger Inactivates Cellular "Police" in Multiple Sclerosis

One of the fundamental mysteries of autoimmune diseases is how normally protective immune responses go bad. A study sheds some light on this issue by showing that a chemical messenger called interleukin 12, or IL-12, allows some white blood cells to proliferate and damage healthy tissues. This finding may lead to new drug treatments for multiple sclerosis (MS) and other autoimmune diseases.

In MS and other autoimmune diseases, certain cells of the immune system—designed to search out and attack disease-causing viruses and bacteria—instead attack healthy tissue in the body. White blood cells called effector T cells are a part of the body's natural defense system and trigger an inflammatory response to fight off foreign substances. Other white blood cells, called T-regulatory cells, police the effector T cells to limit inflammation. "Normally, effector T-cells are under strict control as they circulate through the bloodstream in order to prevent unnecessary inflammation that could be harmful to healthy tissues," says Benjamin Segal, M.D., the neurologist who led the study at the University of Rochester in New York. "However, occasionally, they escape the body's suppression system. We're learning how they do that." The study on the cause of this autoimmune attack, was funded in part by the National Institute of Neurological Disorders and Stroke (NINDS), a component of the National Institutes of Health (NIH), and appeared in the July 15, 2005, issue of the *Journal of Immunology.**

Dr. Segal's research began in Dr. Ethan Shevach's intramural laboratory at the NIH, where he was one of the first scientists to demonstrate that IL-12 played an important role in autoimmune diseases like MS. In studies in the 1990s, Segal and Shevach showed that mice without the IL-12 gene are completely protected against a disease similar to MS. In contrast, exposing normally harmless effector T cells to IL-12 appears to trigger an MS-like disease state.

Dr. Segal and colleagues have shown that the chemical messenger IL-12 inactivates T-regulatory cells, allowing renegade effector T cells to circulate in the central nervous system. The study may explain why people with MS are more likely to suffer a relapse of the disease when they get an infection like the flu. When a person is infected, IL-12 levels rise to allow the person to fight off the infection. This flu-induced IL-12 increase may lead to a relapse by promoting autoimmune effector T cells. These autoimmune T cells are believed to mediate damage to myelin, the fatty covering that wraps around and protects nerve fibers. The researchers hope that understanding this chain of events will lead to the development of better treatments for MS and other autoimmune diseases.

An experimental drug that inhibits IL-12 is being tested by Dr. Segal and others as treatment for patients with relapsing-remitting MS, the most common form of the disease. The scientists believe that IL-12 inhibition could also be useful in other autoimmune diseases such as Crohn disease, psoriasis, and rheumatoid arthritis.

Reference

* King, IL and Segal, BM. "Cutting Edge: IL-12 induces CD4+CD25- T cell activation in the presence of T regulatory cells." The *Journal of Immunology*, July 15, 2005, Vol.175, pp. 641–645.

For More Information

American Autoimmune Related Diseases Association
22100 Gratiot Ave., Eastpointe
East Detroit, MI 48021-2227
Toll-Free: 800-598-4668
Phone: 586-776-3900
Fax: 586-776-3903
Website: http://www.aarda.org
E-mail: aarda@aarda.org

National Institute of Arthritis and Musculoskeletal and Skin Diseases (NIAMS)
1 AMS Circle
Bethesda, MD 20892-3675
Toll-Free: 877-22-NIAMS-(64267)
Phone: 301-495-4484
TTY: 301-565-2966
Fax: 301-718-6366
Website: http://www.niams.nih.gov
E-mail: niamsinfo@mail.nih.gov

National Institute of Neurological Disorders and Stroke (NINDS)
P.O. Box 5801
Bethesda, MD 20824
Toll-Free: 800-352-9424
Phone: 301-496-5751
Fax: 301-402-2186
Website: http://www.ninds.nih.gov
E-mail: braininfo@ninds.nih.gov

National Women's Health Information Center
200 Independence Ave., S.W., Rm. 712 E.
Washington, DC 20201
Toll-Free: 800-994-9662
Phone: 703-289-7923
Fax: 703-663-6942
Website: http://www.womenshealth.gov

Chapter 3

The Central Nervous System

Chapter Contents

Section 3.1

Central Nervous System Overview

This section includes excerpts from "Brain Basics: Know Your Brain," National Institute of Neurological Disorders and Stroke (NINDS), NIH Publication No. 01–3440a, updated May 1, 2007; and an excerpt from "Spinal Cord Injury: Hope Through Research," NINDS, NIH Publication No. 03–160, updated May 21, 2007.

Brain Basics

The brain is the most complex part of the human body. This three-pound organ is the seat of intelligence, interpreter of the senses, initiator of body movement, and controller of behavior. Lying in its bony shell and washed by protective fluid, the brain is the source of all the qualities that define our humanity. The brain is the crown jewel of the human body.

For centuries, scientists and philosophers have been fascinated by the brain, but until recently they viewed the brain as nearly incomprehensible. Now, however, the brain is beginning to relinquish its secrets. Scientists have learned more about the brain in the past decade than in all previous centuries because of the accelerating pace of research in neurological and behavioral science and the development of new research techniques.

The brain is like a committee of experts. All the parts of the brain work together, but each part has its own special properties. The brain can be divided into three basic units: the forebrain, the midbrain, and the hindbrain. The hindbrain includes the upper part of the spinal cord, the brain stem, and a wrinkled ball of tissue called the cerebellum (1). The hindbrain controls the body's vital functions such as respiration and heart rate. The cerebellum coordinates movement and is involved in learned rote movements. When you play the piano or hit a tennis ball you are activating the cerebellum. The uppermost part of the brainstem is the midbrain, which controls some reflex actions and is part of the circuit involved in the control of eye movements and other voluntary movements. The forebrain is the largest and most highly developed part of the human brain: it consists primarily of the cerebrum (2) and the structures hidden beneath it.

When people see pictures of the brain it is usually the cerebrum that they notice. The cerebrum sits at the topmost part of the brain and is the source of intellectual activities. It holds your memories, allows you to plan, enables you to imagine and think. It allows you to recognize friends, read books, and play games.

The cerebrum is split into two halves (hemispheres) by a deep fissure. Despite the split, the two cerebral hemispheres communicate with each other through a thick tract of nerve fibers that lies at the base of this fissure. Although the two hemispheres seem to be mirror images of each other, they are different. For instance, the ability to form words seems to lie primarily in the left hemisphere, while the right hemisphere seems to control many abstract reasoning skills. For some as-yet-unknown reason, nearly all of the signals from the brain to the body and vice-versa cross over on their way to and from the brain. This means that the right cerebral hemisphere primarily controls the left side of the body and the left hemisphere primarily controls the right side. When one side of the brain is damaged, the opposite side

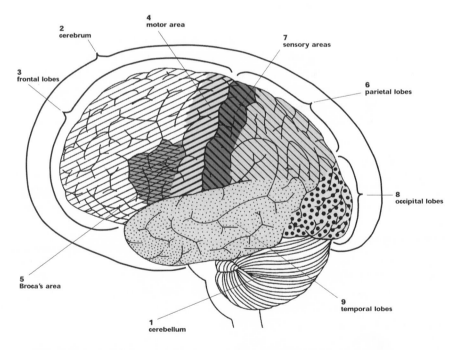

Figure 3.1. Architecture of the Brain (Source: NIH Publication No. 01–3440a, updated May 1, 2007).

35

of the body is affected. For example, a stroke in the right hemisphere of the brain can leave the left arm and leg paralyzed.

The Geography of Thought

Each cerebral hemisphere can be divided into sections, or lobes, each of which specializes in different functions. To understand each lobe and its specialty we will take a tour of the cerebral hemispheres, starting with the two frontal lobes (3), which lie directly behind the forehead. When you plan a schedule, imagine the future, or use reasoned arguments, these two lobes do much of the work. One of the ways the frontal lobes seem to do these things is by acting as short-term storage sites, allowing one idea to be kept in mind while other ideas are considered. In the rearmost portion of each frontal lobe is a motor area (4), which helps control voluntary movement. A nearby place on the left frontal lobe called the Broca area (5) allows thoughts to be transformed into words.

When you enjoy a good meal—the taste, aroma, and texture of the food—two sections behind the frontal lobes called the parietal lobes (6) are at work. The forward parts of these lobes, just behind the motor areas, are the primary sensory areas (7). These areas receive information about temperature, taste, touch, and movement from the rest of the body. Reading and arithmetic are also functions in the repertoire of each parietal lobe. When you look at words and pictures, two areas at the back of the brain are at work. These lobes, called the occipital lobes (8), process images from the eyes and link that information with images stored in memory. Damage to the occipital lobes can cause blindness.

The last lobes on our tour of the cerebral hemispheres are the temporal lobes (9), which lie in front of the visual areas and nest under the parietal and frontal lobes. Whether you appreciate symphonies or rock music, your brain responds through the activity of these lobes. At the top of each temporal lobe is an area responsible for receiving information from the ears. The underside of each temporal lobe plays a crucial role in forming and retrieving memories, including those associated with music. Other parts of this lobe seem to integrate memories and sensations of taste, sound, sight, and touch.

The Cerebral Cortex

Coating the surface of the cerebrum and the cerebellum is a vital layer of tissue the thickness of a stack of two or three dimes. It is called the cortex, from the Latin word for bark. Most of the actual information processing in the brain takes place in the cerebral cortex. When people talk about "gray matter" in the brain they are talking about this thin rind. The cortex is gray because nerves in this area lack the insulation that makes most other parts of the brain appear to be white. The folds in the brain add to its surface area and therefore increase the amount of gray matter and the quantity of information that can be processed.

The Inner Brain

Deep within the brain, hidden from view, lie structures that are the gatekeepers between the spinal cord and the cerebral hemispheres. These structures not only determine our emotional state, they also modify our perceptions and responses depending on that state, and

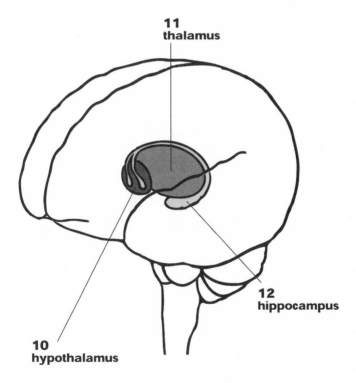

Figure 3.2. Inner Brain (Source: NIH Publication No. 01–3440a, updated May 1, 2007).

allow us to initiate movements that you make without thinking about them. Like the lobes in the cerebral hemispheres, the structures described below come in pairs: each is duplicated in the opposite half of the brain.

The hypothalamus (10), about the size of a pearl, directs a multitude of important functions. It wakes you up in the morning, and gets the adrenaline flowing during a test or job interview. The hypothalamus is also an important emotional center, controlling the molecules that make you feel exhilarated, angry, or unhappy. Near the hypothalamus lies the thalamus (11), a major clearinghouse for information going to and from the spinal cord and the cerebrum. An arching tract of nerve cells leads from the hypothalamus and the thalamus to the hippocampus (12). This tiny nub acts as a memory indexer—sending memories out to the appropriate part of the cerebral hemisphere for long-term storage and retrieving them when necessary. The basal ganglia (not shown) are clusters of nerve cells surrounding the thalamus. They are responsible for initiating and integrating movements. Parkinson disease, which results in tremors, rigidity, and a stiff, shuffling walk, is a disease of nerve cells that lead into the basal ganglia.

Neurological Disorders

When the brain is healthy it functions quickly and automatically. But when problems occur, the results can be devastating. Some 50 million people in this country—one in five—suffer from damage to the nervous system. The NINDS supports research on more than 600 neurological diseases. Some of the major types of disorders include: neurogenetic diseases (such as multiple sclerosis, Huntington disease, and muscular dystrophy), developmental disorders (such as cerebral palsy), degenerative diseases of adult life (such as Parkinson disease and Alzheimer disease), metabolic diseases (such as Gaucher disease), cerebrovascular diseases (such as stroke and vascular dementia), trauma (such as spinal cord and head injury), convulsive disorders (such as epilepsy), infectious diseases (such as AIDS dementia), and brain tumors.

How Does the Spinal Cord Work?

Spine Anatomy

The soft, jelly-like spinal cord is protected by the spinal column. The spinal column is made up of 33 bones called vertebrae, each with a circular opening similar to the hole in a donut. The bones are stacked one on top of the other and the spinal cord runs through the hollow channel created by the holes in the stacked bones. The vertebrae can be organized into sections, and are named and numbered from top to bottom according to their location along the backbone:

- cervical vertebrae (1–7) located in the neck
- thoracic vertebrae (1–12) in the upper back (attached to the ribcage)
- lumbar vertebrae (1–5) in the lower back
- sacral vertebrae (1–5) in the hip area
- coccygeal vertebrae (1–4 fused) in the tailbone

Although the hard vertebrae protect the soft spinal cord from injury most of the time, the spinal column is not all hard bone. Between the vertebrae are discs of semi-rigid cartilage, and in the narrow spaces between them are passages through which the spinal nerves exit to the rest of the body. These are places where the spinal cord is vulnerable to direct injury.

The spinal cord is also organized into segments and named and numbered from top to bottom. Each segment marks where spinal nerves emerge from the cord to connect to specific regions of the body. Locations of spinal cord segments do not correspond exactly to vertebral locations, but they are roughly equivalent.

- Cervical spinal nerves (C1 to C8) control signals to the back of the head, the neck and shoulders, the arms and hands, and the diaphragm.
- Thoracic spinal nerves (T1 to T12) control signals to the chest muscles, some muscles of the back, and parts of the abdomen.
- Lumbar spinal nerves (L1 to L5) control signals to the lower parts of the abdomen and the back, the buttocks, some parts of the external genital organs, and parts of the leg.
- Sacral spinal nerves (S1 to S5) control signals to the thighs and lower parts of the legs, the feet, most of the external genital organs, and the area around the anus.

The single coccygeal nerve carries sensory information from the skin of the lower back.

Spinal Cord Anatomy

The spinal cord has a core of tissue containing nerve cells, surrounded by long tracts of nerve fibers consisting of axons. The tracts extend up and down the spinal cord, carrying signals to and from the brain. The average size of the spinal cord varies in circumference along its length from the width of a thumb to the width of one of the smaller fingers. The spinal cord extends down through the upper two thirds of the vertebral canal, from the base of the brain to the lower back, and is generally 15 to 17 inches long depending on an individual's height.

The interior of the spinal cord is made up of neurons, their support cells called glia, and blood vessels. The neurons and their dendrites (branching projections that help neurons communicate with each other) reside in an H-shaped region called "gray matter."

The H-shaped gray matter of the spinal cord contains motor neurons that control movement, smaller interneurons that handle communication within and between the segments of the spinal cord, and cells that receive sensory signals and then send information up to centers in the brain.

Surrounding the gray matter of neurons is white matter. Most axons are covered with an insulating substance called myelin, which allows electrical signals to flow freely and quickly. Myelin has a whitish appearance, which is why this outer section of the spinal cord is called "white matter."

Axons carry signals downward from the brain (along descending pathways) and upward toward the brain (along ascending pathways) within specific tracts. Axons branch at their ends and can make connections with many other nerve cells simultaneously. Some axons extend along the entire length of the spinal cord.

The descending motor tracts control the smooth muscles of internal organs and the striated (capable of voluntary contractions) muscles of the arms and legs. They also help adjust the autonomic nervous system's regulation of blood pressure, body temperature, and the response to stress. These pathways begin with neurons in the brain that send electrical signals downward to specific levels of the spinal cord. Neurons in these segments then send the impulses out to the rest of the body or coordinate neural activity within the cord itself.

The ascending sensory tracts transmit sensory signals from the skin, extremities, and internal organs that enter at specific segments of the spinal cord. Most of these signals are then relayed to the brain. The spinal cord also contains neuronal circuits that control reflexes and repetitive movements, such as walking, which can be activated by incoming sensory signals without input from the brain.

The circumference of the spinal cord varies depending on its location. It is larger in the cervical and lumbar areas because these areas supply the nerves to the arms and upper body and the legs and lower body, which require the most intense muscular control and receive the most sensory signals.

The ratio of white matter to gray matter also varies at each level of the spinal cord. In the cervical segment, which is located in the neck, there is a large amount of white matter because at this level there are many axons going to and from the brain and the rest of the spinal cord below. In lower segments, such as the sacral, there is less white matter because most ascending axons have not yet entered the cord, and most descending axons have contacted their targets along the way.

To pass between the vertebrae, the axons that link the spinal cord to the muscles and the rest of the body are bundled into 31 pairs of spinal nerves, each pair with a sensory root and a motor root that make connections within the gray matter. Two pairs of nerves—a sensory and motor pair on either side of the cord—emerge from each segment of the spinal cord.

The functions of these nerves are determined by their location in the spinal cord. They control everything from body functions such as breathing, sweating, digestion, and elimination, to gross and fine motor skills, as well as sensations in the arms and legs.

The Nervous Systems

Together, the spinal cord and the brain make up the central nervous system (CNS). The CNS controls most functions of the body, but it is not the only nervous system in the body. The peripheral nervous system (PNS) includes the nerves that project to the limbs, heart, skin, and other organs outside the brain. The PNS controls the somatic nervous system which regulates muscle movements and the response to sensations of touch and pain, and the autonomic nervous system which provides nerve input to the internal organs and generates automatic reflex responses. The autonomic nervous system is divided into the sympathetic nervous system which mobilizes organs and their functions during times of stress and arousal, and the parasympathetic nervous system which conserves energy and resources during times of rest and relaxation.

The spinal cord acts as the primary information pathway between the brain and all the other nervous systems of the body. It receives sensory information from the skin, joints, and muscles of the trunk, arms, and legs, which it then relays upward to the brain. It carries messages downward from the brain to the PNS, and contains motor neurons, which direct voluntary movements and adjust reflex movements. Because of the central role it plays in coordinating muscle movements and interpreting sensory input, any kind of injury to the spinal cord can cause significant problems throughout the body.

Section 3.2

Myelin and Nerve Structure

This section includes an excerpt from "Brain Basics: Know Your Brain," National Institute of Neurological Disorders and Stroke (NINDS), NIH Publication No. 01–3440a, updated May 1, 2007; and "Myelin," from *The MS Information Sourcebook*. Reprinted in full with permission of the National Multiple Sclerosis Society. Copyright © 2006 National Multiple Sclerosis Society. All rights reserved. Material on the National Multiple Sclerosis Society is regularly updated. For the latest version of this information, please visit: www.nationalMSsociety.org.

Brain Basics: Making Connections

The brain and the rest of the nervous system are composed of many different types of cells, but the primary functional unit is a cell called the neuron. All sensations, movements, thoughts, memories, and feelings are the result of signals that pass through neurons. Neurons consist of three parts. The cell body (13) contains the nucleus, where most of the molecules that the neuron needs to survive and function are manufactured. Dendrites (14) extend out from the cell body like the branches of a tree and receive messages from other nerve cells. Signals then pass from the dendrites through the cell body and may travel away from the cell body down an axon (15) to another neuron, a muscle cell, or cells in some other organ. The neuron is usually surrounded by many support cells. Some types of cells wrap around the axon to form an insulating sheath (16). This sheath can include a fatty molecule called myelin, which provides insulation for the axon and helps nerve signals travel faster and farther. Axons may be very short, such

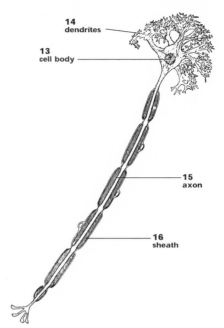

Figure 3.3. Neuron: Primary Functional Unit of the Nervous System (Source: NIH Publication No. 01–3440a, updated May 1, 2007).

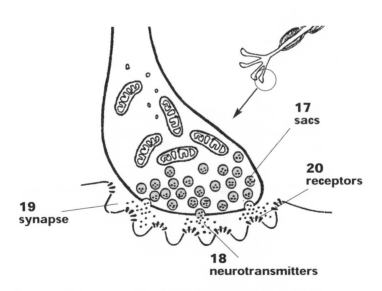

Figure 3.4. Synapse: Where Signals Pass from the Neuron to a Cell (Source: NIH Publication No. 01–3440a, updated May 1, 2007).

as those that carry signals from one cell in the cortex to another cell less than a hair's width away. Or axons may be very long, such as those that carry messages from the brain all the way down the spinal cord.

Scientists have learned a great deal about neurons by studying the synapse—the place where a signal passes from the neuron to another cell. When the signal reaches the end of the axon it stimulates tiny sacs (17). These sacs release chemicals known as neurotransmitters (18) into the synapse (19). The neurotransmitters cross the synapse and attach to receptors (20) on the neighboring cell. These receptors can change the properties of the receiving cell. If the receiving cell is also a neuron, the signal can continue the transmission to the next cell.

Some Key Neurotransmitters at Work

Acetylcholine is called an excitatory neurotransmitter because it generally makes cells more excitable. It governs muscle contractions

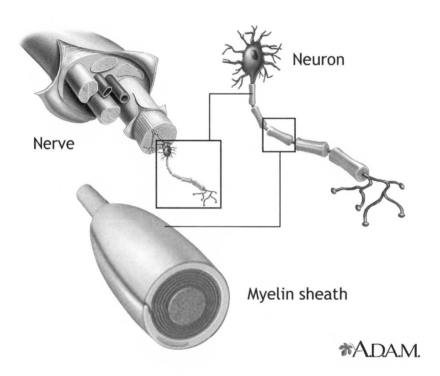

Figure 3.5. *Myelin and Nerve Structure (Source: © 2007 A.D.A.M., Inc. Reprinted with permission.)*

and causes glands to secrete hormones. Alzheimer disease, which initially affects memory formation, is associated with a shortage of acetylcholine.

GABA (gamma-aminobutyric acid) is called an inhibitory neurotransmitter because it tends to make cells less excitable. It helps control muscle activity and is an important part of the visual system. Drugs that increase GABA levels in the brain are used to treat epileptic seizures and tremors in patients with Huntington disease.

Serotonin is an inhibitory neurotransmitter that constricts blood vessels and brings on sleep. It is also involved in temperature regulation. Dopamine is an inhibitory neurotransmitter involved in mood and the control of complex movements. The loss of dopamine activity in some portions of the brain leads to the muscular rigidity of Parkinson disease. Many medications used to treat behavioral disorders work by modifying the action of dopamine in the brain.

Myelin

Myelin is a substance rich in protein and lipids (fatty substances) that forms layers around the nerve fibers and acts as insulation. The nerve can be likened to an electrical cable; the axon, or nerve fiber that transmits the nerve impulse is like the wire, and the myelin sheath is like the insulation around the wire. Myelin is present in both the central nervous system (CNS) and the peripheral nervous system (PNS), but it is only the destruction of CNS myelin that produces the symptoms of multiple sclerosis (MS).

The CNS (the brain, spinal cord and optic nerves) is made up of several different components:

- The gray matter contains the cell bodies of the nerves.

- The white matter contains nerve fibers coated with myelin.

- The supporting cells form a supporting network.

PNS nerve cells perform two major functions:

- Sensory neurons collect information about the body's internal and external environment and convey it to the CNS.

- Motor neurons carry instructions from the CNS to the glands and muscles.

CNS and PNS Myelin Are Produced by Different Cells

CNS myelin is produced by special cells called oligodendrocytes. PNS myelin is produced by Schwann cells. The two types of myelin are chemically different, but they both perform the same function—to promote efficient transmission of a nerve impulse along the axon. The myelin layer is segmented and there are small "nodes" between the segments that are naturally unmyelinated. As chemical ions pass in and out of the axons, the electrical current they generate is conducted down the nerve, jumping from node to node. Myelin prevents the current from leaking out of the nerve at inappropriate points and decreases the electrical resistance of the nerve. This helps make sure the nerve impulse is conducted efficiently.

Abnormal Immune Reaction Believed to Attack Myelin

An abnormal autoimmune reaction in MS is believed to initiate an attack on the myelin, resulting in bare spots and scarred areas along the nerve. Conduction of the nerve impulse is then slowed or halted, producing the neurologic signs and symptoms of MS. Destruction of myelin, a process known as demyelination, can also lead to "cross-talk" between nerves—abnormal nerve-to-nerve signaling, which also may produce symptoms.

The Future of Myelin Repair

Efforts to reverse the damage caused by MS and restore function in people with MS must focus on the repair of myelin, oligodendrocytes, and neurons in the CNS. These efforts will not be successful, however, unless a way is found to stop the immune system from damaging the CNS tissue in the first place.

In October 2002, researchers from around the world met at the International Workshop on Repair of the Central Nervous System (co-sponsored by the National MS Society and the Association pour la Recherche sur la Sclèrose en Plaques) to address issues related to MS-related neural injury and repair.

Some Neural Repair Occurs Naturally

Scientists have discovered that the body heals some lesions naturally, by stimulating oligodendrocytes in the area, or recruiting young oligodendrocytes from further away, to begin making new myelin at the damaged site. Research is now working to identify the molecular signals that are used by the body to activate the oligodendrocytes so that those signals can be mimicked to stimulate additional repair. Scientists are also studying certain proteins known as "growth factors" in order to identify their potential role in myelin repair.

As scientists are working to stimulate myelin repair, they are also focusing their attention on several properties of myelin that work to inhibit this repair. Eventually, therapies may be developed to stop these components of myelin from inhibiting the repair process.

Additional Approaches to Myelin Repair

Scientists are investigating several different strategies for stimulating the repair of myelin.

- Antibodies (immune proteins that attach to specific molecules) have been successfully used to stimulate myelin repair in rodents with an MS-like disease. Based on the outcomes from this research, the antibodies will undergo preliminary testing for safety in people with MS.

- Efforts are also being made to surgically replace damaged oligodendrocytes and nerve cells.

- Scientists are working to identify potential sources of replacement cells for those that are damaged by MS. Possible sources include: skin-derived cells, bone marrow and umbilical cord blood cells, fetal cells, adult brain cells, and Schwann cells from the PNS. The usefulness of these replacement cells will depend on finding or creating the signals needed to stimulate their transformation and growth into healthy new cells.

Chapter 4

Cellular Processes Involved with MS

Early Treatments and Charcot

Years ago treatments were often based upon false hypotheses of what was thought to take place in a person with MS during the progression of the disease. First mentions of an MS-like disease have been traced back to the 1300s, when the disease was often thought to be religious in nature. In this context, people might be suffering for the sins of others, and remissions could be viewed as miracles.

By the 1800s, treatments for this illness included such procedures as flesh-brush rubs, leeches, and skin plasters. Courses of electrical therapy were sometimes given, and prescriptions would include a host of unusual and toxic ingredients, such as mercury, quinine, and strychnine.

Jean-Martin Charcot, a clinician in Paris in the mid-to-late 1800s, provided doctors and patients with the first clinical and pathologic description of the disease. Charcot studied medicine at the University of Paris, where he developed the ability to combine patient experiences and doctors' descriptions, with the autopsy patterns of disease pathology.

By pairing clinical science with a pathologic correlation, Charcot was able to advance the understanding of several chronic diseases, including MS. In his 1868 description of the disease, Charcot describes plaques of demyelination and suggests the involvement of myelin in the development of MS. Charcot is also responsible for giving MS a name: "sclerose en plaque." Although doctors at that time were familiar with this illness, Charcot provided a clear definition of the disease—so other doctors could more readily recognize and understand the condition.

Since this time, researchers have made significant progress in identifying a number of the processes that appear to lead to the development and worsening of MS, with several important findings occurring only within the past decade. Current treatments are based on the cellular changes that are believed to take place within the body of a person with MS. And although many details still remain a mystery, researchers appear to be getting much closer to a cause and cure.

Nerve Impulses, Axons, and Myelin

Nerve impulses serve as messages between the brain and other parts of the body (via the brainstem and spinal cord), delivering instructions on how to perform. Nerve impulses travel along connecting nerve fibers, called axons, which are thin projections from the nerve cells. These vary in length from less than an inch to several feet.

Axons are similar to electrical wires that carry electrical impulses to the objects they are powering. Axons need a protective covering of insulation, just like the wires within your home. Without such insulation, electricity leaks or "shorts" out along the way and is unable to complete its trip to supply power.

Axons are covered with a protective layer called myelin. Composed of fat and protein, myelin acts as insulation for the axons and allows for optimum, uninterrupted flow of nerve impulses. Impulses normally travel at speeds of 225 miles per hour (mph) along these axons. MS affects the central nervous system (CNS), which consists of the brain and spinal cord. This neurological disorder has traditionally been termed a demyelinating disease, which means that the myelin protecting the nerve fibers is damaged or destroyed. Without insulation surrounding an axon, the nerve flow can slow down, become garbled, or "short-circuit" and discontinue entirely. When this happens, messages from the brain arrive at their destination late, confused, or not at all. Activities easily performed in the past may now require more time and may become difficult or even impossible to accomplish.

Until a few years ago, the focus of MS research was primarily on the loss of myelin. Research now shows that the axons in a person with MS appear to become damaged as well. This finding allows researchers to investigate other strategies for treating MS, such as using drugs that can prevent nerve cell death (known as neuroprotective agents) or procedures that may repair damaged nerves.

In relapsing-remitting multiple sclerosis (RRMS), the myelin and axons may not experience permanent or severe damage, and symptoms normally disappear or greatly diminish once the inflammation subsides and the relapse goes into remission. Slight changes to the myelin or axons may occur, slowing down the nerve impulses, but these changes are often not enough to cause symptoms. Nerve impulses traveling along the axons at a reduced speed, however, are thought to contribute to the fatigue often experienced by people with MS.

With the progressive forms of MS, the myelin and axons appear to experience steady damage. Inflammation is not thought to be involved (where cells attack other cells), but instead the cells appear to die on their own, which is known as apoptosis. Sometimes, the magnetic resonance image (MRI) shows ongoing axon damage and brain atrophy early in MS. These findings support the idea of considering MS treatments as soon as possible, and according to the advice of an individual's physician.

Evidence suggests that cells needed to rebuild these axons and myelin may possibly still be present in the areas of damage—and treatments may be found to activate these cells.

Lesions and White Blood Cells

Although researchers have yet to confirm which agents initiate the process leading to myelin and axonal damage, many of the factors involved have been identified. An MS exacerbation begins when the myelin becomes inflamed and swollen. This inflamed area is referred to as a lesion. Tiny vessels in the area dilate and leak activated white blood cells into the tissues of the brain. These inflammatory cells stimulate the secretion of chemicals called cytokines, which activate certain cells (called macrophages) to damage myelin.

White blood cells are essential units of the immune system and are produced by the body to fight foreign substances, which may cause infection or disease. Most researchers believe MS is an "autoimmune disease"—one in which white blood cells are misguided to target and fight the body's own cells.

51

Macrophages

White blood cells originate from the thymus, spleen, and lymph nodes. Two types of white blood cells are relevant to MS: larger cells known as macrophages (Greek for "big eaters") and smaller cells called lymphocytes. Macrophages, also known as scavenger cells, clean up areas by surrounding and consuming debris—in this case, myelin. Macrophages secrete proteases, and these can destroy myelin. Macrophages also produce prostaglandins, some of which promote inflammation and immune functions, while others suppress the same functions. Additionally, macrophages secrete free oxygen radicals. These can also significantly affect immune functions by promoting inflammation and cell destruction.

Lymphocytes

Among the many types of lymphocytes are B-lymphocytes and T-lymphocytes. B-lymphocytes are processed in bone marrow and produce immunoglobulins (also called gamma-globulin)—which are usually antibodies (cells that fight disease and infection). Antibodies are now thought to be able to damage myelin. Treatments aimed at these B-cells and antibodies may be another option for future drug development.

The majority of T-lymphocytes are processed in the thymus gland. Increased numbers of T-lymphocytes may be found in the cerebrospinal fluid (CSF) of a person with MS during an exacerbation. CSF is the fluid that circulates through and nourishes the brain and spinal canal. The many categories of T-lymphocytes include three types of T-cells.

1. T-helper cells—whose numbers increase in cerebrospinal fluid during an exacerbation, modulate the immune response, and are considered "regulatory T-cells" along with T-suppressor cells.

2. T-suppressor cells—researchers find decreased T-suppressor cell activity in blood early in new exacerbations, and as their name suggests, these cells suppress an immune response. T-suppressor cell activity returns to normal following an exacerbation.

3. T-killer cells—are sent to attack and destroy whatever the immune system interprets as being a foreign substance. In conjunction with macrophages, T-lymphocytes are activated when

exposed to a certain stimulus. Once this occurs, T-lympho-cytes become metabolically more active, grow in size, and se-crete a group of chemicals called cytokines. These are protein molecules that facilitate communication between cells and act as mediators for immune responses through interaction with specific cell-surface receptors. The four types of cytokines in-clude:

- interleukins
- lymphokines
- interferons
- tumor necrosis factor

The functions of the cytokines are to (1) increase inflammation and damage (pro-inflammatory) or (2) reduce inflammation (anti-inflammatory). The pro-inflammatory cytokines work by:

- increasing the number of lymphocytes;
- activating macrophages;
- increasing blood flow and edema (swelling from fluid retention) of the tissue; and
- bringing in additional white blood cells.

Th-1 (T-helper 1) cells produce pro-inflammatory cytokines. These are the cells that appear to worsen MS, potentially causing injury to the myelin and axons. These include interferon gamma (IFN-gamma), tumor necrosis factor (TNF-alpha), interleukin 12 (IL-12), IL-6, IL-2, and IL-1. Th-1 cells are thought to increase during an exacerbation.

Th-2 (T-helper 2) cells produce anti-inflammatory cytokines. These may work to stop the inflammation associated with the damaging le-sions in MS. They include interleukin 4 (IL-4), IL-10, and transform-ing growth factor beta (TGF-b). Th-2 cells may decrease during a relapse and increase at the conclusion of the flare-up. Treatments that switch the T-cells from Th-1 to Th-2, such as Copaxone®, are effective in MS.

Plasma Cells

Some lymphocytes entering the brain become plasma cells, which produce large numbers of immunoglobulins (antibodies). They also remain in the CNS for a long time following an exacerbation.

Glial Cells

Glial cells are non-neuronal brain cells, which provide support to neurons. (Neurons are the "thinking cells" of the brain, also known as gray matter.) One type of glial cell relevant to MS is the oligodendrocyte (oligo). Oligos are the cells which produce and nourish myelin. Myelin may sometimes be repaired by the oligos, a process known as "remyelination." When remyelination occurs, a person with MS may experience a recovery or remission. Unfortunately, in most cases of MS, the oligos eventually decrease or are depleted. This results in myelin loss as well as the loss of the ability to make more myelin.

New myelin is normally produced by young oligos. These new myelin cells develop in stages from another type of cell called a stem cell. As a person ages, these stem cells are less able to transform into oligos. Older oligos do not divide or replace themselves. Without young oligos or stem cells to develop myelin, remyelination is often slow and incomplete, if at all.

Researchers are presently working with mechanisms to transplant young oligos or stem cells into people with MS in order to promote remyelination along damaged areas. Although this process would not affect the underlying disease, it does hold the potential for the recovery of nerve function to disabled patients, as well as possible applications for individuals who suffer from spinal cord injuries or other nerve-related afflictions.

In a previous study, glial cells were transplanted into dogs with myelin disorders. These transplants resulted in large-scale remyelination, and for one dog, the remyelination continued to grow and spread for several months.

Another possibility exists in the lesions around the damaged axons of a person with MS. As mentioned earlier, studies suggest that cells capable of remyelination may still exist in these areas, and researchers may be able to find ways to activate these cells.

Insulating myelin may also be found in the two other systems aside from the CNS—the peripheral nervous system (PNS), which consists of the nerves connecting the spinal cord to the arms and legs, and the autonomic nervous system (ANS), which controls involuntary body functions such as breathing, sweating, and beating of the heart.

These systems appear to be unaffected by MS. A few people with MS, however, may experience symptoms related to ANS dysfunction. A phase I trial has taken myelin-building cells from the PNS (known as Schwann cells) and transplanted them into the brain of an MS patient, to see if these cells will produce new myelin in the CNS. More studies are planned depending on the outcome of this groundbreaking trial.

Another type of glial cell playing a role in MS is the astrocyte, a cell that normally supports the axons. Astrocytes increase in number and size when they arrive at the damaged myelin, possibly attaching themselves to the axons and preventing remyelination from taking place. Gliosis is the overgrowth of astrocytes, and this forms scars around the axon.

The Blood-Brain Barrier and Adhesion Molecules

Astrocyte function includes regulating the passage of soluble substances between the blood vessels and other CNS cells. To reach CNS tissue, cells must pass through the blood-brain barrier (BBB). Under normal conditions, the ability of substances to pass through the walls of the blood vessels into the CNS is very limited. This means that many cells, including those that cause harm, are normally unable to pass through the vessel wall and attack CNS cells.

With MS, white blood cells are able to pass through the BBB and target myelin for destruction. Research has shown that the BBB must be altered in order for MS to initially begin and for demyelination to ultimately take place.

Adhesion molecules are protein structures which are believed to assist the white blood cells of the immune system to pass through the BBB. These molecules lie on the surface of white blood cells as well as the cells lining the blood vessels. White blood cells must first adhere (or stick) to the blood vessel lining with the aid of adhesion molecules, before passing through the BBB into the CNS.

Researchers are testing new agents that block these adhesion molecules, thereby preventing the immune system cells from going through the BBB and reaching the myelin. Factors thought to possibly increase BBB permeability include viral infection and vaccination.

Plaques

Once the myelin becomes inflamed and blood leaks into the area (carrying macrophages and lymphocytes), some important changes take place.

- T-suppressor cells (those which suppress an immune response) decrease.

- Th-1 cells (those which initially promote an immune response through cytokines) increase.

- T-killer cells and antibodies are believed to target and attack the myelin and axons, as if they were foreign substances (causing disease or infection).

- The macrophages then "clean up" by consuming and digesting the damaged myelin.

- The oligos, cells which could produce new myelin, decrease or disappear.

- The astrocytes increase in number and size, forming thick, dense tissue together with the other cells in the same area. This process creates firm tissue along the axons and is similar to a scar.

Known as plaques, these areas of thick tissue formed by the astrocytes show up as white patches on MRI exams. The changes in size, number, and location of these plaques may determine the type and severity of the patient's symptoms as well as give the physician a visual chart by which to measure the progression of the disease.

Plaques may affect one axon or span across several. They vary in size from that of a pinhead to more than an inch in length. As plaques accumulate or increase in size, the functioning of the CNS deteriorates.

Interestingly, plaques are often widely distributed throughout the brain and spinal cord, many of which cause no apparent problems. The term multiple sclerosis originates from the discovery of these plaques. Multiple refers to *many*; sclerosis refers to *scars*.

Keep in mind, however, that inflammation does not always result in damage to the myelin and the forming of plaques. Some completely recover with no signs of any interference. What instructs the cells to form the plaque is still unknown. What keeps the plaque from forming in other instances is equally puzzling. Th-2 cells appear and release anti-inflammatory cytokines, which may be one factor in stopping the damage.

Inflammation only occurs in the early stages of secondary-progressive multiple sclerosis (SPMS), and later, primary degeneration causes the myelin and axons to become damaged. At this time apoptosis takes place, and cells simply die off. The latter is true for the other types of progressive MS as well.

Chapter 5

Understanding the Genetics of MS

Multiple sclerosis (MS) is a complex disease influenced by many factors rather than driven by a single cause. Genetic or inherited factors are important but environmental exposure also plays a part. This distinguishes MS from so called "simple" genetic conditions where disease is caused by a deficit in a single gene. The inherited risk of MS is likely to involve several genes (perhaps 5–10) interacting with each other and with environmental factors. Research into the genetics of MS therefore involves the search for genes that contribute to susceptibility and/or to the severity and other aspects of the disease. More recently, genetic research has extended into the study of inherited variations in response to treatment (pharmacogenetics).

How is it known that genes are important in MS?

For many years it has been evident that close family members of a person with MS have a higher risk of having the disease, and the closer they are genetically, the higher the risk. Unrelated family members (such as husband or wife) show no increased risk but the children of marriages where both parents have MS have a particularly high risk. A large study of people with MS who were adopted under the age of one year clearly showed that risk is largely due to genetic factors rather than the environment.

In the 1970s, there was a breakthrough with the discovery of a very strong association between MS and genes that control immune cell function, known as human leukocyte antigens (HLA) genes. For people of northern European origin, about 60 percent with MS have the same HLA gene type, a type found in only 20 percent of the general population. This relationship between MS and a genetic marker, and other associations, make up an important part of what we mean by the "genetics of MS." With the Human Genome Project leading to a complete map of the human chromosomes, and with advances in technologies for rapidly typing many genes, many research groups worldwide are actively involved in genetics research.

How is genetic influence achieved?

Genes contain information that we inherit from our parents and this information is used to produce proteins. Proteins are components of all living cells: some provide essential building materials; some control the breakdown of energy sources and waste products; some act as important messengers; some recognize and destroy bacteria and viruses; others are master regulators that control the activity of genes and their ability to produce other proteins.

Susceptibility to some diseases, in particular those that can be directly transmitted from parent to child, occurs when abnormal genes are copied in either sperm or eggs, thereby leading to the perpetuation of expression of abnormally functioning proteins and, hence, inherited disease. In the case of MS and other complex diseases, it is more likely that subtle changes in the structure and function of a combination of proteins, rather than a devastating mutation in a single protein, are relevant. These combinations act to increase the risk of disease but do not reflect the sole cause. Environmental factors also have a role to play.

Many of the proteins produced by genes exert their effects not in isolation but as part of pathways, akin to cogs in a production line. As in industry, it is possible to compensate for a single, minor problem, but if there are several sequential deficits in a single pathway, or alternatively, deficits in both primary and auxiliary pathways, then more overt susceptibilities emerge; essentially, there is a multiplier effect. In addition, if there are deficits in regulatory proteins, these are likely to exert their influence at either multiple points in a singe pathway or in multiple pathways.

Variable susceptibility to complex diseases among individuals is a consequence of genetic diversity that is driven by two principal factors.

First, the genetic make-up of a child is a mix of that provided by each of its parents. Second, sections of the parents' DNA that were contributed by either of their parents can swap over, or recombine, at the time sperm or eggs form, potentially leading to yet further diversity. More than one minor variation in a gene coding for a given protein might produce increased susceptibility. In addition, different combinations of minor variations in different genes, either in a single pathway or in interacting pathways, could increase susceptibility. These influences may also be exerted in a given cell type or between interacting cells. For example, variations could be at work in either immune cells or in the cells within the brain and spinal cord that they target. This would explain why no one genetic signature confers susceptibility to MS. This also explains why complex diseases such as MS are not usually inherited directly from parent to child but are, instead, driven by the unique genetic mix present in any given individual.

Why is there so much research into the genetics of MS?

The search for MS genes is important because their discovery will provide vital information on which biologic mechanisms influence the disease. This will lead to a better understanding of what causes MS and to the development of new approaches to treatment and prevention. There is a real hope that in the future, genetic tests may predict the likelihood of benefit (or side effects) of a particular treatment, and thereby assist with a more personalized choice of treatment for each person. This already occurs in other diseases although such work is still in its early days.

Which are the best genes to study first in MS?

With perhaps 5–10 genes to find amongst the 30,000 known genes of the human genome, the search may seem impossible. Current knowledge of MS, however, helps researchers to focus in on certain groups of genes.

It is thought that MS is an example of autoimmune disease, a group of disorders that arise when the immune system—so important in protecting against bacteria and viruses—inappropriately targets the body's own tissues. In MS this attack is directed to the brain and spinal cord. It is therefore likely that genes which change the susceptibility to MS include those which influence the immune cells that drive this attack. Genes that influence the level of nervous system damage and its capacity for repair are also likely to be involved.

Are there examples of how genes and the environment might interact?

A current hypothesis holds that low sunlight exposure in childhood could predispose individuals to MS. This predisposition may be exerted through reduced Vitamin D, which is normally produced in the skin by ultraviolet light exposure. Vitamin D is known to dampen immune responses. The genetic influence here could conceivably come through variants in the Vitamin D receptor protein or in other proteins that are activated when Vitamin D binds to this receptor. This would result in an individual variation in the degree of immune system modulation exerted by a given level of sunlight exposure and Vitamin D production. In this way, differences in genetic make-up could contribute to determining individual susceptibility when there is fairly uniform exposure to an environmental trigger, for example low sunlight, by a larger population.

Future Directions in the Genetics of MS

The genetics of MS is not a simple phenomenon that will be unraveled by the analysis of a few individuals. Given the likelihood that multiple genes are involved, each producing a small effect and with none causally involved in all affected individuals, it is clear that studies of many thousands of people with MS, as well as matched controls of similar ethnic background, will be needed in order to detect MS susceptibility genes. To undertake such studies requires an immense effort, which involves recruitment of participants, assessment of the genetic composition of each of the many thousands of recombined segments, or haplotypes, present in each individual followed by detailed statistical analysis. Despite these challenges, in order to achieve fundamental advances in our understanding of MS, this is a genetic puzzle that we must continue to strive to unravel. Research groups in many countries throughout the world are collaborating in this effort.

Chapter 6

Male Experience with MS

Multiple sclerosis (MS) is often regarded as a woman's disease because the risk of contracting the disease is double in females.[1] "It sometimes seems as though males are a forgotten patient population," observes James Bowen, MD, Associate Professor of Neurology at the University of Washington Medical Center and attending physician at the VA Puget Sound Health Care System, both in Seattle.

There are several areas in which men and women differ in their experience of the disease. Men tend to have a later disease onset and shorter disease duration than do women. Men also tend to have more progressive forms of the disease while women have a greater tendency to have relapsing-remitting forms of MS, Dr. Bowen notes. He adds that men often have a less-favorable prognosis and do not respond as well to interferon therapy as do women.[2, 3]

Why Do Men and Women Differ?

While the reasons for these differences are unclear, researchers have set forth several hypotheses focusing on gender-related differences in the structural, chromosomal, endocrine, and immune systems.[4]

"The Male Experience in MS," by Batya Swift Yasgur, *MS Exchange*, November 2004. © 2004 Consortium of Multiple Sclerosis Centers. Reprinted with permission.

Structural Differences

Some proteins manufactured by men differ from those manufactured by women, Dr. Bowen explains. "Although we do not have an example of an actual gender-specific protein that is involved in the MS process, it stands to reason that protein differences might play a role in the different expressions of the disease." Attention has recently focused on myelin proteolipid protein (PLP). This protein accounts for about half of the protein in myelin. Changes in the structure of PLP may lead to an increased immune response, which has been detected in patients with MS.[5] Like myelin basic protein, PLP leads to the development of experimental autoimmune encephalomyelitis (EAE) in animals injected with it. Since PLP is expressed only on the X chromosome, men logically have lower PLP levels.

Chromosomal Differences

Human lymphocyte antigen (HLA) is one of a group of proteins found on the surface of white blood cells and other cells that play a role in the immune response. Abnormalities in certain HLA alleles are known to be associated with MS, says Dr. Bowen. The unique amino acid sequences of HLA alleles determine the immune system's ability to respond to an antigen. Because the HLA system determines whether antigens are presented to immune effector cells as self or non-self tissue, dysfunction in this system can lead to an autoimmune response.

Some HLA alleles are unevenly distributed in men and women, Dr. Bowen explains. In particular, the HLA-DR2 allele is significantly more prevalent in MS patients compared with the general population and is more frequent in women than in men with the disease.[5]

Hormonal Differences

"It is believed that hormones actually change the way the immune system functions, so it is likely that hormones play an important role in gender differences in MS," Dr. Bowen notes.

Female hormones, particularly estriol, appear to cause an earlier onset of disease symptoms, although it is not clear why. Symptoms of MS decrease during late pregnancy, when estriol levels are highest. Studies of EAE in animals have shown estriol to be effective in ameliorating symptoms in both males and females.[6] Female mice that have diminished estrogen levels due to oophorectomy show an increased incidence of acute progressive EAE.[7]

Testosterone seems to provide a protective effect against MS. This may be one of the reasons why MS presents later and in more progressive forms in men.[8] Orchiectomy, which leads to a decrease in testosterone levels, has been shown to modestly decrease time to disease onset and increase acute severity of the disease in EAE mice models.[9]

Yet gender differences persist even after gonadectomy in both sexes, implying that hormones are not the only factor involved in MS susceptibility, severity, progression, and disease type.[9] "The hormonal picture is confusing," admits Dr. Bowen. "There appear to be differences in the immune systems of men and women that are independent of hormones." For example, antigen-presenting cells and lymphocytes taken from females react more vigorously to most antigens than do antigen-presenting cells and lymphocytes taken from males. The addition of estrogen increases the response but is not necessary for the response to occur.[10] "More research is needed for us to understand the mechanisms that affect disease onset, type, and progression in men and women," he adds.

Treatment Issues for Men with MS

Gender differences in MS have an impact on treatment decisions, says Dr. Bowen. "Because the disease progresses so rapidly and is more severe, it is often necessary to take a more aggressive approach to therapy in men with the disease. In general, treatment with interferon should be initiated much earlier in males," he advises.

Men with MS are more likely to have an earlier onset of spinal cord-related symptoms, which also tend to be more severe than those experienced by women, says Dr. Bowen. Spinal cord-related symptoms include difficulties with movement and gait as well as bowel, bladder, and sexual dysfunction. Despite the differences in onset and severity, the same treatments are typically used for both sexes, he adds. "Therapy focuses on strengthening muscles and relieving spasticity, simplifying tasks at work and at home, developing a regular exercise program, and—as the disease progresses—learning to use assistive devices. Likewise, the approach to urinary and bowel difficulties does not differ significantly between men and women, where the goal of treatment is to correct urgency and incontinence issues."

Both men and women experience fatigue associated with MS. Amantadine and modafinil are the most commonly prescribed agents to relieve symptoms of fatigue in both men and women with the disease.

While a reduction in libido commonly occurs in both men and women with MS, a major problem for men is erectile dysfunction, says Dr. Bowen. "Many men have difficulty maintaining an erection and many experience anorgasmia." Some men also experience retrograde ejaculation (when semen backs up and enters the bladder instead of exiting through the urethra).

Agents such as sildenafil and tadalafil can be extremely useful in addressing sexual dysfunction—especially erectile difficulties, Dr. Bowen says. "There are no known interactions between these agents and MS disease-modifying drugs. If these medications fail, other options include penile implants, vacuum erection devices, urethral suppositories, or papaverine injections. A referral to a urologist can be helpful for men with complicated sexual dysfunction, he adds.

"One of the biggest mistakes health care providers make when treating males with MS is not asking about or discussing sexual dysfunction," Dr. Bowen emphasizes. "Men tend to be reticent about discussing sexual problems and may not initiate a discussion. Providers must be comfortable and proactive in bringing up this topic. In my experience, patients who experience sexual dysfunction are often relieved when a clinician asks them about it."

Providing psychosocial support is as important for men as it is for women, although men may be less likely to request this type of intervention, Dr. Bowen says. "Any chronic illness places stress on the patient as well as the family. Individual counseling and/or a support group can be invaluable for men with MS. Couples therapy might be helpful for some patients, particularly those who experience sexual dysfunction."

References

1. Kurtzke JF, Wallin MT. Epidemiology. In: Burks JS, Johnson KP, eds. *Multiple Sclerosis: Diagnosis, Medical Management, and Rehabilitation.* New York:Demos;2000:49–71.

2. Paty DW, SPIMS (Secondary Progressive Interferon beta-1a MS) Study Group. Results of the 3-year, double-blind, placebo-controlled study of interferon beta-1a (Rebif) in secondary-progressive MS. *J Neurol.* 1999;246 (Suppl 1):I/15.

3. Zaffaroni M, Ghezzi A. The prognostic value of age, gender, pregnancy and endocrine factors in multiple sclerosis. *Neurol Sci.* 2000;21(4 Suppl 2):857–860.

4. Duquette P, Pleines J, Girard M, et al. The increased suscepti-bility of women to multiple sclerosis. *Can J Neurol. Sci.* 1992;19: 466–471.

5. Greer JM, Denis B, Sobel RA, Trifilieff E. Thiopalmitoylation of myelin proteolipid protein epitopes enhances immunogenic-ity and encephalitogenicity. *J Immunol.* 2001; 166:6907–6913.

6. Palaszynski KM, Liu H, Loo KK, Voskuhl RR. Estriol treat-ment ameliorates disease in males with experimental autoim-mune encephalomyelitis: implications for multiple sclerosis. *J Neuroimmunol.* 2004;149:84–89.

7. Trooster WJ, Teelken AW, Gerrits PO, et al. The effect of gona-dectomy on the clinical course of chronic experimental allergic encephalomyelitis. *Clin Neurol Neurosurg.* 1996;98:222–226.

8. Voskuhl RR, Palaszynski K. Sex hormones in experimental autoimmune encephalomyelitis: implications for multiple scle-rosis. *Neuroscientist.* 2001;7:258–270.

9. Fillmore PD, Blankenhorn EP, Zachary JF, Teuscher C. Adult gonadal hormones selectively regulate sexually dimorphic quan-titative traits observed in experimental allergic encephalomy-elitis. *Am J Pathol.* 2004;164:167–175.

10. Voskuhl RR, Pitchekian-Halabi H, MacKenzie-Graham A, et al. Gender differences in autoimmune demyelination in the mouse: implications for multiple sclerosis. *Ann Neurol.* 1996;39:724–733.

Chapter 7

African Americans and MS

In recent years, much attention has been given to the importance of racial and cultural sensitivity in clinical practice. This issue is becoming more important in the field of multiple sclerosis (MS) as the diversity of those with the disease appears to increase. Research examining racial issues in MS tends to focus on whether race, ethnicity, or environmental conditions—or a combination thereof—are the most significant risk factors in the development of the disease. Although these are important notions to examine, more research needs to be done on the ways in which MS patients of different races experience the disease and how these differences affect treatment and outcomes.

"One of the biggest challenges facing health care providers when treating African Americans with MS is to identify how race plays a role in the development and course of the disease. Our priority should be to develop strategies for further studying and addressing this issue," stressed Mary D. Hughes, MD, Medical Director of the Augusta MS Center of the Medical College of Georgia, during her talk about African Americans and MS at the 2004 Consortium of Multiple Sclerosis Centers (CMSC) meeting in Toronto. The current literature seems to suggest that differences in the ethnic and racial

"Living with MS: An African-American Perspective," by Krista Binetti, *MS Exchange*, November 2004. © 2004 Consortium of Multiple Sclerosis Centers. Reprinted with permission.

backgrounds of MS patients may have significant implications for the long-term management of the disease.

Disparities in Access to Medical Care

No examination of race and illness can fail to take into account the disparities inherent in a particular health care system. "Health care disparities between African American and Caucasian patients in the United States health care system have been well-documented," said Dr. Hughes. For example, African American patients are less likely to get kidney transplants when warranted, regardless of socioeconomic or insurance status.[1] In addition, she noted, African Americans are more likely to receive limb amputations rather than revascularizations.[2]

"Historically, African Americans are less likely to receive preventive care or to receive care at the appropriate time," she added. For instance, pneumococcal vaccination rates are significantly lower among African Americans than among Caucasians.[3]

The Tuskegee Syphilis Experiment

Another relevant feature of the experience of African American patients seems to be an inherent mistrust of the health care system, according to Dr. Hughes. This may lead to a reluctance to take part in studies that may potentially illuminate the racial differences among people with MS. "Many patients simply do not want to be experimented on," she stated. She suggested that this sentiment might be an indirect result of the Tuskegee Syphilis Experiment. Between 1932 and 1972, the U.S. Public Health Service conducted a study involving over 400 black men from Macon County, Alabama who were infected with syphilis. The purpose of the experiment was to study the natural evolution of the disease and to learn how syphilis affected black individuals. However, participants were not told they had syphilis, were not warned about what the disease might do to them, and were not provided with treatment. At the end of this 40-year study, more than 100 men had died from syphilis or related complications.

"The Tuskegee Experiment is not ancient history," Dr. Hughes pointed out. "It's relatively current history and the memory of it may be an important reason why some African American patients are skeptical about entering into treatment studies." The use of injectable therapies may prove an even greater barrier, she noted, because "there is something about receiving an injection versus taking a pill that makes many patients mistrustful."

Literature on MS in African Americans

Dr. Hughes provided some background information by reviewing the published studies involving African Americans and MS. One of the earliest articles on this topic appeared in *Archives of Neurology* in 1962.[4] The researchers concluded that "little can be said because there are so few reports describing the disease in this race." Not much more would be published about MS in the African American population for the next several decades, Dr. Hughes noted.

A study published in *Neurology* in 1997[5] involving black World War II and Korean Conflict soldiers appeared to provide some early answers. MS risk was found to be significantly higher among African Americans with more education, higher socioeconomic status, and higher service test scores. This does not necessarily mean that these are risk factors for MS, said Dr. Hughes. "One way to interpret this finding," she stated, "is to realize that people who have these characteristics are more likely to have access to health care." In other words, MS may simply be under- or undiagnosed in those without adequate access to medical care.

Differences in Disease Course

Several studies suggest that there may be higher levels of disability among African Americans than among Caucasians with MS. A study in *Archives of Neurology* published in 1998[6] found that among MS patients presenting with optic neuritis, African Americans exhibited significantly more frequent severe visual loss compared with Caucasian study participants at the start of the study and at one year follow-up.

A retrospective study by Alshami and Jeffrey[7] involved 50 MS patients; 25 African American and 25 Caucasian. "The groups were well-matched in terms of age of onset and ratio of males to females," Dr. Hughes explained. "Among African Americans, relapsing-remitting MS was more common than the secondary progressive form of the disease. Also striking was that the duration of the disease was greater in African Americans, as was disability as measured by the Expanded Disability Status Scale (EDSS)." It is important to note that many of the patients who participated in this study were not being treated with disease-modifying therapies.

A study that appeared in the journal *Multiple Sclerosis* in 2003[8] set out to determine the clinical characteristics of MS in African American patients in the New York State Multiple Sclerosis Consortium patient registry. African American participants showed a preponderance of females and a significantly younger age at diagnosis than did Caucasian patients. The authors also found that African Americans with MS had greater disability at similar duration of disease compared with their Caucasian counterparts. In other words, Dr. Hughes explained, it took less time for African Americans with MS to reach higher disability levels.

Treatment Considerations

Dr. Hughes also discussed a subgroup analysis of the EVIDENCE trial.[9] This study involved more than 600 Caucasian Americans with MS and 36 African Americans with the disease. Twenty-four weeks after treatment with interferon beta-1a, African Americans had a greater number of lesions as seen on magnetic resonance imaging (MRI) compared with Caucasians. After 48 weeks, African Americans had 0.31 more relapses than did Caucasian Americans, 0.96 more new T2 lesions, and 0.51 times lower odds of having no new T2 lesions. "On all outcome measures, African American participants did not respond as well to treatment as did the other participants," Dr. Hughes pointed out.

"Overall, the literature seems to suggest that African Americans have significantly higher levels of disability earlier in the disease process than do Caucasians," she noted. Several questions arise as a result of these findings: How should race affect treatment recommendations? Are MS disease-modifying therapies less effective in the African American population? Do health care providers need to begin considering more aggressive therapy for African American MS patients from the beginning? Dr. Hughes admitted that "many of these questions do not have answers at present." The only way of finding answers, she added, is by encouraging black MS patients to participate in clinical studies.

"It's a very exciting time in MS research," she stated. "As we become more aware of issues that are unique to African Americans with MS, we have a greater chance to appropriately respond to these issues." Increased interest in the subject of African Americans with MS might have positive implications for anyone with the disease, regardless of racial or ethnic background, she added. "If we can identify the factors that may predict response to therapy or disease prognosis for a smaller subgroup of patients with MS, we may be able to make generalizations for the larger population."

References

1. U.S. Renal Data System. 1999 Annual Data Report. Bethesda, MD: NIH, NIDDK, April 1999, Appendix, Table F-1.

2. Guadagnoli E, Ayanian JZ, Gibbons G, et al. The influence of race on the use of surgical procedures for treatment of peripheral vascular disease of the lower extremities. *Arch Surg.* 1995; 130:381–386.

3. Centers for Disease Control. Influenza and pneumococcal vaccination levels among persons aged ≥65 years—United States, 2001. *MMWR Morb Mortal Wkly Rep.* 2002;51:1019–1024.

4. Alter M. Multiple sclerosis in the Negro. *Arch Neurol.* 1962;7:83–91.

5. Kurtzke JF, Page WF. Epidemiology of multiple sclerosis in US veterans: VII. Risk factors for MS. *Neurology.* 1997;48:204–213.

6. Phillips PH, Newman NJ, Lynn MJ. Optic neuritis in African-Americans. *Arch Neurol.* 1998;55:186–192.

7. Alshami D, Jeffrey D. American Academy of Neurology 50th Annual Meeting. *Neurology.* 1998;50(4 suppl 4):P04.034.

8. Weinstock-Guttman B, Jacobs LD, Brownscheidle CM, et al. Multiple characteristics in African-American patients in the New York State Multiple Sclerosis Consortium. *Mult Scler.* 2003;9:293–298. Available at: www.multiplesclerosisjournal .com.

9. Cree BC, Goodin DS, Oksenberg JR, et al. Multiple sclerosis disease activity in patients of different ethnic origin: Data from the EVIDENCE trial. American Academy of Neurology 55th Annual Meeting. *Neurology.* 2003;60(suppl 1):P01.120.

Chapter 8

Pediatric MS

Although pediatric-onset multiple sclerosis (MS) has been acknowledged for years, its prevalence and importance are only now being recognized, together with a growing awareness of the special needs of children with this disease. "Children with MS require accurate and prompt diagnosis, coupled with comprehensive, multidisciplinary care," Brenda Banwell, M.D., told attendees at the pediatric MS symposium held at the 2004 Consortium of Multiple Sclerosis Centers (CMSC) meeting in Toronto.

Barriers that impede the prompt diagnosis and treatment of MS in children include the reluctance of clinicians to entertain the diagnosis of MS in a child and the lack of clear clinical and radiographic diagnostic criteria specific to the pediatric population. Yet, approximately 5% of all MS patients experience an onset of symptoms before age 16, said Dr. Banwell, Director of the Pediatric Multiple Sclerosis Clinic at the Hospital for Sick Children in Toronto.

Recognizing MS in Children

According to Dr. Banwell, relapsing-remitting MS (RRMS) is the most common type of MS in children, while primary progressive MS

"Special Considerations in Pediatric MS," by Batya Swift Yasgur, *MS Exchange*, August 2004. © 2004 Consortium of Multiple Sclerosis Centers. Reprinted with permission.

73

is extremely rare in this population.[1] Several disorders are included in the differential diagnosis of acquired pediatric demyelination.[2]

To diagnose MS after a first attack, the clinician must ensure that acute central nervous system (CNS) demyelination is present, Dr. Banwell noted. "For example, if the child goes from well to severely impaired in a matter of hours, one would be more likely to think of vascular problems." Because fever accompanies the first MS attack in 30% to 40% of children, acute infections must also be ruled out, she added.

After determining that the child has demyelination, the next step is to evaluate symptom severity. "Mild symptoms do not necessarily require therapy with acute medications but they obviously require counseling, assessment, and support," Dr. Banwell suggested. Initiation of disease-modifying MS therapies is typically delayed in children until a sustained second attack. Application of the McDonald criteria,[3]—which allow for treatment of adults if magnetic resonance imaging (MRI) scans show new lesions, even in the absence of a second clinical event—requires further study in children.

Treatment of Pediatric MS

The Pediatric MS Clinic in Toronto has cared for more than 50 patients. The mean age at presentation was eleven years and 48% experienced their first demyelinating event at ten years of age or younger. Most patients are receiving, or are about to commence, therapy with a disease-modifying medication, Dr. Banwell reported. Choice of treatment is highly individualized, although the frequency of injection is a major determinant for some children. Dosage is determined by the child's size and typically begins at one-half the target dose. Many children eventually reach the adult dose.

Liver function, complete blood count, kidney function, and electrolytes should be checked at baseline and regularly during therapy. Monthly liver function monitoring is mandatory during the first six months. "We have not seen leukopenia, but we have certainly seen liver enzyme elevations," Dr. Banwell stated.

Management of adverse effects and injection site reactions is similar to that in adults. Fatigue can sometimes be mitigated by encouraging the child to avoid excessively warm environments or to rest briefly after school. Advocacy with the child's school can be helpful—for example, arranging for a second set of textbooks that remain at home so the child does not have to carry a heavy backpack. Medications such as modafinil and amantadine may be useful.

Psychosocial Issues

To carry out a successful treatment protocol in children with MS, one must recognize their special and evolving needs, explained Jennifer Boyd, RN, MHSc, MSCN. "Since children are constantly growing and developing, the approach to care changes at different developmental stages and involves both the child and family," said Ms. Boyd, who is a pediatric MS nurse at the Toronto clinic.

Initially, the parents are often more burdened by this diagnosis, since the child may not understand its implications. "Facilitating adaptation of the parents to the diagnosis will facilitate adaptation of the child," she explained. This involves education as well as support. "Provide current, accurate information; identify resources; offer hope; and refer parents for counseling services as needed," she advised.

Like parents, children require age-appropriate education and support. However, it is important to recognize that many children do not want too much information because they find it overwhelming or even disturbing, Ms. Boyd cautioned. Thus, only "necessary and requested" information should be offered. Clinicians and parents should take their cues from the child's questions, "capitalizing on opportunities to provide education when the child asks questions," she suggested. Children require reassurance that MS is not a death sentence and need encouragement to participate in regular activities with adaptations as needed. Referral to a social worker or psychiatrist at a pediatric facility may be required for additional counseling.

Treatment-Related Issues

Adherence to MS treatment regimens is challenging even for adults but presents particular difficulties in children and adolescents. Younger children may not have the cognitive maturity to understand the rationale for injections and their long-term benefits. Adolescents may not accept the need for therapy or the normal developmental processes of adolescence may compromise their commitment to therapy.

Promoting Adherence in Young Children

Encouraging adherence in young children begins with the very first injection. "We never want a situation where there's a screaming child and a dedicated parent with a needle in hand, determined to help a child who is not on board," Dr. Banwell emphasized. "It is critical that children understand why therapies are being given."

"It is important to make the first injection a positive experience," Ms. Boyd added. To this end, clinicians should involve the whole family when teaching so that parents and siblings can reinforce the message and help educate the child.

Well before the first injection, the clinician and parents should explain to the child on an age-appropriate level the rationale and benefits of treatment, encouraging the child's participation in the planning as much as possible. Letting a child know what to expect before the injection is essential. A teaching doll can be a helpful device for demonstrating injections to children of all ages. Children who are especially afraid of needles might benefit from desensitization treatment—a gradual, step-by-step process in which a child becomes accustomed to a feared object or experience.

Involving the child with decision-making minimizes trauma. Offering choices (manual versus autoinjector, location of the injection) helps the child become an "active participant" rather than a passive recipient of a painful, imposed process.

Part of the clinician's role is also to teach parents how to handle the emotional issues surrounding injections, Ms. Boyd said. "Parents should be encouraged to avoid punishment or removal of privileges if the child doesn't cooperate," Ms. Boyd recommended. Instead, "positive rewards and incentives are preferable as motivators." However, this does not imply a laissez faire attitude. Parents should convey a set of expectations to the child, combined with "a caring, consistent approach."

Children as young as age eight can learn to self-inject and adolescents can learn to administer intramuscular injections, Ms. Boyd noted. The idea of self-injection should be raised early and brought up periodically as the child matures, until he or she is ready to learn the skill. Reviewing the merits of self-injection (autonomy, being "grown up") and encouraging increased involvement can promote commitment on the part of the child. Parental supervision is required until it is clear that the child has mastered the skill and is fully competent, she stressed.

Unique Challenges in Adolescents

Adolescence is a challenging time in all respects and adherence to an MS treatment regimen is no exception. According to Ms. Boyd, several psychosocial factors interfere with adherence in adolescence. Adolescents may question their parents' treatment-related decisions and may refuse to initiate or continue with treatment. Young people who experience a high level of stress or irresolvable conflict with their parents or encounter a lack of support from their peers or lack of respect from health care providers may have difficulty with adherence.

Involving teens in the decision-making process may help to promote adherence in adolescents. Positive, mutually respectful relationships with health care professionals also can provide a boost for adherence. "When we're dealing with teenagers in particular, there are privacy issues," Dr. Banwell noted. Teens need the opportunity to communicate privately with health care providers and to bring up sensitive subjects, such as contraception, without a parent present.

The goal of treatment goes beyond immediate disease management and looks toward the long-term future of children with MS. "Our objective is to increase the chances these young individuals will grow to be socially independent and confident," said Dr. Banwell.

References

1. Boiko A, Vorobeychik G, Paty D, et al. Early onset multiple sclerosis: a longitudinal study. *Neurology.* 2002;59:1006–1010.

2. Banwell BL. Pediatric multiple sclerosis. *Curr Neurol Neurosci Rep.* 2004;4:245–252.

3. McDonald WI, Compston A, Edan G, et al. Recommended diagnostic criteria for multiple sclerosis: guidelines from the International Panel on the diagnosis of multiple sclerosis. *Ann Neurol.* 2001;50:121–127.

Chapter 9

Possible Triggers and Risk Factors of MS

Chapter Contents

Section 9.1

Toxic Agents

Although genetic factors are believed to play an important role in the etiology of multiple sclerosis (MS), evidence also suggests the involvement of environmental (non-genetic) factors. One group of environmental factors that may play a role in triggering MS is toxic agents such as organic solvents, heavy metals, and radiation. Toxic agents have been determined to cause or contribute to a variety of neurological diseases; for example, chronic lead poisoning can result in encephalopathy. Therefore, it is feasible that one or more toxic agents are involved in the development of multiple sclerosis. However, no toxic agent to date has been unequivocally implicated as a risk factor for the disease.

This section summarizes the published research on the involvement of toxic agents in MS, documenting what is known and what is not yet known about the role toxic agents play in this disease. Supporting material for this document can be downloaded from the Accelerated Cure Project website at www.acceleratedcure.org/downloads.

Composition of Toxic Agent

The composition of a toxic agent helps determine its disposition and activity in the body. Therefore, if one or more toxic agents are involved in triggering MS, clues to their nature may be derived from what is known about the pathophysiology of MS. There are two categories of toxic agents that should be considered potential risk factors for MS: toxic substances and radiation.

Substances

Two characteristics of substances (elements and compounds) that greatly affect their potential to be transported throughout the body and cause harm are lipophilicity and size. In MS, a disease of the central nervous system, these two characteristics become important when considering substances that can penetrate the blood-brain barrier (BBB), a tight layer of endothelial cells that protect the brain from harmful cells and molecules. Toxic agents that can pass through this protective wall may be able to cause or contribute to focal demyelinating lesions or more diffuse forms of damage seen in MS.

Generally, although there are exceptions, the ability of a substance to permeate the BBB depends on its size and lipophilicity: the smaller and more hydrophobic a molecule is, the more readily it can enter the brain. Of the individual substances that have been explored for a possible etiological role in MS, several meet the requirements of small size and lipophilicity. For instance, organic solvents (50–150 kilodalton [kDa]) and cyanide (26.03 kDa, a component of cigarette smoke) both meet these criteria. However, none yet has been confirmed as a definite risk factor for MS. In addition, many other substances are known to meet these requirements but have not yet been rigorously assessed for involvement in MS.

Besides directly infiltrating the BBB, toxic substances may also contribute to the development of MS in other ways, such as by making the BBB more permeable to other substances, causing genetic defects that make a person more susceptible to MS, or altering immune system functionality. Toxicity in these cases may not depend on characteristics such as size or hydrophobicity and therefore it is hard to characterize *a priori* the composition of substances that could have these effects.

Radiation

Exposure to radiation may result in damage to deoxyribonucleic acid (DNA) which may initiate tumor formation and other disease processes. Two types of radiation, ionizing radiation (x-rays, alpha particles, and gamma rays) and radon (a radioactive element), have been explored as risk factors for MS, but only a few studies on each type have been performed. Indirect support for the involvement of radiation in MS comes from research suggesting that MS subjects have increased chromosomal breakage, which may be a result of radiation exposure but may due to other causes as well. Interestingly, some researchers hypothesize that ultraviolet radiation may in fact protect people from multiple sclerosis, based on the tendency for the incidence of MS to be lower at lower latitudes. Overall, it has not yet been determined whether and how radiation may contribute to (or guard against) the development of MS.

81

Origin of Toxic Agent

Identifying toxic sources associated with MS may be helpful in understanding why certain geographical locations have higher risks of multiple sclerosis than others. To date, no large scale studies have been conducted to find sources of toxic agents that are more prevalent in areas of high versus low MS incidence. Most of our knowledge about possible sources associated with MS therefore comes from studies of individual toxic agents and our knowledge about their origins.

Toxins

Toxins are specific substances released by biological entities either as a defense mechanism or as an aid in the capture and digestion of food.

- **Infectious agents:** Toxins produced by infectious agents are addressed in Section 9.3 of this chapter.

- **Animal venoms/plant toxins:** No study has directly assessed whether there is a link between MS and history of venomous bites or stings or contact with plant toxins. Because distributions of animal and plant species vary throughout the world, it may be informative to compare geographical prevalence of MS with the presence of toxic species and/or frequency of human exposure to these species.

Endogenous

The endogenous (internal) production of toxic agents may play a role in the pathogenesis of MS. For example, overproduction of nitric oxide (NO), an endogenously produced signaling molecule, has been studied as a factor in the pathogenesis of MS. However, production of endogenous toxic agents generally occurs as a secondary response to other factors such as infections, diet, or genetic factors. Because this section is concerned with finding the primary causes or triggers of MS, we will not discuss endogenous agents in depth.

Toxicants

Toxicants are products or by-products of anthropogenic (human) activities. Most of the individual toxic agents studied in relation to MS fall under this category. Cigarette smoking is a prime example of an anthropogenic activity that may increase the risk of MS. X-rays

82

and ionizing radiation are used in health treatment; organic solvents are used for industrial purposes; and mercury is an essential part of dental amalgam. Until recently, lead was commonly used in gasoline, paint, and pipes. So far, no toxicant or toxicant-producing activity is a clear risk factor for multiple sclerosis; nor has any been studied extensively enough to be ruled out as a trigger of multiple sclerosis.

Earth Naturals

Very few studies have attempted to associate the presence of naturally occurring substances with MS. Although the geographical distribution of MS has been studied extensively, no common geological factors have been identified in regions with elevated rates of MS. A comprehensive large scale comparison between the prevalence of earth naturals and the prevalence of MS in multiple geographic areas would be useful but could prove difficult because of the number of factors that would need to be included.

Therefore, MS studies focusing on earth naturals for the most part have analyzed the levels of specific toxic agents in specific regions. Mercury, radon, and lead are examples of earth natural substances that have been studied as risk factors for MS. Scientists have searched for correlations between MS clusters and areas of unusually high amounts of various elements, but so far no firm conclusions can be drawn from the evidence. Lead has been studied the most extensively, but not all areas with a high prevalence of multiple sclerosis have high lead content. Other trace metals have also been identified in MS clusters, including molybdenum, zinc, and chromium, but whether these have any effect on the risk of MS has not been fully explored.

Vector

No common path of transmission of a toxic agent has been determined to be associated with MS. As with the origin of a toxic agent, it is difficult to identify a common vector without first identifying a specific toxic agent that may be a risk factor. The fact that it is impossible to pinpoint exactly when MS begins to develop in a given person also makes it difficult to determine which vectors may be relevant to the disease. Certain migration studies indicate that the risk of developing MS is dependent on childhood circumstances (although an overview of all migration studies prior to 1995 sheds doubt on this hypothesis, citing small sample sizes and confounding factors). If exposure to MS triggers does occur in childhood, an MS vector would be particularly difficult to identify due to the lapse of time between the initial trigger and clinical onset which typically occurs in adulthood.

Food and Drink

Because foods or beverages can harbor toxic agents either as components or contaminants, it is conceivable that an agent found in food or drink may contribute to the development of MS. Studies of nutritional risk factors in MS have assessed a number of food categories, such as dairy products and products containing saturated fat. So far no specific food or beverage has been conclusively tied to MS, but if future research does strongly implicate one, it may be worth asking whether its involvement is due to the presence of toxic substances it contains rather than nutritional elements.

A number of ecological studies have taken the alternative approach of analyzing soil and water contents in areas with high rates of MS, in search for toxic agents that may end up being ingested. However, it should be noted that abnormal levels of metals in soil do not immediately correspond to high levels in food as the metallic content in plants is dependent on a variety of factors including climate and weather.

Medication

Ionizing radiation, a suggested risk factor for MS, is used in radiological treatments which can be a major source of radiation exposure for humans. Two studies have found that MS patients are more likely to have received radiological treatment than control subjects, but it is unclear whether treatment is a risk factor for MS or whether having MS increases the chance that a person will have radiological treatments.

Epidemiological studies have also examined whether vaccines for other diseases appear to increase the risk of MS. The hepatitis B vaccine has undergone the most intensive scrutiny, with some studies finding no evidence for its involvement in MS and others finding support for a role, although possibly a small one. In addition to a hepatitis B antigen, the vaccine contains an adjuvant (aluminum hydroxy-phosphate sulfate) and yeast proteins; in the past it also contained thimerosal, which is a mercury-based preservative. Whether any of these components could increase the susceptibility to MS and how this would occur have not yet been determined.

Finally, a few studies have also looked at whether oral contraceptives affect the risk of MS, but none has found a positive correlation.

Substance Abuse

A few epidemiological studies have found that people with MS are more likely than non-MS controls to have been smokers and that higher levels of smoking can result in increased risk, although not every study on this topic has detected an association. One study explored whether alcohol, drug, tobacco, or medication abuse affected the risk of MS. In a case-control study of 108 MS patients, subjects completed a questionnaire on history of substance abuse. Only drug abuse was associated with a significantly increased risk of MS, but no specific drug was identified.

Domestic Uses

Little research has been performed on whether exposures to toxic agents used in domestic settings increase the risk of MS. Two studies examined the correlation between MS and the use of herbicides and pesticides but no link was found. It is also unclear whether the exposure was due to occupational or domestic use of these products.

Occupational Exposure

Specific occupations, such as metalworking, have been linked with an increased risk of MS. However, these studies do not tend to investigate any specific toxic agents that are used in these respective industries and that could affect risk of MS through occupational exposure.

Other studies have investigated the effect on risk of MS of occupational exposure to a specific agent, namely organic solvents. Organic solvents have been linked to multiple sclerosis in several studies although most of them do not assess actual exposure but likelihood of exposure. Organic solvent exposure has been documented in various occupations, including automobile assembly, printing, typography, carpentry, cabinetmaking, shoe and leather production, and painting.

Environmental Exposure

A multitude of toxic substances are released into the environment through vehicle exhaust, industrial waste, and other human activities such as cigarette smoking. However, no study has comprehensively categorized all toxic agents present in the environment in high prevalence MS clusters.

A few individual toxic agents that may be encountered through environmental exposure have been studied in MS. For example, researchers have studied lead levels in areas with high prevalence of MS; however, these studies typically have concentrated on soil levels as opposed to airborne lead. Again, no concrete evidence exists that indicates environmental exposure to one or more specific agents is a significant risk factor for MS.

An alternative approach involves determining whether people with MS, prior to onset, were more likely to be living in environments with a generally high level of toxicants. In other diseases such as asthma, exposure to high levels of toxicants such as air pollutants has been found to increase a person's susceptibility. Some researchers have examined whether living in an urban versus a rural setting may be associated with MS (people in urban settings are presumably more likely to come in contact with certain types of toxicants such as vehicle exhaust than those in rural areas). So far no definite relationship has been determined between MS and urban life; studies have found positive correlations between the risk of multiple sclerosis and both urban and rural settings. For example, in one study of Southern Hesse, Lauer, et al., found that people with MS were more likely to have lived in rural areas as children than would be expected based on population distributions. However, other studies have linked MS with urban environments, such as a study of U.S. veterans which associated urban residence at the time of entrance into the military with a higher risk of MS for white males.

Animal Bites

This has not been assessed. As mentioned, no studies have explored whether there is a connection between MS and venomous animal bites. Numerous studies looking into infectious triggers of MS have assessed whether exposure to household pets is associated with risk of MS, with inconclusive results overall. Even if domestic animal exposure is a risk factor for MS, it has not been proposed that this could occur through transmission of toxic agents via bites.

From Nature

Whether people who develop MS have had greater exposure overall to toxic agents found in nature has not been assessed. Specific agents produced by natural sources have been studied, such as radon which is present throughout the earth in varying concentrations and is the main source of radiation exposure for most people. Mercury and lead are also present in nature in varying amounts but in quantities lower than toxic levels. As stated before, no specific toxic agent including these has yet been strongly linked with risk of MS.

Entrance

Toxic agents can be introduced into the body in a variety of ways, and these modes of entrance can greatly influence their level of toxicity. No specific studies have tried to characterize specific entry mechanisms as risk factors for MS. Rather, any inferences that can be made about entry site(s) that may be involved in MS are based on investigations of specific toxic agents and their known entrance routes.

For some of the toxic agents that have been studied with respect to MS, entrance into the body is well-defined. For example, cigarette smoke is inhaled through the lungs. On the other hand, there are some toxic agents, such as organic solvents, that could enter the body through multiple paths. In these cases, researchers often do not attempt to identify the mode of entrance, but rather only consider exposure levels. Following are sites of entry that toxic agents may take into the body.

Skin

No studies have assessed whether the skin (intact or broken) is a key entrance site for toxic agents that increase susceptibility to MS. In terms of specific toxic agents, dermal entry is a likely pathway for organic solvents to enter the body. However, MS studies that analyze organic solvent exposure do not report whether or not subjects were in direct contact with the substance. Since the skin is exposed to innumerable substances every day, identifying entrance through this path might be difficult.

Lungs (Inhalation)

This is a mode of entrance for several of the toxic agents that have been investigated in MS. Cigarette smoke and vapors from organic solvents are absorbed through the lungs. Also, before being banned from gasoline, high levels of lead were present in the air in heavily populated areas. Mercury is a volatile substance and may be inhaled, for instance through accidental or occupational exposure.

Gastrointestinal (GI) Tract (Ingestion)

Food or beverages containing lead, mercury, or other toxic agents not yet studied in MS, may be ingested and enter the body through the GI tract. It is possible that studies of dietary patterns in people with multiple sclerosis may one day identify toxic risk factors that enter through this route.

Eyes

This mode of entry has not been assessed. Toxic agents could enter through this route via eye drops, contact solution, and eye ointments, but no studies have correlated any of these substances with an increased risk of MS. Studies on past eye irritation or inflammation in MS patients could provide information on whether or not this route was an entrance for a toxic agent.

Suppositories

This mode of entry also has not been assessed.

Intravenous or Other Injections

This has not been assessed directly. Vaccines (which are usually injected) have been investigated as possible risk factors for MS, but their involvement has not yet been determined. As for other types of injections, medical records with information on injections or histories of drug abuse may clarify whether or not MS subjects had been exposed to toxic agents through this route.

Implants

Because of their high mercury content, dental amalgams are the only implants that have been studied repeatedly for an effect on risk of MS. Implants may be more feasible to study in relation to MS than other modes of entrance since they are generally recorded in medical files and are often easily detectable.

A number of studies have assessed whether people with MS are more likely to have dental amalgams than non-MS subjects. So far, no conclusion can be reached on whether or not dental amalgams play a role in the pathogenesis of multiple sclerosis.

Radiation

Radon and ionizing radiation can enter the body without direct contact. Only a few studies have assessed exposure to radiation as a risk factor for MS, but each of these reported evidence for a link between radiation and MS.

Pharmacokinetics: Disposition of Toxic Agent

Pharmacokinetics refers to how the body handles the toxic agent to which it has been exposed, including how it absorbs, distributes, transforms, stores, and excretes the agent. This section reviews the evidence present in MS that may reflect processing of a toxic agent.

Local Toxicity

Local toxicity covers a range of effects that are produced at the site of entry of a toxic agent into the body. Some of these effects (such as hair loss and corrosion) are acute in nature and/or easily identifiable and therefore potentially feasible to research. However, to date no studies have been published that explore the correlation of local toxicity effects with multiple sclerosis. The potentially long separation in time between the initial triggers of MS and the development of MS would complicate any efforts to associate local toxicity events with MS. In addition, not all toxic exposures cause noticeable local effects.

Absorption

The main sites of absorption are the GI tract, lungs, and skin. No evidence that associates absorption through these sites with development of MS has been found independent of specific substances previously mentioned, which may tend to be absorbed in particular sites.

Distribution

The distribution of toxic agents throughout the body, including to the brain, occurs primarily through the blood. However, many substances do not remain in the blood stream for extensive lengths of time, except in the case of ongoing chronic exposures. Instead, they are stored or excreted, so implicating a toxic agent as a cause of MS by testing the blood of MS patients may prove difficult. One small study investigating the potential for lead poisoning in MS did analyze blood samples from five MS subjects; each was found to have normal lead levels.

89

Systemic Toxicity

The central nervous system and the immune system both exhibit damage or alteration of function in MS and thus are candidate targets for systemic effects of toxic agents. However, actual evidence linking any particular toxic agent with systemic effects in MS is sparse. Several toxic agents that have been studied in MS have been shown to be capable of entering the central nervous system (CNS) and causing damage. For example, lead has a high affinity for cerebral endothelial cells and can accumulate in high amounts in the brain. Mercury also accumulates in CNS cells such as microglial cells, neurons, and epithelial cells. However, no analyses of CNS tissue have shown conclusive evidence of systemic toxicity: for instance, post-mortem brain analysis of multiple sclerosis patients revealed no significant increases in either lead or mercury compared with control subjects.

In addition to the CNS and immune system, other organs or systems are often impaired during the course of MS, but this impairment is generally secondary to the loss of nervous system function. However, it is possible that a toxic agent that is involved in triggering MS could also be distributed to, and cause harmful effects in, other organs or tissues which could be detected. For example, if an agent that increases the risk of MS also impairs reproductivity, then loss of fertility would likely be documented in MS subjects. Therefore, recording and analyzing other conditions experienced by MS subjects either before or after MS onset may reveal common patterns that would point toward a toxic trigger.

Modification

Modification of toxic agents has not been extensively studied in MS patients because no correlation between a toxic agent and the disease has been strong enough to warrant further investigation.

- **Biotransformation:** The biotransformation of toxic agents has not been studied in relation to MS, although this may be an important area to research. It is possible that MS patients are unable to transform certain toxic agents into less harmful metabolites, making them more susceptible to toxic effects. This impairment could be a result of a genetic defect, for instance.

- **Interaction:** Evidence suggests that cigarette smoke and indoor radon have a synergistic effect on lung cancer rates when encountered in combination. Since both substances are also hypothesized to be risk factors for MS, it is possible that their interaction may further increase the risk of MS. However, no specific studies on the synergistic, additive potentiate, or antagonistic effects of toxic agents in relation to multiple sclerosis have been published.

Storage

The main storage sites of toxic agents include plasma, adipose tissue, bone, the liver, and kidneys. Very few studies have analyzed these tissues in MS subjects to assess the presence of toxic agents. As mentioned, Westerman, et al., studied the lead levels in the bones and blood of five MS subjects, but found no significant differences from controls. Interestingly, fat can sequester lipophilic toxic agents and therefore concentrations of those agents in other tissues can decrease as a person's amount of body fat increases. Likewise, these agents can be released into the bloodstream and made available to other tissues as fat is mobilized. It may therefore be useful to investigate whether there is any correlation between body weight changes and risk of MS.

Excretion

A common method of determining exposure to toxic agents is to analyze bodily excretions for high concentrations of substances of concern. However, because the body attempts to excrete toxic agents as quickly as possible, it may not be possible to detect transient exposure to a toxic agent that triggers a disease like MS in which onset may occur years after exposure. Nevertheless, a few attempts have been made to measure levels of toxic agents in the excretions of MS subjects and controls.

In one study (Perry, et al.), scientists studied urine samples from 12 MS subjects and 12 control subjects. The controls were chosen from the same households as the MS subjects to eliminate environmental and dietary factors as confounders. Researchers found no significant difference between MS subjects and controls in excretion of trace metals, including lead, tin, nickel, silver, copper, iron, molybdenum, and zinc. Westerman, et al., also studied the urinary lead content of MS subjects and found normal levels compared with control subjects. In a study of dental amalgams, researchers found that MS patients had significantly higher hair mercury levels compared to control subjects. However, it is unclear how many of the cases and controls had dental amalgams in place at the time of the study.

Excretion of substances through other routes such as in feces or via exhalation has not yet been assessed in MS subjects. Cerebrospinal fluid, which removes toxic agents from the CNS, has been assessed in numerous studies of MS, but not for the presence of toxic agents.

Pharmacodynamics

Toxic agents exert their effects on the human body through numerous types of biochemical or physiological mechanisms. This section focuses on three potential mechanisms by which toxic agents could contribute to the development of MS: increasing permeability of the blood-brain barrier, alteration of the immune system, and demyelination. To date, no comprehensive list of all toxic agents known to cause these physiological changes has been compiled together with an analysis of their potential relationship to MS. However, some of the agents that have been analyzed for a role in MS are known or suspected to be capable of exerting these types of changes. The available evidence regarding the role of toxic agents in these aspects of MS pathogenesis follows.

Alteration of the Immune System

Multiple sclerosis is often labeled an autoimmune disease because of the presence of inflammatory cells (T and B lymphocytes, monocytes, and macrophages) as well as cytokines, antibodies, and complement components in MS lesions. Both immune system stimulators and suppressors have been hypothesized to play a role in the pathogenesis of MS, although how they cause or exacerbate the disease remains to be determined.

- **Lead:** There is no direct evidence that lead alters the immune system in a way that can increase the risk of MS. However, researchers have found that lead may stimulate the immune response in mice by enhancing the immunogenicity of molecules of neural proteins. For example, in one study, myelin basic protein and glial fibrillary acidic protein were incubated with lead before being injected into mice. Mice receiving the lead-altered protein generated significantly more autoantibodies against the neural proteins than mice receiving only native protein. Researchers hypothesized that lead could exacerbate neurological diseases such as MS by increasing the levels of antibodies against myelin protein. Another study found that adding lead to the diet of mice with lead enhanced their T-cell response to certain mitogens such as concanavalin A.

- **Mercury:** Mercury may have immunomodulatory or immunotoxic effects on humans as shown primarily through experiments on animals. For instance, in certain animals, mercury has been shown to induce an autoimmune response. Its effects on MS subjects have not been extensively researched, although one study analyzed blood samples from MS subjects who had amalgams at the time of the study with MS subjects who had their amalgams removed. The study found that CD8+ T cell levels were increased in the subjects who had their amalgams removed compared with those who still had the implants, indicating that mercury may suppress these regulatory cells.

- **Nicotine:** Cigarette smoke has immunosuppressive effects, and recent research suggests nicotine may be the major component responsible for this change. For example, studies have shown that T-cell and antibody responses are inhibited in rats chronically exposed to nicotine; another study has shown that exposure to nicotine alters the differentiation of human dendritic cells. More information can be found in Sopori and Kozak's 1998 review on the immunomodulatory effects of cigarette smoke.

- **Tobacco glycoprotein:** This substance, present in cigarette smoke, has been shown to have stimulatory effects on the immune system, for instance by causing the proliferation of T cells as demonstrated in an in vitro study of human lymphocytes.

Demyelination

During the course of the disease in MS, myelin in the central nervous system is damaged or destroyed. There is no direct evidence that demyelination in MS is caused by toxic agents; however, the following toxic agents have been shown to cause demyelination in other circumstances.

- **Cyanide:** Demyelination of the nervous systems of animals given large doses of cyanide has been well-documented. However, modest demyelination has also been demonstrated with smaller exposures. For example, in one experiment, rats given small doses of cyanide or thiocyanate in conjunction with a restricted diet showed signs of myelin degeneration in their spinal cords.

- **Lead:** Accidental lead poisoning has been shown to cause demyelination as seen in the postmortem analysis of brain tissue from nonhuman primates. However, another study to test the results of direct exposure to lead and other metals found that lead pellets implanted in the brains of rats failed to cause significant necrosis after 21 days.

- **Mercury:** Mercury poisoning has numerous effects on the nervous system (both central and peripheral) which include demyelination, neuronal loss, brain atrophy, and astrocytosis. Chang 1977, and Atchinson and Hare 1994, both review the range of neurotoxic effects due to mercury poisoning.

- **Organic solvents:** A few studies have documented changes in the white matter of brains of people exposed to organic solvents, indicating alteration of the myelin sheath. Organic solvents may not be directly responsible for these changes, but instead may allow other toxic or demyelinating factors to enter the brain by altering the blood-brain barrier.

- **Radiation:** One study suggests that ionizing radiation may aggravate lesions in the brain and increase the rate at which demyelination occurs. The study describes a sharp deterioration in the clinical status in four of five patients with various demyelinating neurological diseases after receiving radiation treatment.

Increasing Permeability of the Blood-Brain Barrier

The blood-brain barrier is a dense wall of endothelial cells which prevents macromolecules from crossing from the bloodstream into the brain. Normally only small molecules such as oxygen and carbon dioxide can pass through. However, in multiple sclerosis, permeability of the blood-brain barrier is enhanced, allowing T-lymphocytes and other blood cells to pass through more readily to the brain. It is hypothesized that the breakdown of the blood-brain barrier is an early step in the development of multiple sclerosis lesions.

Several elements and compounds have been shown to disrupt the blood-brain barrier, including aluminum, nitrobenzene, and pyridostigmine bromide (a nerve gas antidote). Of the toxic agents specifically investigated for a role in MS, the following are known or suspected to disrupt the blood-brain barrier.

- **Lead:** The blood-brain barrier is a target for lead toxicity. Studies have shown that lead interferes with many different functions of the barrier, including transport and metabolic processes.

- **Mercury:** Numerous studies have shown that mercury alters the blood-brain barrier in animals, although most of them involved the administration of relatively high doses. In 1977, Chang summarized the findings in this field in a paper on the neurotoxic effects of mercury. A more recent overview cited additional studies demonstrating the alteration of blood-brain barriers by inorganic mercuric chloride, but does not discuss the implications this research has for MS.

- **Nicotine:** Researchers have demonstrated that nicotine increases microvascular blood flow within certain areas of the brain, including visual-auditory, sensorimotor-cortical, and interpeduncular systems. This may result in greater influxes of toxic agents or other factors across the blood-brain barrier.

- **Organic solvents:** The small size and hydrophobic nature of organic solvent molecules allow them to penetrate the blood-brain barrier with relative ease; they may also affect and impair the function of the blood-brain barrier. At least two studies have found increased concentrations of macromolecules (for example, albumin) in the cerebral spinal fluid (CSF) of people exposed to organic solvents compared with controls, indicating that this exposure may have increased the permeability of the blood-brain barrier. One study did not find significant overall differences in CSF albumin levels in solvent-exposed subjects compared with controls, but cited evidence of slight blood-CSF barrier damage in a subset of the subjects with recent occupational exposure.

Other

A few studies have proposed more indirect methods on how toxic agents could play a role in the development of multiple sclerosis.

- **Genetic:** Both radiation and chemical agents may cause genetic mutations that could lead to multiple sclerosis in susceptible individuals.

- **Increased nitric oxide levels:** Recent evidence has suggested that nitric oxide may play a significant role in the progression of MS. Nitric oxide is an endogenous signaling molecule with a variety of functions and may be involved with inflammation in

MS. Research has shown that cigarette smoke may increase blood levels of nitric oxide in the body, but not all data concurs with this hypothesis.

- **Increased vulnerability to disease:** One study found that the risk of current, past, or chronic *Chlamydia pneumoniae* infection (another potential MS risk factor) was positively associated with cigarette smoking.

Epidemiological Effects

The following factors can influence a person's exposure to toxic agents or the effects produced by these agents. As a result, they can increase or decrease susceptibility to the diseases associated with toxic agents.

- **Age:** MS typically manifests itself in adulthood, although it can also be diagnosed in children and adolescents. However, since subclinical development of the disease may precede clinical symptoms by a substantial period of time, it is impossible to know exactly when MS disease processes are initiated in an individual. This makes it difficult to determine what specific age groups are most likely to be exposed to or affected by any environmental factors involved in MS. Some studies of migration of people between areas of lower and higher MS prevalence suggest that childhood or adolescence may be times when people are exposed to risk factors for MS, although these studies do not explore which risk factors may be involved. No information is available on exposure of people with MS to toxic agents before birth, which may also be important because the placenta is permeable to certain toxic agents and therefore the diet and habits of the mother could be risk factors for the baby.

- **Gender:** Multiple sclerosis affects roughly twice as many females than males. However, no toxic agents studied in relation to MS have been shown to exert more harmful effects in females compared with males. It may be that due to societal and occupational factors, females may have greater exposure to certain toxic agents. For example, in many societies, females spend a majority of time inside the home, increasing their potential exposure to radon.

- **Genetics:** Certain genetic polymorphisms may affect a person's ability to neutralize toxic agents. It is possible, although this has not been extensively researched, that some individuals with MS are more susceptible to intoxication because of genetic defects. Landtblom, et al., studied two enzyme systems (GSTM1 and CYP2D6) that metabolize organic solvents, but found no differences in the genetic predisposition of MS subjects who had been exposed to organic solvents and MS subjects who had not been exposed. Agundez, et al., likewise found no correlation between polymorphisms in the CYP2D6 gene and risk of MS when comparing 118 MS subjects to 200 controls.

- **Socioeconomic status:** Several studies have investigated possible associations between MS and socioeconomic status, which may affect exposure to certain toxic agents such as medication. In a review of the social epidemiology of MS, Lowis reported that studies provide mixed results on whether MS is linked with socioeconomic status. There is no direct evidence to support the hypothesis that an increased risk of MS for higher income classes, if there is one, is due to increased exposure to toxic agents.

- **Diet:** Because food and drink are vectors for toxic agents, diet could play an important role in exposure to toxic risk factors for MS. For example, mercury levels in water are amplified in fish, lead, and other metals present in soil can build up in vegetation, and drinking water can contain a multitude of toxic agents. This area has not been researched extensively and the research that has been completed is unclear.

- **Health status:** Weakened health status may make a person more susceptible to the effects of toxic agents. Documenting the health status and medical history of people with MS prior to onset may therefore provide clues about the involvement of toxic risk factors in MS.

- **Occupation:** Several case-control or cohort studies have been conducted attempting to find correlations between particular occupations and the risk of MS. Certain industries such as metal working and chemical industries have been linked with an increased risk of MS, but the evidence implicating them generally comes from only a few studies. Furthermore, little information can be found on specific toxic agents for which exposure is increased in any given occupation.

- **Environment and geographical location:** As mentioned previously, several scientists have characterized the soil, air, and water properties of areas with high prevalence of MS, but no toxic agents have been consistently present in MS cluster sites. Most of the studies have focused on specific toxic agents, but no overall consensus has emerged, for example, no one toxic agent has been highlighted across studies of multiple clusters. In 2002, Pugliatti, et al., published a review that maps the prevalence of MS in different areas of the earth. A global study of various environmental factors such as geology and trace metal prevalence may help identify correlations between high prevalence MS clusters and corresponding environmental concentrations, but so far none has been published.

Section 9.2

Nutritional Factors

Multiple sclerosis (MS) is a demyelinating disease of the central nervous system. Currently, little is known about what causes this disease. Evidence that the incidence of MS is increased in blood relatives of people with MS suggests the role of genetic factors. However, epidemiological data indicating variations in MS prevalence across geographic regions as well as the incomplete concordance of MS between identical twins imply that an environmental component is also important in the etiology of MS.

Nutrition has been implicated as a possible etiological factor in MS. Like the prevalence of MS, diet can vary depending on ethnicity or location and may change upon migration to another country or environment. The finding of one or more dietary risk factors for MS would be a significant accomplishment in understanding how the disease develops, and could lead to measures useful for preventing or ameliorating the disease.

This section reviews published research focusing on potential nutritional triggers of MS. Supporting material can be found in "MS Nutritional Studies," which is a database summarizing the details of the studies referred to in this section. A separate document, "Analysis of specific nutritional factors in the development of MS," reviews and assesses the research conducted to date on the nutrients that have been most thoroughly studied for a role in MS. These documents can be downloaded from the Accelerated Cure Project website at http://www.acceleratedcure.org/curemap/docs.php.

Nutrient Properties

Although any type of nutrient could conceivably play a role in the development of MS, to date, vitamins, minerals, and lipids have received the most attention in the MS scientific literature. The evidence for these and other types of nutrients as risk factors for MS are briefly discussed here.

Vitamins

Fat-soluble vitamins such as A, D, E, and K have specific roles in body functions such as myelin formation and immune system function; disruptions of these functions due to nutritional imbalances could possibly therefore increase the risk of MS. Of these four vitamins, the strongest evidence for a correlation with MS exists for vitamin D deficiency. Evidence that vitamin D deficiency may predispose a person to MS comes from a variety of sources: ecological studies that evaluate exposure to vitamin D sources like sunlight, fish, and supplements; studies reporting associations between lesion activity and low vitamin D levels or sunlight exposure; and studies of bone density and vitamin D levels. The results of vitamin D supplementation studies in ameliorating MS have been inconclusive, however.

A few studies have investigated vitamin A (retinol or carotenoid) levels or intake in MS and non-MS controls, but most reported no associations. Evidence is mixed concerning the involvement of vitamin E in MS. Although some studies have reported lower levels of vitamin E in the serum or cerebrospinal fluid (CSF) of MS subjects compared with controls, others were not able to detect any significant differences. Furthermore, intake of vitamin E supplements has not been shown to protect against MS, although it has been suggested that vitamin E therapy may be beneficial in inhibiting the disease course of people with MS with signs of significant oxidative stress. Vitamin K has not yet been assessed for a possible role in MS.

99

Water-soluble vitamins are broadly distributed throughout the body and include vitamins B_1 (thiamin), B_2 (riboflavin), B_3 (niacin), B_5 (pantothenic acid), B_6 (pyridoxine), B_7 (biotin), B_9 (folic acid), B_{12} (cobalamine), and C (ascorbic acid). Most of the B-complex vitamins have not yet been assessed with respect to MS, although some of them such as niacin, pyridoxine, and biotin are known to play a role in the nervous system and/or can result in neurological deficits if too much or too little is consumed. Thiamin and riboflavin have only been assessed in MS by one study using a 164-item food frequency questionnaire, which found a protective influence for each.

The only B-complex vitamin that has been studied extensively for involvement in MS is cobalamine (B_{12}), a cofactor for myelin synthesis. Like MS, vitamin B_{12} deficiency is characterized by demyelination and axonal degeneration, and causes symptoms such as weakness, paresthesia, and unsteady gait. Indeed, vitamin B_{12} deficiency and MS can be difficult to differentiate because they can share a similar clinical disease presentation as well as similar magnetic resonance imaging (MRI) findings. Therefore it is not unreasonable to conjecture that lack of vitamin B_{12} might be a trigger of MS. However, evidence is mixed concerning whether vitamin B_{12} deficiency does increase the risk of MS. Some studies have reported an association between MS and low vitamin B_{12} levels while others show no correlation. Studies of serum methylmalonic acid (MMA) and homocysteine (HCY) concentrations, which tend to indicate severe intracellular B_{12} deficiency, also present inconclusive evidence. Trials of high doses of vitamin B_{12} in MS have shown only minor benefits.

Evidence regarding the effect of dietary vitamin C intake on the risk of MS is limited. One case-control study using a food frequency questionnaire mentioned a negative association between higher intake of vitamin C and the risk of MS. However, a prospective study of two large cohorts of women reported that higher intake of vitamin C was unrelated to reduced risk of MS, even after long-term intake lasting more than 10 years. The effects of vitamin C supplementation in existing MS have only been assessed in a small, uncontrolled study in which several nutrients were administered simultaneously.

Minerals

Due to their size and electrochemical properties, minerals tend to play very specific roles in the functioning of the body. Their functions can be closely related; in fact, some minerals can substitute for another when there is a deficiency. Imbalances can also occur between two or more minerals and may appear as a deficiency. Perhaps for these reasons, MS studies evaluating the involvement of individual minerals are uncommon. Instead, most studies assess the presence of a variety of minerals at once. For example:

- A multi-trace element analysis of scalp-hair samples mentions significantly lower concentrations of copper, iodine, manganese, sulfur, and vanadium and a significantly higher selenium level in scalp-hair samples of MS subjects. No difference was observed for several other elements including aluminum, calcium, chlorine, and zinc.

- An investigation of daily urinary excretions of trace elements in MS subjects revealed no significant difference in metals (lead, nickel, silver, copper, iron, molybdenum, and zinc) between MS cases and controls. Since no significant differences were noted, the authors conclude that it is unlikely that a metabolic imbalance of trace metal or environmental metal toxicity causes MS. This study, however, was very small, consisting of only 12 MS subjects and 12 controls.

- A study of an MS cluster focus (area of increased MS prevalence) concluded that an environment predisposing to MS may consist of soil low in copper, iron, and/or vanadium and high in lead, nickel, and/or zinc, as well as water high in chloride, chromium, molybdenum, nitrate, and/or zinc and low in selenium and/or sulfate.

Macrominerals: Most macrominerals, including sulfur, phosphorus, potassium, sodium, and chlorine remain generally unexplored as potential etiological factors for MS, with the exception of the studies mentioned above and a food frequency study that found a potential protective effect for potassium.

Calcium and magnesium have each been evaluated in a few studies. The scalp-hair analysis previously mentioned found no difference in magnesium or calcium concentrations in samples from MS subjects and controls, and a study of serum and CSF reported no statistically significant difference in magnesium levels between MS and non-MS subjects. However, a food frequency study found a protective effect for calcium with respect to MS, and a study of autopsy samples reported significantly lower magnesium content in visceral organs and central nervous system (CNS) tissues, particularly white matter and demyelinated plaques, in MS subjects compared with controls. A small, uncontrolled study of the effects of dietary supplementation with calcium, magnesium, and vitamin D reported a decreased relapse rate of MS.

Trace minerals: In comparison with macrominerals, trace minerals tend to have been investigated more extensively for a possible role in MS, with several having been analyzed using a variety of sample types. Iron, for instance, has been assessed not only in blood and urine (with no significant differences found in MS samples compared with controls) but also brain tissue, with one study finding evidence for iron deposits around demyelinated plaques and another failing to find such deposits. Zinc has been evaluated in studies of blood (plasma, serum, whole blood, and erythrocytes), CSF, urine, and scalp hair. Studies using blood products have reported mixed results with some finding higher and others finding lower or normal zinc levels in MS subjects. One study reporting higher zinc levels in whole blood in MS subjects noted that zinc increases in whole blood are also seen in other CNS diseases. Studies using other tissues have found no significant differences in zinc concentrations between cases and controls.

Results for copper are also mixed. Although most studies report only insignificant differences in blood, CSF, and urine copper levels between MS cases and controls, one study reported significantly elevated CSF copper levels in MS cases and two other studies reported lower serum copper concentrations in MS cases. Another study also detected significantly lower copper concentrations in the scalp hair of MS cases versus controls. In a similar fashion, studies of selenium and glutathione peroxidase (GSH-Px) activity have varied in their results and conclusions regarding this element's possible involvement in the etiology of MS. In terms of intervention studies, one such effort reported increased GSH-Px activity following supplementation with selenium, vitamin C, and vitamin E, but clinical effects were not reported in this study. Another study which noted signs of significant oxidative stress (in the form of reduced erythrocyte GSH-Px) in MS subjects suggested antioxidant supplementation with selenium to compensate but did not actually test out the recommendation.

A few other trace minerals, including molybdenum, nickel, chromium, iodine, and manganese, have been assessed in MS but only in a limited fashion.

Ultra-trace minerals: Aside from arsenic, which was found in normal quantities in scalp hair samples of four MS subjects, and vanadium, which was explored in a study of soil in an MS cluster, ultra-

trace minerals such as fluorine, silicon, boron, lithium, and germa-
nium have not been assessed.

Carbohydrates

Carbohydrates are a favored energy source in humans. In the MS
literature, they are generally described in terms of the foods in which
they are found, such as the starch in gluten grains or the sugars in
sweets.

Gluten is a mix of elastic proteins found in wheat, rye, barley, and
other cereal grains. Gluten proteins can cause immune responses, and
thus have been postulated to play a role in autoimmune diseases.
Studies examining whether MS subjects consumed above-average
amounts of cereal and bread have produced mixed results.

Although gluten-free diets have helped reduce symptoms of other
autoimmune diseases, such as celiac disease, only one pilot study has
been reported in MS, and gluten antibodies do not appear to be frequently present in MS subjects. Immunologic cross-reactivity and
molecular similarities between gluten and self-antigens have been
reported in studies of celiac disease; no such relationships have been
reported in MS, although one study of autism subjects detected antibody cross-reactivity between a gluten peptide (gliadin) and cerebellar antigens.

Aside from food frequency studies that inquired about consumption of sweets such as chocolate, no effort has been made to specifically investigate a potential etiological role in MS for sugars. Likewise,
the role of glycogen in MS has not been discussed.

Lipids

Lipids serve as an energy storage medium, provide structure to
cells, and can be converted into other types of chemicals such as hormones and vitamins. Myelin is composed primarily of lipids, and these
nutrients, particularly saturated and polyunsaturated fatty acids
(PUFA), factor significantly in the MS medical literature.

Essential fatty acids (EFA) are polyunsaturated fatty acids that
must be obtained from the diet since they are not synthesized in the
body. The two EFA are omega-6 (linoleic acid), and omega-3 (linolenic
acid). EFA are important to the nervous, immune, cardiovascular, and
reproductive systems. EFA also produce prostaglandins, which regulate inflammation and body functions such as heart rate and blood
clotting.

A few studies have reported lower levels of omega-3 fatty acids in various tissues of people with MS compared with controls, although one failed to find any differences in red blood cells. Other studies have linked lower fish intake with increased MS risk, which also suggests that omega-3 may protect against MS since fish oil is high in omega-3 fatty acids, although again not all studies are consistent. Omega-3 supplementation trials have not shown sufficient clinical benefit to add weight to the hypothesis that omega-3 deficiency is involved in MS etiology.

Omega-6 fatty acid levels, particularly linoleic acid levels, have been observed to be significantly lower in the blood and brain of MS subjects compared with both normal and neurological controls. Decreased concentrations of linoleic acid have also been reported in MS subjects in serum lipids, total plasma, and CSF. Lower linoleate concentrations in serum lipids could be due to an altered rate of linoleic acid entry into or removal from the blood or a defective metabolic pathway that is necessary in the absence of large amounts of linoleate. Analysis of the absorption of safflower and sunflower oil in MS cases indicated that lowered fatty acid levels in the CSF and serum of MS subjects are not due to dysfunctional intestinal absorption.

Linoleate supplementation, which has been studied extensively, has yielded mixed results. Several studies have found increased linoleic acid levels in both MS cases and controls after supplementation, but various double-blind, controlled trials have reported different effects of supplementation on relapses and disability associated with MS, or have detected no therapeutic effect at all. In general, larger clinical studies are needed to assess the effects of omega-6 dietary intervention.

Saturated fats have been studied fairly extensively in the MS literature, with mixed results. Several epidemiological studies have suggested a positive association between MS and consumption of saturated and animal fat (meat, milk, butter, and eggs). In contrast with epidemiological studies, however, many population-based case-control studies have failed to confirm the relationship between fat intake and MS risk. Some studies have observed that MS subjects and controls did not differ significantly in frequency of fat intake before the onset of MS, suggesting that fat consumption is not associated with increased MS risk. A few studies have assessed the clinical effect of a reduction in dietary saturated fat (combined with an increase in polyunsaturated fat intake); each reported some degree of clinical benefit, but it should be noted that these trials were all uncontrolled.

Trans fatty acids have been addressed in only one study on the role of milk in MS, which discusses the trans fatty acid vaccenic and its potential to increase MS susceptibility. Trans fatty acids may alter membrane structure, accelerating demyelination and allowing easier access through the blood brain barrier, though evidence is mixed about whether or not vaccenic acid can enter the brain.

Monounsaturated fats come from many of the same sources as polyunsaturated fats, such as olive oil, canola oil, and nuts. Oleic acid, a nonessential fatty acid with one double bond, is the most common monounsaturated fat found in the diet. Oleic acid supplementation of MS subjects has often been used as a placebo control in experiments involving linoleic acid, an omega-6 EFA, but has not been specifically discussed as a factor that may affect the risk of MS.

Phospholipids have not been extensively assessed. An evaluation of a low-fat diet treatment also analyzed other lipids, noting no significant differences in phospholipid content of MS subjects and controls.

Triglycerides, which exist in butterfat, animal lard, and oils, have also not been extensively assessed. A study of nonenzymatic antioxidants of the blood found a significantly lower ratio of vitamin E to cholesterol plus triglyceride during exacerbation, but reported no significant differences in plasma triglyceride levels between MS subjects and controls.

Steroids in the form of corticosteroids are often used to treat relapses in MS patients. The influence of corticosteroids on the risk of developing MS has not yet been assessed. However, their use may affect the concentrations of other nutritional elements in the body which may affect the results of nutritional studies. For example, in a small study of trace element status in MS subjects with and without corticosteroid treatment, elevated red blood cell (RBC) zinc-copper ratios were found in MS subjects compared with controls; ratios were particularly enhanced in those subjects receiving steroid treatment. These results suggest that a copper and zinc imbalance may either cause or result from MS and can be affected by corticosteroid therapy.

Another type of steroid that has been studied with respect to MS is cholesterol. An evaluation of a low-fat diet treatment noted no significant differences in the cholesterol content of MS subjects compared with controls; similar findings were reported in a study examining anti-oxidant levels in MS.

Amino Acids

Individual amino acids (such as lysine, glycine, and tyrosine) as derived from food have not been discussed in the MS literature as potential factors influencing the risk of MS.

Peripheral Chemicals (Phytochemicals)

Of the various types of peripheral chemicals, only phytoestrogens, carotenoids, and flavonoids have been mentioned briefly in the MS literature. Catechins, lactoferrin, isothiocyanates, diallyl-sulfides, and monoterpenes have not been assessed.

Phytoestrogens: According to one review, because women with MS tend to have less frequent relapses during pregnancy and more frequent relapses in the months after delivery, estrogen is thought to slow disease progression. The same review mentions a recent study observing an ameliorating effect of quercetin, a flavonoid phytoestrogen, on the progression of the animal model experimental autoimmune encephalomyelitis (EAE) as well.

Carotenoids: Provitamin A carotenoids can be converted into vitamin A and function as antioxidants. Two small studies have analyzed plasma or serum levels of beta-carotene in MS subjects and healthy controls; one found decreased levels in MS subjects (along with decreased levels of other antioxidants) while the other found no significant differences. A prospective study using a food frequency survey indicated that higher intake of dietary carotenoids was unrelated to a reduced risk of MS. Therefore, at this time, evidence does not suggest that carotenoids play a significant role in the etiology of MS.

Flavonoids: Experiments have shown that flavonoids can protect axons and oligodendrocytes from oxidative damage and phagocytosis; however, no connection between flavonoid deficiency and MS has been demonstrated.

Water

The role of water as a result of its function in the body has not been discussed in the MS literature. Water as a nutrient vector, however, has been mentioned briefly.

Basis of Nutritional Disease

An appropriately balanced diet is necessary to avoid deficiency, toxicity, imbalance, and misuse of nutritional factors and to maintain good health. At the extremes of the nutritional spectrum, inadequate amounts of a nutrient in the body signify a state of deficiency, while excessive amounts characterize toxicity; imbalance combines features of both. Misuse describes the improper buildup of nutrients in the body due to altered biochemical mechanisms. Each of these states could potentially lead to disease, either directly or indirectly.

MS does not provide any overt clues about which, if any, of these nutritional states may be involved in its etiology. For example, no reports have been made of MS prevalence rates consistently rising following sudden shortages of particular nutrients in particular populations, or of MS frequency being elevated in people following certain extreme diets. Therefore, all possible states must be considered. The MS literature describes the use of several different types of experiments to determine whether subjects with MS have abnormal exposures to or concentrations of certain nutrients. Common experimental techniques include food frequency questionnaires, ecological studies of food usage in different geographical regions, and evaluation of serum and CSF samples for nutrient levels. Studies that alter the diets of people with MS to determine whether any beneficial effect can be detected can also provide information about nutritional contributions to MS.

Following are short summaries of the evidence generated for each of the four nutritional disease states (deficiency, toxicity, imbalance, misuse) as a risk factor for MS.

Deficiency

A variety of nutritional deficiencies have been investigated for a possible role in MS, including deficiencies of vitamin D, vitamin E, vitamin B_{12}, calcium, manganese, and essential fatty acids. At this point, although evidence has been produced linking MS with certain deficiencies, findings are often mixed or based on limited results. Furthermore, remaining to be explained is how any of these deficits might contribute to the pathological processes that initiate MS.

- **Vitamin D:** As noted, several types of studies (including ecological studies and prospective intake surveys) have reported an association between lower levels of vitamin D and the development of

107

MS. These deficiencies may come about through dietary practices or lack of exposure to sunlight, and may affect the immune system in a way that increases the risk of MS. More study is needed to confirm and explain these findings.

- **Vitamin B$_{12}$** deficiency and MS share many neurological symptoms, including weakness and fatigue. It is reasonable to suggest that vitamin B$_{12}$ deficiency could increase the risk of MS, and in fact many (although not all) studies of vitamin B$_{12}$ levels in serum and CSF show a decrease in people with MS compared with controls.

- **Vitamin E:** Severe vitamin E deficiency can also damage nerves and cause symptoms similar to those seen in MS, such as impaired sensations, lack of coordination, and muscle weakness. As with vitamin B$_{12}$, evidence from case-control and prospective cohort studies is mixed regarding whether MS is associated with lower levels of vitamin E.

- **Calcium:** There is evidence, although limited and inconclusive, that lower levels of calcium are associated with MS. Calcium depletion may also help account for the bone loss and osteoporosis often observed in MS subjects.

- **Zinc:** A few studies have reported zinc deficiency in the plasma of MS subjects, although many other studies of blood products and other tissues found no evidence of deficiency. Possible explanations for low zinc levels in MS include malabsorption, disease activity, chronic inflammation, or abnormal zinc regulation.

- **Manganese:** A few studies of various tissues (such as CSF and scalp hair) have reported that manganese levels are decreased in MS cases, but, as is the case with most trace elements, not enough evidence exists to make a definite conclusion.

- **Essential fatty acids:** Several studies, including serum and CSF measurements and food intake studies, suggest that MS subjects are deficient in both omega-3 and omega-6 fatty acids. Omega-6 fatty acid levels have been found to be significantly lower in the brain and blood of MS subjects and can be corrected by sunflower oil or evening primrose oil supplementation. Since the Western diet already consists of much more omega-6 than omega-3, however, increasing n-3 fatty acid intake while maintaining n-6 intake may provide the most appropriate balance of the two EFA.

Toxicity

Of all the nutrients studied in MS, saturated fat is the only one for which an increase in intake has been repeatedly linked with MS. Since the myelin sheath is composed mainly of lipids, it has been proposed that excess saturated fat intake could alter myelin sheath stability. Low-fat treatments, such as the Swank diet, have been devised to correct the toxicity. Positive results in terms of clinical outcomes of people with MS have been reported from studies of these diets, but it should be noted that these studies were not controlled and randomized.

Imbalance

MS risk could potentially be influenced by a state of imbalance between a number of nutritional factors, including saturated and polyunsaturated fats, omega-6 and omega-3 essential fatty acids, zinc, and copper.

- **Saturated and unsaturated fats:** A study of essential fatty acids in the serum and CSF suggests that MS subjects have an imbalance between saturated and unsaturated fatty acids, which may be pronounced during acute MS exacerbation. A diet with excess saturated fat could produce a relative deficiency of EFA, creating a lipid imbalance that could affect cell fluidity, myelination, and synthesis of immunoregulatory compounds. Alternatively, instead of just creating a deficiency in EFA, saturated fats may actually antagonize the functions of eicosapentaenoic (EPA) and docosahexaenoic acids (DHA), two omega-3 unsaturated fatty acids, which may lead to an inflammatory leukotriene response.

- **Omega-3 and omega-6 fatty acids:** In the Western diet, the ratio of omega-6 to omega-3 fatty acid intake is close to 20:1. MS rates tend to be higher in regions where Western diet practices are observed, suggesting that an omega-6 to omega-3 imbalance could play a role in MS. According to one review, omega-3 EFA from fish oil are immunosuppressing nutrients that help prevent EAE disease progression, while large amounts of omega-6 EFA inhibit the effects of omega-3 EFA. Therefore, deficiencies in omega-3 fatty acids with respect to omega-6 EFA could alter immune regulation in a way that leads to MS.

- **Zinc and copper:** A possible zinc-copper imbalance may be a cause or consequence of MS. A study with a small sample size observed decreased copper content and elevated zinc-copper ratio in the red blood cells of MS subjects compared with controls.

Misuse

Misuse (failure of the body to properly process, use, or excrete a nutrient, as is seen in phenylketonuria, for instance) has not been explicitly assessed in the MS literature.

Nutrient Vectors

Nutritional vectors are the means by which nutrients enter the body. In MS, the vectors that have been most frequently assessed are food and sunlight. No unusual disruptions in or overuses of a particular vector have been prominently associated with MS. However, vector preferences and availability are different among populations and individuals; therefore, any such differences that can be associated with MS may help reveal nutrients involved in the etiology of the disease.

Food

Food is the major vector for nutrient entry into the body. Exposures to different types of food are primarily assessed by ecological studies of food consumption and case-control food frequency studies. Studies show that meat and other animal products, dairy, and fish oil have potentially significant roles in MS, while other foods such as fruits, vegetables, and sweets appear to play a minor role, if any at all.

Meat and other foods of animal origin: Many studies cite an association between MS and the intake of meats that are high in saturated fat as well as nutrients such as proteins and amino acids. Several epidemiological studies have suggested a positive association between MS and high saturated and animal fat consumption. For instance, one study of 22 countries for which data on MS prevalence and diet were available reported a significant, positive correlation between MS prevalence and animal fat intake. An epidemiologic study of nutrient intake and death rates revealed that mortality from MS was correlated with consumption of meat, milk, butter, and eggs. In an ecologic study, significant correlations were found between MS prevalence and fat intake, total meat intake, and pork consumption. Beef consumption, however, was not significantly correlated, even though beef and pork have the same fat composition.

In contrast with epidemiological studies, however, many population-based case-control studies fail to detect a relationship between fat intake and MS risk. These studies have observed that MS subjects and controls did not differ significantly in frequency of meat and fat intake before onset of MS, indicating that fat consumption is not associated with increased MS risk.

Dairy: Evidence is also mixed regarding the influence of dairy product consumption on the risk of MS. While ecologic studies report a strong positive correlation between MS and dairy food consumption, many case-control studies report no difference in intake between MS cases and controls. However, a few case-control studies have found that greater dairy intake was associated with MS. Living on a farm has also been reported as a risk factor, especially in comparing the high incidence of MS in farming regions as opposed to coastal regions. However, a number of confounding factors, such as socioeconomic status, an agricultural lifestyle, or climate may affect the validity of these conclusions.

Some speculations have been made about specific dairy products or components that could be responsible for an increase in MS risk. Fresh cow milk intake is more closely correlated with MS than cream, butter, and cheese, suggesting the presence of a factor in cow milk, such as an oxidative product of dairy called butyrate, which may trigger the development of MS. In addition, fresh unpasteurized milk could be a potential risk factor for MS by acting as a vector for bacterial or viral agents. The high concentration of saturated fatty acids in many dairy products could also help explain the higher risk of MS. Calcium in milk has also been discussed as a potential factor in MS etiology.

Breast milk and infant formula: Breast feeding of infants has been proposed to reduce their future risk of MS, either by providing essential nutrients such as unsaturated fatty acids found in breast milk, by affecting the immune system of the infant, or by reducing the intake of cows' milk or other substances that may increase susceptibility to MS. Two studies supporting this hypothesis found that MS subjects reported being breastfed as infants for shorter periods of time on average than controls. However, previous studies found no association between formula or breast feeding and MS. The impact of breast feeding on MS needs further study before any conclusions can be drawn.

Fish and fish oil: Fish and fish oil intake is of particular interest in MS research because fish oil is high in omega-3 fatty acids. Some studies have reported lower rates of MS in regions where fish intake is high, and differences in fish intake have been proposed as an explanation for lower MS rates in coastal versus inland regions in certain countries such as Norway. However, an analysis of data from the *Nurses' Health Study* revealed no protective effect of consumption of omega-3 fatty acids from fish. The clinical effects on MS of fish oil supplements have also been analyzed. Results suggest that such treatment may lead to reduced exacerbation rate and decreased disability. However, these studies tend to have limitations such as small numbers of participants or lack of a control arm.

Cereals and breads: A few case-control studies of dietary practices have assessed intake of cereals and breads in MS and control subjects. Results have been contradictory, with one study concluding that high consumption of cereal-derived products correlated positively with MS, another finding instead a protective effect of higher cereal and bread intake, and a third finding no significant relationship between cereal and bread intake and risk of MS.

Fruits and vegetables: Usually, fruits and vegetables are mentioned only as one of a variety of factors assessed in food frequency studies. From the few studies that are available, there is a general consensus that frequency of fruit and vegetable consumption is not related to the risk of MS.

Sweets: A few studies mention an association between consumption of sweets and risk of MS. One population-based study observed no significant differences in diet except slight differences in intake of sweets such as cake, cocoa, and chocolate. Similarly, one food frequency survey found an increased risk of MS, in females only, with consumption of sweets such as candy, jam, jelly, and chocolate. Another similar case-control study observed a positive correlation between high incidence of MS and frequent consumption of coffee, tea, and cocoa. One hypothesis states that an allergic reaction to cocoa products may cause MS.

Drinking Water

Drinking water has not been discussed independently of other factors in any MS study. Rather, drinking water is usually mentioned as one of a number of environmental factors surveyed in questionnaires. Of a few case control studies of exposure to various exogenous factors, two studies indicated that a higher percentage of MS subjects compared with controls drank from a piped water supply. Two different studies, however, found no difference in source of water or drinking habits of MS subjects and controls. In a study of a high-risk MS cluster, the water contained large amounts of chloride, chromium, molybdenum, nitrate, and zinc and only trace amounts of selenium and sulfate, suggesting the possible contribution of an environmental factor to MS.

Supplements

Supplements are primarily used to treat or prevent the deficiency of a nutritional factor. In a prospective study of two large cohorts of women (*Nurses' Health Study I and II*), it was concluded that vitamin C, E, and multivitamin supplementation were unrelated to the risk of MS. However, in a follow-up analysis, the same authors concluded that there was a 40 percent reduction in risk of MS among women who use supplemental vitamin D, typically in the form of multivitamins. The authors noted that they faced limitations in separating the effects of vitamin D intake from other components of multivitamins (vitamin E, folic acid, zinc, B_1, B_2, B_6, and B_{12}).

Air

Air as a vector (for example, oxygen) has not been assessed in any study relating nutrition to MS.

Sunlight

Sunlight is the means by which ultraviolet radiation (UVR) is carried to the earth's surface. Exposure of skin to sunlight catalyzes the production of vitamin D_3; the precursor of the stored and active forms of vitamin D. Lack of UVR may play a causal role in MS by creating a vitamin D deficiency, thus potentially accounting for the latitude gradient of MS incidence (increasing MS prevalence with increasing latitude).

The relationship between sunlight exposure and MS has been investigated through regional comparisons of MS distribution rates to average annual hours of sunlight, case-control studies assessing amounts of outdoor activity and sunlight exposure, and studies of MS disease activity during different seasons. Most studies suggest a protective effect of sunlight exposure on MS, with high sun exposure corresponding with a reduced risk of MS. Some discrepancies do exist, however. One population-based epidemiologic study indicates that MS subjects actually spent more time outdoors in the summer and did not tend to have occupations with less outdoor exposure, thus contradicting the hypothesis of the protective effect of sunlight.

Pharmacokinetics and Pharmacodynamics of Nutrients

Pharmacokinetics

Pharmacokinetics describes what the body does to a nutrient, that is, how the nutrient is processed. In general, how the pharmacokinetics of nutrients relate to MS has not been widely assessed in the scientific literature.

Digestion: Although individual vectors and properties have been addressed in great detail, the organs necessary for digestion and the processes by which nutrient vectors such as food are broken down to vitamins and minerals are not generally covered.

Absorption–organs: The small intestine, which includes the duodenum, jejunum, and ileum, is responsible for absorption. Defects in intestinal absorption could potentially alter nutrient concentrations in MS subjects.

- The duodenum is responsible for fatty acid absorption. It has been suggested that lower linoleate concentrations in serum lipids could be due to an altered rate of linoleic acid entry into or removal from the blood or a defective metabolic pathway. However, studies of absorption of safflower and sunflower oil in MS cases have indicated that lowered fatty acid levels in the CSF and serum of MS subjects are not due to dysfunctional intestinal absorption.

- Hypotheses concerning MS and the absorption of zinc by the jejunum have been conflicting. While malabsorption has been cited as a possible explanation for low serum zinc levels, other studies of blood zinc levels suggest that altered zinc levels are probably not the result of zinc malabsorption or nutritional abnormalities but rather reflect chronic inflammatory activity or abnormalities in control mechanisms. Biopsy studies of the jejunum in MS subjects also provide mixed results, with some reporting structural and biochemical abnormalities and others reporting none.

114

- Malabsorption of vitamin B_{12} by the ileum is one cause of B_{12} deficiency, which has been detected in some MS subjects. However, no evidence exists showing that people with MS have any dysfunction in this organ.

Malabsorption of the various nutrients absorbed by the colon has not been assessed.

Absorption–processes: Studies of MS and nutrition have not gone into detail about the specific processes, including active transport, passive diffusion, facilitated diffusion, and phagocytosis, through which absorption can occur.

Distribution: The mechanisms by which most nutrients are distributed throughout the body have not yet been fully assessed for potential involvement in MS. However, a few studies have investigated the role of protein carriers which transport certain minerals and vitamins, and which could therefore influence the concentrations of these nutrients in the tissues of people with MS. For example, copper is transported by ceruloplasmin, an enzyme that also plays a role in modulating lipid peroxidation. A small study of trace element status, however, found no deficiency in plasma ceruloplasmin in MS subjects.

An alteration in the primary protein carriers for zinc in the blood could indicate zinc deficiency in people with MS. Various studies have found abnormalities in MS subjects in terms of zinc or zinc carrier (for example, albumin, alpha-2 macroglobulin) concentrations although discrepancies exist within these findings.

One study found elevated levels of a vitamin B_{12} transport protein called R-binder in MS subjects compared with normal and other neurological disease (OND) controls, but the significance of this finding was not known.

Transformations: Though individual nutrient vectors and properties have been studied extensively, the steps by which these nonspecific nutritional factors are converted into usable form for highly specific functions in the body have not been assessed in terms of MS.

Storage: In general, improper storage of nutrients has not been extensively studied in connection with MS. Some studies have detected increased iron deposition in MS brain tissue which may contribute to tissue damage. However, it is unclear how these deposits are formed (one hypothesis is that deposition is mediated by upregulation of heme

115

oxygenase-1 in astroglia). Another small study that observed significantly elevated copper levels in the CSF of MS subjects postulated that MS causes changes in the brain that alter metal uptake, distribution, and storage that are then detectable in the CSF.

Excretion: Analysis of excretions can help investigators assess the intake as well as the appropriate processing of certain nutritional factors. For example, an investigation of daily urinary excretions of trace elements in MS subjects revealed no significant difference in metals (lead [Pb], nickel [Ni], silver [Ag], copper [Cu], iron [Fe], myoglobin [Mb], zinc [Zn]) between MS cases and controls. It has not yet been suggested, however, that excretion abnormalities are involved in the development of MS.

Pharmacodynamics

Pharmacodynamics describes the effect that a nutrient has on the body. Deficiency, toxicity, imbalance, and misuse of nutritional factors can have different effects that could be involved in the etiology of MS. The mechanisms by which various nutrients could play a role in MS are still under investigation. Proposed mechanisms of nutrient actions important in MS include regulation of the immune response, myelination/demyelination, and function of the blood brain barrier (BBB).

Regulation/stimulation of the immune response includes:

- **Vitamin D and Ultraviolet (UVR):** Ultraviolet radiation appears to have immunosuppressive effects on T helper 1 (Th1) cell immune responses, which may modulate autoimmune attacks in MS. This effect may be mediated by the impairment of antigen-presenting cells, the induction of regulatory T cell activity, and/or the suppression of melatonin, which enhances the release of Th1 cytokines. Vitamin D, which is synthesized via UVR exposure as well as ingested through the diet, is also thought to inhibit Th1 activity and promote regulatory T cell function.

- **Calcium:** According to one study, calcium and $1,25\text{-}(OH)_2D_3$ work together to regulate the immune system, as has been demonstrated in experiments involving experimental allergic encephalitis (EAE), a T-helper cell-dependent autoimmune disease. Altered concentrations of either nutrient could affect immune system response.

- **Trace metals:** Dietary intake of metals such as zinc has been shown to influence the responsiveness of the immune system.

Elevated levels of lead, nickel, and zinc in the soil of a high-risk MS cluster focus suggest that these trace elements may stimulate an immune response, perhaps by interacting with or altering the function of self-constituents.

- **Polyunsaturated fats (PUFA):** PUFA, especially n-3 fatty acids, produce various immunomodulatory and antiinflammatory factors, which may affect the course of MS. Modulatory effects of n-3 supplementation on immune function may involve altering the immune cell membrane and regulating metabolic pathways related to immune activation, such as cytokine or eicosanoid production. An immunosuppressive function of PUFA in existing MS is suggested by studies showing that linoleic acid supplementation may reduce the duration and severity of acute exacerbations.

- **Dairy or gluten products:** The idea that food antigens could trigger an immune response leading to the development of MS has been investigated just a few times. One study showed an abnormal T cell response in MS subjects to cow milk proteins, similar to the response demonstrated by diabetes subjects. However, no abnormal response to gluten proteins was found in another study.

Myelination or demyelination includes:

- **Vitamin B$_{12}$** deficiency can lead to alterations in the lipid composition of myelin and therefore could play a role in the poor remyelination seen in MS. Defective synthesis of the myelin sheath may also trigger an autoimmune response which contributes to MS pathogenesis.

- **Zinc** is an essential part of carbonic anhydrase, which is a part of the myelin sheath. Decreased carbonic anhydrase activity as a result of zinc deficiency could change myelin metabolism and increase MS susceptibility.

- **Fatty acids:** Since the myelin sheath is composed mainly of lipids, an imbalance in the composition of fatty acids available in the body could alter its function and stability. The composition of fatty acids and lipids in MS brain tissue (normal appearing white matter and plaques) has been analyzed in a few studies, with some finding alterations compared with control brain tissue and others finding no significant differences.

- **Calcium:** It has been hypothesized that low milk intake during an adolescent growth spurt may lead to inadequate levels of calcium with adverse effects on myelin lipid synthesis. Therefore, high childhood consumption of milk followed by a sudden decrease in adolescence could be related to MS incidence in young adulthood.

- **Antioxidants:** An excess of free radicals in the CNS can cause lipid peroxidation and induce protein and myelin sheath damage. Increased radical production with decreased antioxidant defense in the CNS may therefore help to promote the myelin damage seen in MS.

Permeability of blood brain barrier includes:

- **Saturated fat:** Several mechanisms have been proposed by which saturated fat could weaken the blood brain barrier, increasing the risk of MS. Swank's hypothesis (and the rationale for his low saturated fat diet) is that aggregation of blood cells following consumption of fats results in sludging of the blood, reduced oxygen availability in the brain, and increased vascular permeability in the central nervous system. Another theory is that dietary lipid imbalances can alter cell membrane function, leading to defects in the blood brain barrier.

- **Polyunsaturated fat:** Hutter has proposed that an excess of the omega-6 arachidonic acid and deficiency of omega-3 EPA and DHA leads to the overproduction of inflammatory leukotrienes which increase the permeability of the blood brain barrier.

Individual and Group Factors Influencing Nutritional Disease

Individual and group factors such as genetics, modernization, health status, geography, and cultural norms may alter a person's susceptibility to certain diseases. The following section discusses these factors and their possible relevance to a nutritional basis for MS.

Age

It has been postulated that development of MS is influenced by the occurrence of events at specific ages (such as adolescence). For instance, one study observed an association between age of migration and risk of MS in Asian immigrants moving to England, where the incidence of MS is considerably higher. Asian immigrants who entered England at an age younger than 15 had a higher risk of developing MS than those who entered after, suggesting that the childhood to adolescent years before age 15 are critical to the risk of developing MS. Similar findings have been reported by other investigators (although it should be noted that not all migration studies find associations between migration age and MS risk).

Although it stands to reason that nutrition during childhood or adolescence may influence the risk of MS, only a few nutritional studies have actually investigated age-dependent differences between MS and non-MS cases. Two studies have found that plasma and serum levels of zinc and copper are lower in younger MS subjects compared with controls (but not significantly different in older subjects), but whether this relates to conditions at onset of MS is not known. Another study found a strong inverse association between sun exposure in childhood and adolescence and risk of MS. It has been hypothesized that inadequate concentrations of nutrients such as calcium and phosphate during growth spurts (at the fetal stage and puberty) could potentially disturb myelin synthesis and cause MS. Other studies observed no notable differences in childhood diet or vitamin E levels in different case/control age groups.

Genetics

A few studies have looked for possible associations between MS and genetic variants that affect the utilization of nutrients, in particular the metabolism and function of vitamin D. For example, several studies have assessed the vitamin D binding protein gene and the vitamin D receptor gene, with mixed results. One study also examined the 25(OH)D2 1alpha-hydroxylase gene but found no evidence for linkage or association with MS.

Modernization

The documented prevalence of MS has increased greatly since its original identification in 1868. Undoubtedly, this is at least partly due to increased awareness of the disease and better diagnostic techniques, but some have wondered whether changes occurring in modern society, including increases in standards of living, may also have increased the risk of MS.

Socioeconomic status: Not all studies agree that socioeconomic status is related to MS, but studies that do report a correlation often suggest that higher socioeconomic status is associated with higher risk of MS. Greater affluence allows for better nutrition with higher meat consumption, which could potentially increase the risk of MS through intake of nutrients such as saturated fats. (Conversely, it has been suggested that the association between high animal fat intake and MS could merely reflect the relationship between MS risk and high socioeconomic level. However, this has been deemed unlikely since total calories and total protein have not been similarly associated with MS risk, as would be expected if a factor directly related to socioeconomic class was the causal agent.)

As a counterpoint to the supposition that high socioeconomic status is associated with MS, an investigation of MS incidence in New Zealand found instead a significantly higher proportion of MS subjects who had lived in rural areas before age 21 and probably came from lower socioeconomic backgrounds. Though contradictory to trends in the U.S., these results were consistent with the childhood milk intake patterns in New Zealand, where fresh milk is cheapest and most available to those of lower socioeconomic backgrounds.

Food processing: It has been suggested that milk processing may destroy a factor that is related to the clinical appearance of MS and is present in unpasteurized cow's milk, since fresh cow milk intake has been more closely correlated with MS in certain studies than cream, butter, and cheese. A proposed factor is butyrate, an oxidative product of dairy products.

Fortification: Fortification of foods with minerals and vitamins has not been assessed for a possible effect on the risk of MS.

Health Status

Intake and processing of nutrients can be greatly altered by a person's health status, and can therefore lead to further changes in health.

Trauma, illness, or addiction: Although trauma, illnesses, and addiction have been studied as possible risk factors for MS, with varying results, discussions of their involvement have not included their effects on nutritional health.

Fitness: It has been reported that obesity occurs more frequently among MS cases due to immobility and an inactive lifestyle following diagnosis. However, whether fitness level influences risk of developing MS in the first place has yet to be assessed.

Occupation: Occupation can influence a person's health in a number of ways, for instance by increasing or limiting his or her exposure to certain nutritional factors. Living on a farm has been reported as a risk factor, especially in comparing the high incidence of MS in farming regions as opposed to coastal regions, although not all studies have found rural residence to increase the risk of MS. Other occupations have been studied with respect to risk of MS, including metal processors, electricians, health service workers, and so on, but typically from a toxic agent exposure rather than a nutritional point of view.

Sunlight exposure is another nutritional factor that may affect the risk of MS and may be affected by choice of occupation. Many studies postulate a protective effect of sunlight, suggesting that occupations that offer greater exposure to sunlight decrease the risk of MS. For example, one such case-control study found a negative association between mortality from MS and residential and occupational exposure to sunlight. However, not all studies have found that MS subjects tended to have occupations with less outdoor exposure.

Geography

The availability of foods and nutrients is shaped by the environment in which a person lives; it is possible that geographic patterns of MS prevalence are at least somewhat influenced by nutritional factors.

Flora and fauna: Differences in disease prevalence among geographic regions are sometimes due to differences in the plants and animals available there. The reported associations between MS and coastal or rural environments which may be due to food intake have already been mentioned. A review of ecological data by Lauer also found correlations in several countries between MS and the cultivation of oats (but not wheat).

Geology: Only a few attempts have been made to relate MS prevalence to the minerals present in soil. One example is the previously-mentioned study that characterized the soil and water contents in a region with high MS prevalence.

Climate: Most studies that mention climate indicate that latitudes closer to the poles, colder temperatures, and/or a lower amount of sunlight received are associated with a higher incidence of MS, although one study could not find an independent effect on MS risk apart from latitude for solar radiation, temperature, or other climatic factors. One hypothesis suggests that cold stress increases energy consumption and thus the need for fat and protein, leading to biochemical imbalances that may lead to MS.

Cultural Practices

Cultural practices affecting nutrition that may affect the risk of MS have not been addressed extensively. However, the consumption of a local dish in the Orkney and Shetland Islands of Scotland, a region that maintains the highest MS rates ever reported, was associated with MS. The dish, called potted head or pig's brain, was the only one of six unusual food items that had any association with MS. The six food items included: potted head, raw fish, sea bird's eggs, undercooked meat, unpasteurized milk, and raw eggs. Other local specialties have occasionally been associated with an increased risk of MS (for example, horse meat in an Italian case control study), but to date no strong influence of cultural dietary practices on MS prevalence has been documented.

Section 9.3

Infectious Diseases

Analysis of Specific Pathogens as Possible Triggers of MS

Multiple sclerosis (MS) is believed, based on familial concordance data, to be a multifactorial disorder, requiring the presence of both genetic and environmental factors to initiate the mechanisms that lead to demyelination and neural damage. Although the environmental factors that trigger MS are still being determined, infectious agents such as bacteria and viruses have long been speculated to play a role in the etiology of MS. Scientists have investigated many different pathogens as candidate triggers of MS, using a variety of experimental techniques that have evolved over time as knowledge about infectious agents and disease has grown.

This section surveys a number of pathogens that have been evaluated for a role in MS, summarizing the results of the experiments that have been conducted to identify possible associations. It does not provide an exhaustive analysis for each pathogen; detailed reviews already exist for a number of them. Instead, it attempts to give an overview of the spectrum of infectious agents explored in MS, and provide a sense of what is known and not known regarding the involvement of these potential infectious triggers of MS.

Each pathogen discussed in this section is presented with a brief description of the pathogen being evaluated and an opinion given as to the strength of the evidence associating the pathogen with the risk of MS. For most of the pathogens listed, few conclusions can be drawn about their possible involvement in MS. A common finding is that positive results provided by one or more studies are contradicted by another study or group of studies. There are several possible reasons for this situation, including:

- differences and/or deficiencies in the experimental methods and techniques used

- differences in choices of cases and control subjects and differences in recruitment methods used

- small sample sizes resulting in a lack of statistical power

- inherent difficulties in detecting or isolating certain pathogens (such as *Chlamydia pneumoniae*), which may prevent replication of results from lab to lab

- non-specific findings implicating multiple pathogens (none, one, or some of which may be true susceptibility factors)

- lengthy time spans between the age of initial infection, the age of MS onset, and the age at which tissues or data are collected for analysis; the infection-to-analysis span can be especially long for studies examining MS autopsy brain tissue

- the possibility that MS may be a etiologically heterogeneous disease and therefore evidence for any given infectious trigger may be subtle or modest, or not even present in a given population under study

- the possibility that differences detected between MS and non-MS subjects may be artifacts of the disease process (for instance, the presence of pathogens in the central nervous system in MS subjects may be an artifact of blood-brain barrier leakage)

Indeed, because of time lapses, disease heterogeneity, and other factors, it is probably difficult to conclusively exclude the involvement of any particular pathogen of interest in any type or form of MS. Still, we believe there is value in presenting the available data as it will help to highlight areas where additional research could more conclusively indicate whether infections trigger MS and if so, which pathogens are involved.

Viruses

Adenovirus

Description: Adenoviruses are common human pathogens that can cause respiratory infections, conjunctivitis, and occasionally gastroenteritis. These viruses most frequently infect children although outbreaks in adult groups are also possible. Adenoviruses persist in human tonsils and are capable of integrating their genome into the host deoxyribonucleic acid (DNA), making them candidate vectors for gene therapy.

Conclusion: Only a few studies were found that explore a causal role for this virus in MS. The correlation found between adenovirus titers, upper respiratory infections, and subsequent relapses could indicate a possible interaction between the presence and activity of adenoviruses and MS disease mechanisms.

Canine Distemper Virus (CDV)

Description: CDV is a virus that infects dogs and other animals, including wildlife, and can result in encephalomyelitis. It is closely related to the measles virus. Humans can be infected with CDV asymptomatically, but the measles vaccine protects humans against CDV infection. A vaccine against CDV was introduced in the 1960s and is now widely available for pet dogs.

Conclusion: There is no strong evidence at this time to support a role for CDV as a cause of MS. If CDV were an important trigger of MS, it would be expected that control of this virus would produce an eventual reduction in the incidence of MS, but such a reduction has not yet been documented.

Coronavirus

Description: Human coronaviruses (HCV) are responsible for approximately 20 percent of colds in humans. Incidence of coronavirus infection peaks in the winter. Immunity does not persist and individuals can be periodically reinfected. There are two main serotypes of HCV, OC43 and 229E. While human coronaviruses typically infect respiratory epithelial cells, they have been found in brain tissue as well, and the coronavirus murine hepatitis virus (MHV) is known to cause a chronic demyelinating disease similar to MS in mice.

Conclusion: At this time no strong evidence has emerged to support a causal role for coronavirus in MS. Once the role of MHV in demyelination is better understood, it may be possible to compare it with HCV to determine which of MHV's pathogenic factors are also present in HCV.

Cytomegalovirus

Description: Human cytomegalovirus (CMV or HCMV) is a member of the herpes family and is a common pathogen worldwide. It causes three types of clinical syndromes: (1) congenital infection can cause hepatosplenomegaly, retinitis, rash, and central nervous system (CNS) involvement, although 90% of infected infants are asymptomatic; (2) primary infections in older children and adults can cause mononucleosis, although 90% of primary infections at this age are asymptomatic, and (3) primary or reactivated infections in immunocompromised individuals (for example, people with acquired immunodeficiency syndrome [AIDS]) can develop into a life-threatening systemic infection involving the central nervous system (CNS), lungs, gastrointestinal (GI) tract, liver, and retinas. Transmission occurs via contact with infected secretions such as saliva or breast milk. HCMV can persist in and be chronically excreted by a variety of tissues, including salivary glands and blood cells.

Conclusion: Although its persistence and potential for CNS involvement make it a plausible candidate for an MS trigger, at this time little evidence exists to support a specific role for HCMV in causing MS.

Epstein-Barr Virus

Description: Epstein-Barr virus (EBV) is a ubiquitous member of the herpes family; 95% of the world's population is thought to have been infected with this virus. Primary EBV infection can be asymptomatic or can manifest as infectious mononucleosis (IM), especially in adolescents and young adults. (Primary infection in children is often mild or asymptomatic.) Development of IM during primary infection is associated with large expansions of T cells in the blood. Why IM develops in some people but not others is not known, but it may be due to host factors and/or characteristics of the infection. EBV is trophic for B cells and is thought to cause lymphoproliferation in immunocompromised individuals. EBV persists in B cells and epithelial cells as a latent infection that periodically reactivates, and is primarily exchanged through transmission of saliva.

Conclusion: A variety of evidence exists to suggest a possible role for EBV in causing MS, including several findings that suggest possible etiological mechanisms. Some evidence (for example, increased antibody titers in MS cases versus controls) may result from MS disease processes rather than reflect a cause of MS. However, the existence of multiple types of evidence supporting a causal role, particularly the increased seroprevalence of EBV in pediatric MS cases, is striking and makes EBV a pathogen of particular interest in MS.

Herpes Simplex Virus

Description: Herpes simplex virus (HSV) 1 and 2 are closely related neurotropic viruses whose primary symptoms are oral lesions (HSV-1) and genital lesions (HSV-2). Other manifestations of HSV infection include lesions at other skin sites, meningitis, encephalitis, and disseminated disease. HSV is transmitted by oral and sexual contact. Infection is established through replication of the virus in epithelial cells and movement up the peripheral sensory nerve to the dorsal ganglia, where it can further replicate, move back down the sensory nerves to form a new lesion, or assume a state of latency.

Conclusion: The results of case or control studies do not strongly support a role for HSV in causing MS. However, antiviral treatment studies showing a reduction in MS lesion formation or relapses may suggest a role for HSV or other herpesviruses in stimulating disease activity.

Human Herpesvirus 6

Description: Human herpesvirus 6 (HHV-6) is a common virus that infects most people in early childhood, most likely through salivary transmission. It is tropic for CD4 T cells but also has been shown to inhabit CNS tissue, and like many of the viruses described in this section has been detected in the CNS tissue and/or cerebral spinal fluid (CSF) of subjects with neurological conditions such as encephalitis. Two strains have been identified: HHV-6A and HHV-6B. The B strain is associated with the childhood disease exanthem subitum, also known as roseola; both strains have been found to be neurotropic.

Conclusion: It is possible that HHV-6 is involved in triggering MS. There is some evidence that HHV-6 is preferentially found in plaque tissue of MS subjects but the significance of this is unknown. Some studies have also identified differences in the antibody response to HHV-6 between MS subjects and controls.

Human Immunodeficiency Virus (HIV)

Description: Human immunodeficiency virus (HIV), also referred to in older texts as HTLV-III, is the human retrovirus that causes AIDS (acquired immune deficiency syndrome). HIV infects CD4 T cells and macrophages, and AIDS is characterized by depletion of CD4 T cells which leads to opportunistic infections and tumors as well as dementia and other neurological abnormalities. HIV is chiefly transmitted through sexual contact, through contact with blood (for example, transfusion of contaminated blood), and perinatally.

Conclusion: No strong evidence exists for an association between MS and HIV. However, there is evidence for possible increased reactivity to retroviral components.

Human T-Cell Leukemia (or T-lymphotropic) Virus (HTLV)

Description: There are two known strains of HTLV: HTLV-1 and HTLV-2. HTLV-1 is an exogenous human retrovirus that is prevalent to varying degrees in different parts of the world and is particularly common in southwestern Japan and the Caribbean. Most HTLV-1 infected individuals have an asymptomatic infection, but a small percentage develop an associated disease such as adult T-cell leukemia or lymphoma. Approximately 0.25% of infected people develop HTLV-I-associated myelopathy/tropical spastic paraparesis (HAM/TSP), a demyelinating disease that resembles MS in many aspects. Transmission of the virus typically occurs through sexual contact, contact with contaminated blood, or breast feeding. HTLV-2 is a closely related virus that has not yet been conclusively associated with any human disease.

Conclusion: At this time the evidence does not indicate a causal role of HTLV-1 in MS. However, the existence of a similar demyelinating disease (HAM/TSP) that is thought to be caused or triggered by HTLV-1 suggests that the involvement of retroviruses should continue to be studied in MS.

Human Endogenous Retroviruses (HERV)

Description: HERV are retrovirus-like elements that make up as much as 8% of the human genome and are found in both coding and non-coding regions. Most are unable to replicate because of genetic defects, but many HERV are capable of encoding retroviral proteins.

Expression of HERV ribonucleic acid (RNA) may be increased at sites of inflammation; HERV may also be transactivated by herpesviruses. Several different HERV have been investigated in MS. One, multiple sclerosis-related virus (MSRV, previously called LM7), is particularly noteworthy because it was first isolated from cells from people with MS.

Conclusion: No conclusion can yet be drawn about the involvement of endogenous retroviruses in MS. The increase in MSRV expression activity in MS subjects, combined with its production of proteins that may be harmful to oligodendrocytes or act as super-antigens, suggest a role for this virus. However, it should be noted that increased MSRV expression activity is not specific to MS but has also been seen in other diseases.

JC Virus

Description: JC virus (JCV) is a relatively common virus that is found worldwide, with prevalence varying according to geographic region. In some areas the majority of the adults studied have been found to be seropositive for JCV. Normally the virus establishes a latent, asymptomatic infection in the kidneys (and possibly other sites in the body), which is kept under control by the immune system. However, if the immune system is suppressed, JCV may travel to and/or become activated in the brain, where it can cause a demyelinating disease called progressive multifocal leukoencephalopathy (PML). Notably, PML has been diagnosed in a small number of subjects receiving the new MS drug Tysabri.

Conclusion: Although the similarities between PML and MS might suggest a causal role for JCV in MS, there is currently no strong evidence to support this idea.

Measles

Description: The measles virus is a paramyxovirus that, in an unvaccinated person, can cause a disease involving rash, fever, runny nose, conjunctivitis, and other complications. The disease is marked by a viremia that spreads to the lymphatic system, skin, respiratory system, intestines, and urinary tract. The virus may also spread to the brain where it occasionally results in encephalitis. It can persist in the brain and at a later time reactivate to cause an inflammatory, demyelinating disease called subacute sclerosing panencephalitis (SSPE). Measles ribonucleic acid (RNA) can be detected in the brain tissue of people with SSPE. Note that an effective vaccine to measles became available in the U.S. in 1963; since the implementation of public health vaccination programs, the incidence of measles in the U.S. and other countries has been dramatically reduced.

Conclusion: Higher prevalence and titers of anti-measles antibodies have been found in MS subjects versus controls; however, similar findings have also been reported for other pathogens. Due to vaccination programs, measles infection has nearly been eliminated in many countries where MS prevalence rates are the highest (for example, the U.S.). This would suggest that, were the measles virus an important trigger of MS, incidence rates should have begun to decline in these countries unless the vaccine itself can also trigger MS.

Mumps

Description: The mumps virus is a paramyxovirus that is found throughout the world and transmitted through close person-to-person contact. Mumps epidemics can occur where vaccination is not practiced. Distribution of the virus from the respiratory system through the bloodstream results in systemic infection involving target organs such as the salivary glands, testes, ovaries, and the pancreas. The central nervous system can also be affected through the development of mumps meningitis, or more rarely, mumps encephalitis. Approximately one-third of mumps infections are subclinical. A vaccine for mumps was licensed in the U.S. in 1967; since then the incidence of reported clinical mumps infection in this country has declined by 99%.

Conclusion: There is no strong evidence to support involvement of the mumps virus in the development of MS. Later age of mumps infection was associated with MS in multiple studies, but this was often also found true for other types of infections in these same studies. Similarly, the immunological differences between MS and control subjects found concerning the mumps virus have also been reported for other pathogens.

Parainfluenza and Related Paramyxoviruses (6/94 Virus, Sendai Virus)

Description: In addition to measles and mumps, other paramyxoviruses have been investigated for a role in MS. These include strains of the human parainfluenza virus (which cause primarily respiratory system symptoms), animal viruses such as Sendai, simian virus 5, Newcastle disease virus, and canine distemper virus (described separately in this section), and the 6/94 virus which was originally isolated from MS brain tissue.

Conclusion: The available evidence does not strongly support the involvement of these paramyxoviruses in MS. Follow-up investigations of indications connecting one of these viruses with MS have generally failed to replicate the findings or have shown them not to be specific to the particular virus or to MS.

Rubella (German Measles)

Description: Rubella is a togavirus that causes German measles, a disease characterized by rash and lymphadenopathy. Rubella infection can be transmitted transplacentally and can cause birth defects in a developing fetus. The incidence of rubella infection in the U.S. has declined by approximately 99% since the introduction of the rubella vaccine in 1969.

Conclusion: The available evidence does not strongly suggest a role for rubella in causing MS. Immune abnormalities involving rubella, such as intrathecal synthesis of anti-rubella antibodies, have also been detected for other viruses and may be a nonspecific feature of the disease.

Vaccinia

Description: The vaccinia virus is a poxvirus that is used to vaccinate people against smallpox. Serious complications from vaccination are rare but can include CNS effects, most notably encephalitis. Routine smallpox vaccination was ended in the U.S. in 1972, but the vaccinia virus is still used to prepare recombinant vaccines for other diseases.

Conclusion: Although vaccinia antibodies have been detected more frequently and at higher levels in MS cases than controls, this is also true of other viruses. The fact that routine vaccinia vaccination was discontinued in 1972 but unvaccinated people continue to be diagnosed with MS also points away from a significant causal role for this virus in MS.

131

Varicella Zoster

Description: Varicella zoster virus (VZV) is the cause of chickenpox and historically has been encountered by most susceptible individuals in childhood, although a vaccine has been introduced to prevent infection. In unvaccinated people, the initial infection develops and resolves over a period of a few weeks. The course of the infection includes initial replication in the oropharynx, dissemination throughout the body by viremia, and development of a characteristic rash. VZV may subsequently persist in the dorsal root ganglia. If reactivated, VZV can cause herpes zoster, also known as shingles; this mainly occurs in older adults.

Conclusion: No strong evidence has been presented to suggest a role for VZV in causing MS. People with MS often manufacture intrathecal antibodies to VZV, but this is true of other viruses as well. Longitudinal patterns of MS and varicella infection appear to be similar, but this could have a variety of explanations.

Bacteria

Borrelia Burgdorferi

Description: *Borrelia burgdorferi* is a Gram-negative spirochete that causes Lyme disease, a disease that can affect multiple organ systems including the central nervous system. In fact, the neurological symptoms of chronic Lyme disease can closely resemble those of MS, which creates challenges in the differential diagnosis of these diseases. Diagnosis is also complicated by the possibility of false positives and false negatives in detecting antibody responses to *B. burgdorferi* which is the standard diagnostic approach for Lyme disease. In the U.S., *B. burgdorferi* is transmitted by the bite of hard ticks such as the deer tick in the northern and midwestern U.S. and the western black-legged tick in western states. Lyme disease is endemic to those regions inhabited by these ticks, notably wooded areas in the northeast U.S., the Great Lakes region, and the Pacific Northwest.

Conclusion: Because it is endemic only to certain geographic locations, *B. burgdorferi* is unlikely to be an MS trigger in all cases. However, assuming that MS is an etiologically heterogeneous disease, in individuals who are predisposed to MS, it is plausible that *B. burgdorferi* infection may initiate certain pathogenic events leading to MS.

Chlamydia Pneumoniae

Description: *Chlamydia pneumoniae* (Cpn) is a common obligate intracellular bacterium that causes respiratory tract infections and is transmitted by respiratory secretions. It has been implicated as a risk factor in other diseases, most notably heart disease, but also other neurological disorders such as Alzheimer disease.

Conclusion: The available evidence concerning Cpn and MS is quite mixed. Although some studies have linked the presence of Cpn DNA or antibodies in CSF to MS, not all have shown such a connection. Furthermore, the one prospective study conducted to analyze Cpn antibodies prior to MS onset showed no clear association between seropositivity and risk of MS. Investigations of anti-chlamydial treatments in MS have been limited.

Other Pathogens Investigated in MS

In addition to the pathogens presented in this section, a number of other pathogens have been evaluated for an etiological role in MS but to a lesser degree. For each of the following listed pathogens, only a few studies (often only one or two) could be found that evaluated experimental evidence for its involvement in MS.

Accelerated Cure Project's infectious agents studies spreadsheet (which can be downloaded at www.acceleratedcure.org/downloads/phase2-infectiousagents-studies.xls) contains a listing of the studies found to date for each of these pathogens.

Viruses

- acute human encephalomyelitis virus
- adult T-cell leukemia (ATL) virus
- BK virus
- Borna disease virus
- bovine leukemia virus (BLV)
- caprine arthritis encephalitis virus
- hepatitis C
- hepatitis G
- human herpesvirus 7

- human herpesvirus 8
- human papilloma virus (HPV)
- Inoue-Melnick virus
- Influenza virus
- Lipovnik virus
- Maedi-Visna virus
- Marek disease virus
- Parvovirus B19
- poliovirus
- respiratory syncytial virus (RSV)
- simian immunodeficiency virus
- simian virus 40
- Spumavirus
- vesicular stomatitis virus

Bacteria

- Acinetobacter
- bacillus Calmette-Guérin
- Bifidobacterium
- *Bordetella pertussis*
- *Clostridium tetani*
- *Corynebacterium diphtheriae*
- Enterococcus
- *Escherichia coli*
- *Helicobacter pylori*
- *Haemophilus influenzae*
- microsporidia
- *Mycobacterium bovis*
- *Mycobacterium leprae*
- *Mycobacterium tuberculosis*
- *Mycoplasma pneumoniae*

- *Pseudomonas aeruginosa*
- Staphylococcus/*Staphylococcus S. aureus*
- Streptococcus

Fungi

- *Candida albicans*

Protozoa

- *Toxoplasma gondii*

Conclusion

The information presented in this section shows that although many different infectious agents have been studied, some quite extensively, for a potential role in MS, currently no specific pathogen can be conclusively labeled as an MS trigger. There are many challenges inherent in identifying the triggers of a disease which may take many years to manifest itself and which may require the contributions of multiple etiological factors. Assuming that MS is a multifactorial and heterogeneous disease, it is likely that the evidence implicating infectious triggers of MS will not be clear cut, will be opposed by conflicting findings, and will require careful interpretation. It is also possible that identifying and confirming infections triggers of MS will require the use of new investigative techniques and expanding the scope of research to pathogens not previously evaluated in MS.

For Additional Information

Accelerated Cure Project, Inc.
300 Fifth Ave.
Waltham, MA 02451
Phone: 781-487-0008
Fax: 781-487-0009
Website: http://www.acceleratedcure.org
E-mail: info-web0107@acceleratedcure.org

Chapter 10

MS Exacerbation: Attack, Relapse, or Flare

An exacerbation (also known as an attack, a relapse, or a flare) is a sudden worsening of a multiple sclerosis (MS) symptom or symptoms, or the appearance of new symptoms, which lasts at least 24 hours and is separated from a previous exacerbation by at least one month. The most common disease course in MS, called relapsing-remitting MS, is characterized by clearly defined acute exacerbations, followed by complete or partial recovery with no progression of the disease between attacks.

True Exacerbations Generally Last from Days to Weeks

A true exacerbation of MS is caused by an area of inflammation in the central nervous system. This is followed by demyelination—the destruction of myelin, which is the fatty sheath that surrounds and protects the nerve fibers. Demyelination results in the formation of an abnormal area called a plaque and causes the nerve impulses to be slowed, distorted, or halted, producing the symptoms of MS. One example of an exacerbation of MS would be the development of optic neuritis, an inflammation of the optic nerve that impairs vision.

An exacerbation may be mild or may significantly interfere with the individual's daily life. Exacerbations usually last from several days to several weeks, although they may extend into months. It is generally accepted that a short course of corticosteroids will cause an exacerbation to be shorter and/or less severe.

Pseudoexacerbation Temporarily Aggravates MS Problems

Sometimes an increase in symptoms has nothing to do with the underlying MS, but is caused by factors such as fever, infection, or hot weather that can temporarily aggravate MS problems. This is referred to as a pseudoexacerbation. Once the triggering event is past—for example, when the body temperature returns to normal, the symptoms subside as well. Some people with MS report a worsening of their symptoms during or after periods of intense stress. Researchers are exploring the effects of stress on the immune system and its possible involvement in MS.

Remission

A remission does not mean that all the symptoms of MS disappear, but rather that a person with MS returns to the baseline that existed before the last exacerbation began.

Additional Information

National Multiple Sclerosis Society
733 Third Ave., 6th Fl.
New York, NY 10017-3288
Toll-Free: 800-344-4867 (FIGHTMS)
Phone: 212-986-3240
Fax: 212-986-7981
Website: http://www.nationalmssociety.org
E-mail: nat@nmss.org

Chapter 11

Disease Progression in MS

Clinical and Biological Features

Multiple sclerosis (MS) literally means "many scars," which refers to the lesions that accumulate in the brain and spinal cord throughout the course of the disease. These scars, or lesions, consist mostly of dead nerve cells, whose axons have been denuded of the myelin sheaths that normally protect them and permit the conduction of nerve impulses. MS is a chronic, degenerative disease that usually begins in young adulthood and most visibly destroys muscular control, although many other brain functions are affected. Most people will live with MS for decades after their diagnosis. MS reduces life expectancy after onset (as measured by current diagnostic criteria) by only about 10–15 years, and about half of the patients survive 30 years or more from onset.

Disease Activity and Progression

MS, as defined by ongoing central nervous system (CNS) lesion formation and increasing cumulative damage, is now recognized as a disease that is active in most patients most of the time. Disease

Excerpts from "Multiple Sclerosis: Current Status and Strategies for the Future," Board on Neuroscience and Behavioral Health, Institute of Medicine. Reprinted with permission from the National Academies Press, Copyright 2001 National Academy of Sciences. Reviewed in June 2007 by Dr. David A. Cooke, M.D., Diplomate, American Board of Internal Medicine.

activity has reversible and irreversible sequelae; irreversible sequelae ultimately lead to progressive impairment and disability in most patients. MS takes a variety of forms, distinguished by the clinical pattern of disease activity. Accumulated deficit can produce sustained worsening in both relapsing and progressive MS. In relapsing MS, worsening occurs in most patients during acute attacks with incomplete recovery. In progressive MS, the dominant pattern is a gradual accumulation of neurologic deficits, with slow clinical worsening.

Disease activity and progression have both clinical and subclinical components. Clinical disease activity and progression are judged by observation and neurologic examination. Subclinical components refer to pathological changes that are not observable in a clinical examination but are observed using a variety of laboratory tests, predominantly neuroimaging parameters.

Varieties of MS

Asymptomatic MS: Autopsy studies indicate there are individuals without any known clinical history that have neuropathologic changes typical of MS. It is difficult to get an accurate estimate of subclinical disease, but one recent review suggested asymptomatic MS might account for up to 25% of all cases.

Relapsing-remitting MS: This is the major MS subtype. Approximately 85% of patients with a diagnosis of MS start out with relapsing MS. Overall, this subtype accounts for 55% of MS. Relapsing MS patients show a high rate of inflammatory lesion activity (gadolinium-enhancing lesions).

Benign relapsing MS: This category represents a subset of relapsing patients who have few attacks and make an excellent recovery. They show minimal impairment and disability, even after 20–30 years. The proportion of MS patients with benign disease is controversial. Reasonable studies suggest 10–20% of people with MS fit into this category.

Primary progressive MS: This subtype accounts for 10% of MS. Patients show gradual worsening from onset, without disease attacks. These patients tend to be older and often present with a spinal cord dysfunction without obvious brain involvement. This subtype is the least likely to show inflammatory lesion activity on MRI (gadolinium-enhancing). Unlike the other subtypes of MS, men are as likely as women to develop primary progressive MS.

Progressive relapsing MS: This subtype accounts for 5% of MS. Patients show slow worsening from onset, with superimposed attacks. Recent studies suggest these patients are similar to primary progressive patients.

Secondary progressive MS: This is the major progressive subtype and accounts for approximately 30% of MS. Relapsing MS patients usually transition to secondary progressive disease. They show gradual worsening, with or without superimposed relapses. Natural history studies of untreated relapsing MS indicate 50% of patients will be secondary progressive at 10 years and almost 90% by 25 years. This form of MS shows a lower rate of inflammatory lesion activity than relapsing MS, yet the total burden of disease continues to increase. This most likely reflects ongoing axonal loss.

Acute MS: Also referred to as Marburg variant MS, this is the most severe form of MS. Significant disability develops much more rapidly than usual, over weeks to months. Pathologic changes are widespread and destructive. These cases are rare and generally occur in young people.

Clinically isolated syndromes: This refers to patients who present with an isolated central nervous system (CNS) syndrome (optic neuritis, incomplete transverse myelitis, brainstem or cerebellar lesion), which is often the first MS attack. Clinical, magnetic resonance imaging (MRI), and cerebrospinal fluid (CSF) studies indicate that such patients with normal brain MRI and CSF have a low risk of developing MS. In contrast, those with abnormal MRI have a high risk of developing MS.

Initial Signs and Symptoms of MS

Common signs and symptoms of MS include:

- sensory problems (numbness or tingling of a body part)
- weakness
- difficulty walking
- monocular decreased vision
- poor coordination

Uncommon signs and symptoms of MS include:

- bladder problems

- bowel problems
- sexual dysfunction
- cognitive difficulties
- pain

Clinical Activity

Relapses

Relapses are variously referred to as acute attacks, exacerbations, or disease flare-ups. They involve the acute, or sudden onset, of focal neurological disturbances. Examples of typical MS relapses include blurring of vision in one eye (optic neuritis), persistent numbness or tingling of a body part (sensory system relapse), weakness of a body part (motor system relapse), or loss of coordination (cerebellar system relapse). Early in the MS disease process, relapses are likely to involve sensory, motor, cerebellar, or visual system abnormalities. Later in the disease process, relapses are likely to involve bladder, bowel, cognitive, and sexual function abnormalities. Acute disease attacks are a characteristic feature of the relapsing-remitting MS subtype. Relapses also occur in patients with progressive relapsing disease and in a number of patients with secondary progressive disease. The only clinical disease subtype in which relapses never occur is primary progressive MS.

Relapses generally consist of three phases. There is a period of worsening, with onset of new deficits or increasing severity of old deficits. This is followed by a period of stability, with no change in deficits. The final phase is the period of recovery, with variable degrees of improvement in deficits. Most patients recover within six weeks, although for some, improvements can continue over months. Recovery can be complete return to baseline status, partial return, or no improvement. However, some degree of improvement is typical, particularly early in the disease. Relapsing patients then remain clinically stable until the next disease attack.

To be considered a relapse, deficits must persist for a minimum of 24 hours. This avoids confusion with deficits lasting only minutes to hours, which are believed to be a consequence of impaired nerve conduction through old lesion areas rather than the formation of a new lesion. Alternatively, new abnormalities that last seconds to minutes, such as Lhermitte sign (a tingling sensation radiating down the arms, neck, or back on neck flexion), or paroxysmal attacks (stereotypic

142

neurologic deficits occurring multiple times a day that last less than a minute) are also considered relapses if they occur repeatedly over several weeks. Sequential relapses are considered distinct only when they occur at least 30 days apart with a month of clinical stability in between. Although clinical relapses always produce changes in a patient's condition, they are not always associated with changes on neurologic examination. Maximal deficit in an MS relapse typically develops over several days but in some cases can develop much faster, over hours or even minutes, or much more slowly, over a period as long as several weeks.

Physiologic factors such as temperature, pH, or electrolyte balance can temporarily disrupt nerve conduction and produce neurologic abnormality. A relapse must be distinguished from a pseudoexacerbation, which is a neurologic deterioration associated with a physiologic change such as infection or fever. This condition can last for days, mimicking a true relapse. Pseudoexacerbation deficits disappear once the precipitating factor has been corrected. They reflect a temporary disruption in nerve conduction, rather than the formation of a new lesion.

Approximately 85 percent of MS patients begin with relapsing-remitting disease. MS relapses can involve a single neural system, as in optic neuritis, or several anatomically distinct systems at the same time, for example, combined motor and sensory problems. Attacks involving single neural systems are somewhat more common in the first MS relapse.

Most patients experience their second attack within two to three years of the first, but five percent of patients remain free of relapses for 15 years or more. In most cases, there is substantial recovery from the first relapse; only four percent of patients show no improvement. The average relapse rate is one to two attacks a year, but this rate normally declines over time. The longer a person has MS, the less likely it is that relapses will be followed by complete recovery and the more likely it is that relapses will be associated with residual deficits and increasing disability.

Relapse features have prognostic significance (Table 11.1). In the first few years after disease onset, the number and type of relapses, as well as the degree of recovery, help predict future disease course. Relapses that involve visual, sensory, or brainstem systems have a better prognosis than those that involve cerebellar, motor, or sphincter systems. In the first two years of disease, a low relapse rate with excellent recovery indicates a better prognosis than a high relapse rate with poor recovery. Relapses restricted to single neural systems are prognostically better than those involving multiple systems. The relapse rate also has prognostic significance in the later stages of MS. With disease duration of five or more years, an increasing relapse rate, polyregional relapses that involved multiple systems, and incomplete recovery from relapses, indicate a worse prognosis.

Table 11.1. Prognostic Relapse Indicators

Feature	Favorable Prognosis	Unfavorable Prognosis
Relapse rate in first 2 years	Less than 5 relapses	5 or more relapses
Relapse rate after 5 years	No increase	Increasing
Duration between relapses	Long	Short
Number of neural systems involved	One	Multiple
Relapse recovery	Complete	Incomplete
Type of systems involved	Visual, sensory, brainstem	Motor, cerebellar, bowel or bladder

Progression

The relapsing form of MS is characterized by acute disease exacerbations. In contrast, progressive MS is characterized by slow deterioration and increasing neurological deficits. There are three forms of progressive MS. Approximately 15 percent of MS patients show slow deterioration from onset. In the second form, 10 percent have either primary progressive MS and never experience acute disease attacks or progressive relapsing MS (five percent), and have occasional subsequent attacks. The third form, secondary progressive MS, is the major progressive subtype. These are relapsing patients who begin to slowly worsen five to fifteen years after the first relapse. Once relapsing patients enter a progressive phase, they either stop having relapses or continue to experience exacerbations superimposed on slow worsening.

Documentation of a progressive course requires at least six months of observation. Observation over a year or two is often necessary to be confident of progression, since deficits can accumulate at a very gradual rate. The major defining feature of progressive MS is slow deterioration that occurs independently of acute disease relapses and does not reflect residual deficits from acute disease attacks. An analysis of the disease course among 1,844 patients indicated that the presence or absence of relapses during the progressive phase does not significantly affect the progression of irreversible disability (four percent of patients in this study had been treated for up to one year with beta-interferon, but this did not affect the study results). Progressive MS patients can be clinically stable for up to several years at a time and can even show slight improvement for a period of time. Ultimately, however, all progressive MS patients develop disability with limited ability to walk. Progressive MS is a more severe form than benign or relapsing-remitting MS and has a worse prognosis.

Subclinical Disease Activity and Progression

Clinical parameters such as relapses and progression underestimate the actual damage to tissue that occurs in MS. When macroscopically normal-appearing brain tissue is looked at under the microscope, one can detect inflammation, gliosis (scarring), and myelin damage. Chemical studies of normal-appearing brain tissue often reveal changes in organelles such as lysosomes, in enzymes, and in myelin constituents. In addition, a number of the new research neuro-imaging techniques can detect changes in brain and spinal cord areas that appear free of lesions on conventional magnetic resonance imaging (MRI). Some of these abnormalities are detectable several months to years before they can be seen with conventional MRI. Changes in normal-appearing brain tissue are generally pronounced in MS patients with severe impairment. As a group, secondary progressive MS patients show more abnormalities in normal white matter and brain tissue than relapsing patients. (White matter corresponds to brain regions where axons are ensheathed in myelin; gray matter corresponds to brain regions that are rich in cell bodies.) Primary progressive patients often show subtle but diffuse changes in normal-appearing brain areas.

Even conventional MRI indicates that most new lesion formation is clinically silent, meaning that clinical exam does not reveal any corresponding symptoms. Approximately 80 to 90 percent of new brain lesions do not produce identifiable relapses. They might, however, be associated with subtle cognitive changes or other neuropsychological changes that are not detected in clinical examination. The total lesion burden increases in MS patients, on average, five to ten percent per year, reflecting in large part the development of clinically silent

145

lesions. Atrophy of both brain and spinal cord can be detected even in patients with minimal symptoms. Atrophy can progress without obvious lesion formation, most likely reflecting loss of axons. MS patients show an accelerated rate of age-related brain and spinal cord atrophy that is three- to tenfold higher than the rate in control populations.

Spinal cord lesions are generally similar to those in the brain except for the absence of "black holes." Spinal MS lesions rarely cover more than half of the cross-sectional area of the cord or exceed two vertebral segments in length. They are found more often in the cervical spinal cord (neck region) than thoracic region (midback) and are most common in the midcervical region. Disease activity is much less frequent in the spine than in the brain.

In summary, the clinical manifestations of MS possibly represent only the tip of the iceberg, with most of the CNS damage occurring much earlier and being detectable only when the accumulated damage overwhelms the ability of the CNS to compensate.

Chapter 12

Diseases That Mimic MS

It is hardly unusual to hear stories of people who have been misdiagnosed several times before finally being diagnosed with multiple sclerosis (MS). Others remain in limbo for years, wondering if they will ever get a definite MS diagnosis. This is partly because there is no single diagnostic test to establish a definite MS diagnosis, and also because there are many diseases which manifest symptoms similar to MS. These are called MS mimics.

Why Mimics Matter

Familiarizing yourself with MS mimics and the ways in which they compare to MS can demystify much of the diagnostic process. Sometimes, the process of elimination is the only way to a MS diagnosis. Therefore, the more you know about MS mimics, the quicker you and your doctor can eliminate them as possibilities. Today, with MS specialists advocating early, aggressive treatment, the sooner a MS diagnosis can be confirmed, the better.

"If you are diagnosed with MS, you want to be sure that the diagnosis is correct," states Dr. Jack Burks, Clinical Professor of Neurology at the University of Nevada School of Medicine and senior editor of the book *Multiple Sclerosis: Diagnosis, Medical Management, and Rehabilitation*. "Certainly, other diseases can look like MS, but the treatments are not the same."

What Is Devic Disease?

Until recently, Devic disease (also known as neuromyelitis optica or NMO) was thought to be an unusual variant of MS. However, recent discoveries have shown that MS and Devic are not the same disease. Devic disease is characterized by immune attacks of the optic nerve and spinal cord. Symptoms include loss of vision, weakness, numbness, and bladder/bowel problems. But Devic disease is different from MS in a number of ways.

How Does Devic Disease Differ from MS?

Devic tends to strike only the optic nerves and spinal cord. Other symptoms are rare, although certain symptoms (including uncontrollable vomiting and hiccups) are now recognized as specific to Devic disease. In Devic disease, a spine magnetic resonance image (MRI) usually shows areas of inflammation, while brain MRIs generally show minimal changes. The cerebrospinal fluid in Devic disease differs from that of typical MS in that it usually has a large number of white blood cells, no oligoclonal bands, and normal intrathecal immunoglobulin G (IgG) synthesis.

Is Treatment the Same?

The immunomodulatory therapies used for MS, such as the interferons and glatiramer acetate do not effectively treat Devic disease. Devic is generally treated with immunosuppressant therapy, such as Rituxan and Imuran. (Interestingly, in 2005, there was a published Japanese study that showed that IFN-beta was just as effective in treating Devic as treating MS. However, there has been some confusion about Devic in the West versus in Japan. The Japanese tend to use the term *opticospinal MS* for Devic disease. It is possible that Devic manifests differently in Asians, possibly accounting for a different response to beta interferons.) Consequently, it is important to distinguish between Devic disease and MS in order to treat accordingly.

Differentiating Devic Disease from MS

The recent discovery of an antibody in the blood of individuals with Devic disease provides doctors with a reliable biomarker to distinguish Devic disease from MS. The antibody (known as NMO-IgG) seems to be present in about 70 percent of those with Devic disease and is not present in people with MS.

If your doctor is having a hard time distinguishing which disease you have, let them know that there is now an NMO antibody test that can be ordered through the Mayo Clinic that may help confirm the diagnosis.

Autoimmune Diseases That Mimic MS

Acute disseminated encephalomyelitis (ADEM) is a demyelinating, neurological disease characterized by inflammation of the brain and spinal cord. Symptoms may include headache, seizure, stiff neck, ataxia, optic neuritis, vomiting, weight loss, lethargy, delirium, and sometimes paralysis of a single limb or one side of the body.

ADEM differs from MS in that it is often clearly triggered by an immunization, or viral infection. The most common cause is prior measles infection, usually in children. ADEM runs a monophasic course, which means that there is one episode.

Systemic lupus erythematosus (SLE), is a chronic, inflammatory disease that may affect the skin, joints, blood, and kidneys. Symptoms include achy, swollen joints, extreme fatigue, anemia, skin rash, sun or light sensitivity, hair loss, seizure, and Raynaud phenomenon where fingers turn white or blue in the cold.

Sometimes called the great imitator, lupus commonly displays symptoms associated with another disease, such as MS. Lupus and MS can be diagnosed simultaneously, although that is less common than being diagnosed with one disease, and then later, diagnosed with the other.

An antinuclear antibody (ANA) test can help to confirm a lupus diagnosis, but other diseases, including MS, can also produce positive ANA results. In addition, even a person who has lupus will not always produce positive results on this test. A urinalysis or kidney biopsy may be performed to check for signs of possible kidney problems. MRI, computed tomography (CT) scan, echocardiography, x-rays, and other diagnostic criteria are also used. Sometimes, MS lesions on the spinal cord can be a distinguishing factor, or first-trimester miscarriages, which are quite common in women with lupus, but not women with MS.

Sjögren syndrome is a chronic disease in which white blood cells attack the moisture-producing glands. It is a systemic disease, which means that it affects the entire body. Symptoms include dry eyes and mouth, difficulty swallowing and speaking, fatigue, joint pain, decreased sensation, and numbness. Sjögren can plateau, worsen, or go into remission, and some people will experience mild symptoms, while others will be greatly debilitated.

Nerve conduction velocity (NCV) tests can be helpful in differentiating between MS and Sjögren syndrome because nerve damage in MS is central, but nerve damage in Sjögren syndrome is peripheral. However, this is not always the case. Occasionally, Sjögren syndrome affects the central nervous system, causing cognitive impairment and spinal cord involvement. "Some researchers believe that Sjögren syndrome is somehow linked to MS," Burks says. "But this opinion remains highly controversial."

Myasthenia gravis (MG) is a disease in which weakness occurs when the nerve impulse responsible for initiating movement fails to reach the muscle cells. Individuals with MG have an increased risk of developing other autoimmune diseases.

MG symptoms tend to fluctuate throughout the day, often worsening at night. Droopy eyelids, facial weakness, impaired eye coordination, weakness of the limbs, neck, shoulders, hips, and trunk muscles are all typical. Muscle fatigue is common, and heat, overexertion, or increased stress can aggravate this symptom. MG can occur at any age, although young women and older men are the most commonly affected. Those with MG experience no loss or change in sensation, and they don't normally experience generalized fatigue. Instead, they experience localized fatigue in overtired muscles.

"A very specific test for MG is a blood test for serum antibodies to acetylcholine receptors," Burks explains. "Eighty percent of all patients with MG will have abnormally elevated serum levels of these antibodies."

Sarcoidosis typically appears between the ages of 20 and 40. Usually, the disease appears briefly and heals naturally. However, between 20 and 30 percent of sarcoidosis patients are left with some permanent lung damage, and in 10 to 15 percent of the patients, the disease can become chronic. Symptoms include dry mouth, excessive thirst and fatigue, skin rash, vision abnormalities, chronic arthritis, shortness of breath, enlarged lymph glands, cough, and fever. A chest x-ray is one of the most helpful diagnostic tools.

Infectious Diseases That Mimic MS

Lyme disease (LD) is an infection caused by *Borrelia burgdorferi*, a bacterium carried by deer ticks. Untreated, the bacterium travels through the bloodstream, causing severe fatigue, a stiff, aching neck, tingling or numbness in the extremities, and facial palsy. The primary symptom is usually a rash that radiates from the tick bite. Diagnosis should be made on the basis of symptoms and evidence of a tick bite, not blood tests, which can often give false results if performed in the first month after infection. Those who live or work in residential areas surrounded by tick-infested woods, or enjoy hiking, camping, fishing, and hunting, or live in endemic areas, are at increased risk for this disease.

Human T-cell lymphotrophic virus-1 (HTLV-1) is associated with progressive spinal cord dysfunction. Symptoms include spasticity, partial paralysis of the lower limbs, bladder and bowel incontinence, and impotence. HTLV-1 can be ruled out with a titer, which is a type of elevated antibody test. "HTLV-1 affects the spinal cord and does appear similar to primary progressive MS," Burks explains. "But HTLV-1 primarily occurs in the Caribbean, so it is important to ask about travel to endemic areas. Besides the Caribbean, these areas include Southern Japan and less commonly, the Pacific Coast of South America, Equatorial Africa and the Southern United States. HTLV-1 is also common among intravenous drug users."

Neurosyphilis, the advanced form of syphilis, can cause visual problems, cognitive changes, and sensory or motor tract dysfunction. As with HTLV-1, testing the production of antibodies can eliminate syphilis and neurosyphilis from the list of possible diagnoses. "Neurosyphilis is not as common as it once was," Dr. Burks explains. "This is because syphilis, the forerunner of neurosyphilis, is so readily treatable today."

Vascular Diseases That Mimic MS

Stroke symptoms include sudden trouble with vision in one or both eyes, sudden trouble walking, dizziness, loss of coordination, sudden severe headache, confusion, trouble speaking or understanding, sudden nausea, fever, vomiting, or loss of consciousness.

"Strokes can be caused by bleeding in the brain or by blood clots that cut off the blood supply to an area of the brain," Burks explains. "The result is that neurons in the brain die. Major strokes cause very obvious losses in function and are unlikely to be confused with MS. However, smaller strokes can produce changes or loss in function that can look similar to a MS attack. Many people with MS have first been misdiagnosed with stroke."

Central nervous system (CNS) angitis, an inflammation of the blood vessels of the brain, can produce headache, confusion, and other neurologic deficits that slowly progress.

Dural arteriovenous fistulas are abnormal structures of blood vessels along the spinal cord that deprive the spinal cord of blood, resulting in weakness, bladder and bowel changes, and sensory symptoms, all of which appear in a relapsing or progressive manner. MRI of the spinal cord or spinal angiography may be required to confirm diagnosis.

Binswanger is a cerebrovascular disease usually seen in older patients with high blood pressure. Demyelination of the white matter surrounding the brain, similar to white matter lesions seen in MS, can appear with this disease.

Other Mimics

Other diseases are occasionally confused with MS. These include fibromyalgia and vitamin B_{12} deficiency, muscular dystrophy (MD), amyotrophic lateral sclerosis (ALS or Lou Gehrig's disease), migraine, hypothyroidism, hypertension, Behçet disease, Arnold-Chiari deformity, and mitochondrial disorders, although your neurologist can usually rule them out quite easily.

Fibromyalgia involves pain and fatigue of the muscles, ligaments, and tendons. Muscular pain can be shooting or throbbing. Burning, stiffness, fatigue, face and head pain, cognitive impairment, numbness, tingling, dizziness, and impaired coordination are common. Changes in weather, hormonal fluctuations, stress, or depression can all contribute to symptom flare-ups. "Although fibromyalgia does mimic MS, it will not show up on an MRI or even be observable at an exam," Burks says. "Fibromyalgia is very nonspecific."

Vitamin B_{12} deficiency may cause demyelination, numbness and tingling of the hands and feet, fatigue, weakness, and in extreme cases, change in mental status. "There is a theory that vitamin B_{12} can actually produce more myelin, so people with MS may assume that they need more of it," Burks says. "But B_{12} is only beneficial if you have a deficit to begin with."

A Final Word

"While MS may have many mimics, a neurologist can usually make a correct diagnosis early in the disease by taking a careful history, doing a complete neurological exam, looking at the MRI, and sometimes, evaluating the spinal fluid," Dr. Burks states. "If you are concerned about your diagnosis, you can discuss your concerns with your neurologist and possibly get referred for a second opinion from a MS expert at a comprehensive MS center. The Multiple Sclerosis Foundation can help you locate a MS center in your area."

Additional Information

Multiple Sclerosis Foundation
6350 N. Andrews Ave.
Ft. Lauderdale, FL 33309-2130
Toll-Free: 888-MSFOCUS (673-6287)
Phone: 954-776-6805
Fax: 954-351-0630
Website: http://www.msfocus.org
E-mail: support@msfocus.org

Chapter 13

Other Demyelinating Disorders

Chronic Inflammatory Demyelinating Polyneuropathy (CIDP)

Chronic inflammatory demyelinating polyneuropathy (CIDP) is a neurological disorder characterized by progressive weakness and impaired sensory function in the legs and arms. The disorder, which is sometimes called chronic relapsing polyneuropathy, is caused by damage to the myelin sheath (the fatty covering that wraps around and protects nerve fibers) of the peripheral nerves. Although it can occur at any age, and in both genders, CIDP is more common in young adults and in men more so than women. It often presents with symptoms that include tingling or numbness (beginning in the toes and fingers), weakness of the arms and legs, loss of deep tendon reflexes (areflexia), fatigue, and abnormal sensations. CIDP is closely related to Guillain-Barré syndrome and it is considered the chronic counterpart of that acute disease.

Is there any treatment?

Treatment for CIDP includes corticosteroids such as prednisone, which may be prescribed alone or in combination with immunosuppressant

This chapter includes excerpts from the following National Institute of Neurological Disorders and Stroke (NINDS) documents: "Guillain-Barré Syndrome Fact Sheet," February 2007; "Chronic Inflammatory Demyelinating Polyneuropathy (CIDP) Information Page," February 2007; "Leukodystrophy," February 2007; and "Schilder's Disease Information Page," February 2007.

drugs. Plasmapheresis (plasma exchange) and intravenous immuno-globulin (IVIg) therapy are effective. IVIg may be used even as a first-line therapy. Physiotherapy may improve muscle strength, function, and mobility, and minimize the shrinkage of muscles and tendons and distortions of the joints.

What is the prognosis?

The course of CIDP varies widely among individuals. Some may have a bout of CIDP followed by spontaneous recovery, while others may have many bouts with partial recovery in between relapses. The disease is a treatable cause of acquired neuropathy and initiation of early treatment to prevent loss of nerve axons is recommended. However, some individuals are left with some residual numbness or weakness.

Guillain-Barré Syndrome

Guillain-Barré (ghee-yan bah-ray) syndrome is a disorder in which the body's immune system attacks part of the peripheral nervous system. The first symptoms of this disorder include varying degrees of weakness or tingling sensations in the legs. In many instances the weakness and abnormal sensations spread to the arms and upper body. These symptoms can increase in intensity until certain muscles cannot be used at all and, when severe, the patient is almost totally paralyzed. In these cases the disorder is life threatening—potentially interfering with breathing and, at times, with blood pressure or heart rate—and is considered a medical emergency. Such a patient is often put on a respirator to assist with breathing and is watched closely for problems such as an abnormal heart beat, infections, blood clots, and high or low blood pressure. Most patients recover from even the most severe cases of Guillain-Barré syndrome, although some continue to have a certain degree of weakness.

Guillain-Barré syndrome can affect anybody. It can strike at any age and both sexes are equally prone to the disorder. The syndrome is rare afflicting only about one person in 100,000. Usually Guillain-Barré occurs a few days or weeks after the patient has had symptoms of a respiratory or gastrointestinal viral infection. Occasionally surgery or vaccinations will trigger the syndrome.

After the first clinical manifestations of the disease, the symptoms can progress over the course of hours, days, or weeks. Most people reach the stage of greatest weakness within the first two weeks after symptoms appear, and by the third week of the illness 90 percent of all patients are at their weakest.

What causes Guillain-Barré syndrome?

No one yet knows why Guillain-Barré—which is not contagious—strikes some people and not others. Nor does anyone know exactly what sets the disease in motion. What scientists do know is that the body's immune system begins to attack the body itself, causing what is known as an autoimmune disease. Usually the cells of the immune system attack only foreign material and invading organisms. In Guillain-Barré syndrome, the immune system starts to destroy the myelin sheath that surrounds the axons of many peripheral nerves, or even the axons themselves (axons are long, thin extensions of the nerve cells; they carry nerve signals). The myelin sheath surrounding the axon speeds up the transmission of nerve signals and allows the transmission of signals over long distances.

In diseases in which the peripheral nerves' myelin sheaths are injured or degraded, the nerves cannot transmit signals efficiently. That is why the muscles begin to lose their ability to respond to the brain's commands, commands that must be carried through the nerve network. The brain also receives fewer sensory signals from the rest of the body, resulting in an inability to feel textures, heat, pain, and other sensations. Alternately, the brain may receive inappropriate signals that result in tingling, "crawling-skin," or painful sensations. Because the signals to and from the arms and legs must travel the longest distances they are most vulnerable to interruption. Therefore, muscle weakness and tingling sensations usually first appear in the hands and feet and progress upwards.

When Guillain-Barré is preceded by a viral or bacterial infection, it is possible that the virus has changed the nature of cells in the nervous system so that the immune system treats them as foreign cells. It is also possible that the virus makes the immune system itself less discriminating about what cells it recognizes as its own, allowing some of the immune cells, such as certain kinds of lymphocytes and macrophages, to attack the myelin. Sensitized T lymphocytes cooperate with B lymphocytes to produce antibodies against components of the myelin sheath and may contribute to destruction of the myelin. Scientists are investigating these and other possibilities to find why the immune system goes awry in Guillain-Barré syndrome and other autoimmune diseases. The cause and course of Guillain-Barré syndrome is an active area of neurological investigation, incorporating the cooperative efforts of neurological scientists, immunologists, and virologists.

How is Guillain-Barré syndrome diagnosed?

Guillain-Barré is called a syndrome rather than a disease because it is not clear that a specific disease-causing agent is involved. A syndrome is a medical condition characterized by a collection of symptoms (what the patient feels) and signs (what a doctor can observe or measure). The signs and symptoms of the syndrome can be quite varied, so doctors may, on rare occasions, find it difficult to diagnose Guillain-Barré in its earliest stages.

Several disorders have symptoms similar to those found in Guillain-Barré, so doctors examine and question patients carefully before making a diagnosis. Collectively, the signs and symptoms form a certain pattern that helps doctors differentiate Guillain-Barré from other disorders. For example, physicians will note whether the symptoms appear on both sides of the body (most common in Guillain-Barré) and the quickness with which the symptoms appear (in other disorders, muscle weakness may progress over months rather than days or weeks). In Guillain-Barré, reflexes such as knee jerks are usually lost. Because the signals traveling along the nerve are slower, a nerve conduction velocity (NCV) test can give the doctor information to aid the diagnosis. In Guillain-Barré patients, the cerebrospinal fluid that bathes the spinal cord and brain contains more protein than usual. Therefore, a physician may decide to perform a spinal tap, a procedure in which the doctor inserts a needle into the patient's lower back to draw cerebrospinal fluid from the spinal column.

How is Guillain-Barré treated?

There is no known cure for Guillain-Barré syndrome. However, there are therapies that lessen the severity of the illness and accelerate the recovery in most patients. There are also a number of ways to treat the complications of the disease.

Currently, plasma exchange (sometimes called plasmapheresis) and high-dose immunoglobulin therapy are used. Both of them are equally effective, but immunoglobulin is easier to administer. Plasma exchange is a method by which whole blood is removed from the body and processed so that the red and white blood cells are separated from the plasma, or liquid portion of the blood. The blood cells are then returned to the patient without the plasma, which the body quickly replaces. Scientists still don't know exactly why plasma exchange works, but the technique seems to reduce the severity and duration of the Guillain-Barré episode. This may be because the plasma portion of the blood contains elements of the immune system that may be toxic to the myelin.

In high-dose immunoglobulin therapy, doctors give intravenous injections of the proteins that, in small quantities, the immune system uses naturally to attack invading organisms. Investigators have found that giving high doses of these immunoglobulins, derived from a pool of thousands of normal donors, to Guillain-Barré patients can lessen the immune attack on the nervous system. Investigators do not know why or how this works, although several hypotheses have been proposed.

The use of steroid hormones has also been tried as a way to reduce the severity of Guillain-Barré, but controlled clinical trials have demonstrated that this treatment not only is not effective but may even have a deleterious effect on the disease.

The most critical part of the treatment for this syndrome consists of keeping the patient's body functioning during recovery of the nervous system. This can sometimes require placing the patient on a respirator, a heart monitor, or other machines that assist body function. The need for this sophisticated machinery is one reason why Guillain-Barré syndrome patients are usually treated in hospitals, often in an intensive care ward. In the hospital, doctors can also look for and treat the many problems that can afflict any paralyzed patient—complications such as pneumonia or bed sores.

Often, even before recovery begins, caregivers may be instructed to manually move the patient's limbs to help keep the muscles flexible and strong. Later, as the patient begins to recover limb control, physical therapy begins. Carefully planned clinical trials of new and experimental therapies are the key to improving the treatment of patients with Guillain-Barré syndrome. Such clinical trials begin with the research of basic and clinical scientists who, working with clinicians, identify new approaches to treating patients with the disease.

What is the long-term outlook for those with Guillain-Barré syndrome?

Guillain-Barré syndrome can be a devastating disorder because of its sudden and unexpected onset. In addition, recovery is not necessarily quick. As noted, patients usually reach the point of greatest weakness or paralysis days or weeks after the first symptoms occur. Symptoms then stabilize at this level for a period of days, weeks, or, sometimes, months. The recovery period may be as little as a few weeks or as long as a few years. About 30 percent of those with Guillain-Barré still have a residual weakness after three years. About three percent may suffer a relapse of muscle weakness and tingling sensations many years after the initial attack.

Guillain-Barré syndrome patients face not only physical difficulties, but emotionally painful periods as well. It is often extremely difficult for patients to adjust to sudden paralysis and dependence on others for help with routine daily activities. Patients sometimes need psychological counseling to help them adapt.

Leukodystrophy

Leukodystrophy refers to progressive degeneration of the white matter of the brain due to imperfect growth or development of the myelin sheath, the fatty covering that acts as an insulator around nerve fiber. Myelin, which lends its color to the white matter of the brain, is a complex substance made up of at least ten different chemicals. The leukodystrophies are a group of disorders that are caused by genetic defects in how myelin produces or metabolizes these chemicals. Each of the leukodystrophies is the result of a defect in the gene that controls one (and only one) of the chemicals. Specific leukodystrophies include metachromatic leukodystrophy, Krabbe disease, adrenoleukodystrophy, Pelizaeus-Merzbacher disease, Canavan disease, childhood ataxia with central nervous system hypomyelination or CACH (also known as vanishing white matter disease), Alexander disease, Refsum disease, and cerebrotendinous xanthomatosis. The most common symptom of a leukodystrophy disease is a gradual decline in an infant or child who previously appeared well. Progressive loss may appear in body tone, movements, gait, speech, ability to eat, vision, hearing, and behavior. There is often a slowdown in mental and physical development. Symptoms vary according to the specific type of leukodystrophy, and may be difficult to recognize in the early stages of the disease.

Is there any treatment?

Treatment for most of the leukodystrophies is symptomatic and supportive and may include medications; physical, occupational, and speech therapies; and nutritional, educational, and recreational programs. Bone marrow transplantation is showing promise for a few of the leukodystrophies.

What is the prognosis?

The prognosis for the leukodystrophies varies according to the specific type of leukodystrophy.

Schilder Disease

Note: Schilder disease is not the same as Addison-Schilder disease (adrenoleukodystrophy).

Schilder disease is a rare progressive demyelinating disorder which usually begins in childhood. Symptoms may include dementia, aphasia, seizures, personality changes, poor attention, tremors, balance instability, incontinence, muscle weakness, headache, vomiting, and vision and speech impairment. The disorder is a variant of multiple sclerosis.

Is there any treatment?

Treatment for the disorder follows the established standards in multiple sclerosis and includes corticosteroids, beta-interferon or immunosuppressive therapy, and symptomatic treatment.

What is the prognosis?

As with multiple sclerosis, the course and prognosis of Schilder disease are unpredictable. For some individuals the disorder is progressive with a steady, unremitting course. Others may experience significant improvement and even remission. In some cases, Schilder disease is fatal.

Additional Information

American Autoimmune Related Diseases Association
22100 Gratiot Ave., Eastpointe
East Detroit, MI 48021-2227
Toll-Free: 800-598-4668
Phone: 586-776-3900
Fax: 586-776-3903
Website: http://www.aarda.org
E-mail: aarda@aarda.org

GBS/CIDP Foundation International
The Holly Building
104 ½ Forrest Ave.
Narberth, PA 19072
Phone: 610-667-0131
Fax: 610-667-7036
Website: http://www.gbsfi.com
E-mail: info@gbsfi.com

Hunter's Hope Foundation [A Leukodystrophy Resource]
P.O. Box 643
Orchard Park, NY 14127
Toll-Free: 877-984-HOPE (4673)
Phone: 716-667-1200
Fax: 716-667-1212
Website: http://www.huntershope.org
E-mail: info@huntershope.org

National Organization for Rare Disorders (NORD)
P.O. Box 1968
Danbury, CT 06813-1968
Toll-Free: 800-999-NORD (6673)
Phone: 203-744-0100
Fax: 203-798-2291
Website: http://www.rarediseases.org
E-mail: orphan@rarediseases.org

National Tay-Sachs and Allied Diseases Association
2001 Beacon Street, Suite 204
Brighton, MA 02135
Toll-Free: 800-90-NTSAD (68723)
Phone: 617-277-4463
Fax: 617-277-0134
Website: http://www.ntsad.org
E-mail: info@ntsad.org

Neuropathy Association
60 East 42nd St., Suite 942
New York, NY 10165-0999
Phone: 212-692-0662
Fax: 212-692-0668
Website: http://www.neuropathy.org
E-mail: info@neuropathy.org

United Leukodystrophy Foundation
2304 Highland Drive
Sycamore, IL 60178
Toll-Free: 800-728-5483
Phone: 815-895-3211
Fax: 815-895-2432
Website: http://www.ulf.org
E-mail: office@ulf.org

Part Two

Symptoms of
Multiple Sclerosis

Chapter 14

Overview of MS Symptoms

Symptoms of multiple sclerosis (MS) may be mild or severe, of long duration or short, and may appear in various combinations, depending on the area of the nervous system affected. Complete or partial remission of symptoms, especially in the early stages of the disease, occurs in approximately 70 percent of MS patients.

The initial symptom of MS is often blurred or double vision, red-green color distortion, or even blindness in one eye. Inexplicably, visual problems tend to clear up in the later stages of MS. Inflammatory problems of the optic nerve may be diagnosed as retrobulbar or optic neuritis. Fifty-five percent of MS patients will have an attack of optic neuritis at some time or other, and it will be the first symptom of MS in approximately 15 percent. This has led to general recognition of optic neuritis as an early sign of MS, especially if tests also reveal abnormalities in the patient's spinal fluid.

Most MS patients experience muscle weakness in their extremities and difficulty with coordination and balance at some time during the course of the disease. These symptoms may be severe enough to impair walking or even standing. In the worst cases, MS can produce partial or complete paralysis. Spasticity—the involuntary increased tone of muscles leading to stiffness and spasms—is common, as is fatigue. Fatigue may be triggered by physical exertion and improve with rest, or it may take the form of a constant and persistent tiredness.

Excerpted from "Multiple Sclerosis: Hope Through Research," National Institute of Neurological Disorders and Stroke (NINDS), NIH Publication No. 96-75, updated April 16, 2007.

Most people with MS also exhibit paresthesias, transitory abnormal sensory feelings such as numbness, prickling, or "pins and needles" sensations; and uncommonly, some may also experience pain. Loss of sensation sometimes occurs. Speech impediments, tremors, and dizziness are other frequent complaints. Occasionally, people with MS have hearing loss.

Approximately half of all people with MS experience cognitive impairments such as difficulties with concentration, attention, memory, and poor judgment, but such symptoms are usually mild and are frequently overlooked. In fact, they are often detectable only through comprehensive testing. Patients themselves may be unaware of their cognitive loss; it is often a family member or friend who first notices a deficit. Such impairments are usually mild, rarely disabling, and intellectual and language abilities are generally spared.

Cognitive symptoms occur when lesions develop in brain areas responsible for information processing. These deficits tend to become more apparent as the information to be processed becomes more complex. Fatigue may also add to processing difficulties. Scientists do not yet know whether altered cognition in MS reflects problems with information acquisition, retrieval, or a combination of both. Types of memory problems may differ depending on the individual's disease course (relapsing-remitting, primary-progressive, etc.), but there does not appear to be any direct correlation between duration of illness and severity of cognitive dysfunction.

Depression, which is unrelated to cognitive problems, is another common feature of MS. In addition, about ten percent of patients suffer from more severe psychotic disorders such as manic-depression and paranoia. Five percent may experience episodes of inappropriate euphoria and despair—unrelated to the patient's actual emotional state—known as "laughing/weeping syndrome." This syndrome is thought to be due to demyelination in the brainstem, the area of the brain that controls facial expression and emotions, and is usually seen only in severe cases.

As the disease progresses, sexual dysfunction may become a problem. Bowel and bladder control may also be lost.

In about 60 percent of MS patients, heat—whether generated by temperatures outside the body or by exercise—may cause temporary worsening of many MS symptoms. In these cases, eradicating the heat eliminates the problem. Some temperature-sensitive patients find that a cold bath may temporarily relieve their symptoms. For the same reason, swimming is often a good exercise choice for people with MS.

The erratic symptoms of MS can affect the entire family as patients may become unable to work at the same time they are facing high medical bills and additional expenses for housekeeping assistance and modifications to homes and vehicles. The emotional drain on both patient and family is immeasurable. Support groups and counseling may help MS patients, their families, and friends find ways to cope with the many problems the disease can cause.

Possible symptoms of multiple sclerosis include:

- muscle weakness
- spasticity
- impairment of pain, temperature, touch senses
- pain (moderate to severe)
- ataxia
- tremor
- speech disturbances
- vision disturbances
- vertigo
- bladder dysfunction
- bowel dysfunction
- sexual dysfunction
- depression
- euphoria
- cognitive abnormalities
- fatigue

A number of other diseases may produce symptoms similar to those seen in MS. Other conditions with an intermittent course and MS-like lesions of the brain's white matter include polyarteritis, lupus erythematosus, syringomyelia, tropical spastic paraparesis, some cancers, and certain tumors that compress the brainstem or spinal cord. Progressive multifocal leukoencephalopathy can mimic the acute stage of an MS attack. Physicians will also need to rule out stroke, neurosyphilis, spinocerebellar ataxias, pernicious anemia, diabetes, Sjögren disease, and vitamin B_{12} deficiency. Acute transverse myelitis may signal the first attack of MS, or it may indicate other problems such as infection with the Epstein-Barr or herpes simplex B viruses. Recent reports suggest that the neurological problems associated with Lyme disease may present a clinical picture much like MS.

Investigators are continuing their search for a definitive test for MS. However, until one is developed, evidence of both multiple attacks and central nervous system lesions must be found before a diagnosis of MS is given.

Are Any MS Symptoms Treatable?

While some scientists look for therapies that will affect the overall course of the disease, others are searching for new and better medications to control the symptoms of MS without triggering intolerable side effects.

Many people with MS have problems with spasticity, a condition that primarily affects the lower limbs. Spasticity can occur either as a sustained stiffness caused by increased muscle tone or as spasms that come and go, especially at night. It is usually treated with muscle relaxants and tranquilizers. Baclofen (Lioresal), the most commonly prescribed medication for this symptom, may be taken orally or, in severe cases, injected into the spinal cord. Tizanidine (Zanaflex), used for years in Europe and now approved in the United States, appears to function similarly to baclofen. Diazepam (Valium), clonazepam (Klonopin), and dantrolene (Dantrium) can also reduce spasticity. Although its beneficial effect is temporary, physical therapy may also be useful and can help prevent the irreversible shortening of muscles known as contractures. Surgery to reduce spasticity is rarely appropriate in MS.

Weakness and Ataxia

Weakness and ataxia (incoordination) are also characteristic of MS. When weakness is a problem, some spasticity can actually be beneficial by lending support to weak limbs. In such cases, medication levels that alleviate spasticity completely may be inappropriate. Physical therapy and exercise can also help preserve remaining function, and patients may find that various aids—such as foot braces, canes, and walkers—can help them remain independent and mobile. Occasionally, physicians can provide temporary relief from weakness, spasms, and pain by injecting a drug called phenol into the spinal cord, muscles, or nerves in the arms or legs. Further research is needed to find or develop effective treatments for MS-related weakness and ataxia.

Vision Problems

Although improvement of optic symptoms usually occurs even without treatment, a short course of treatment with intravenous methylprednisolone (Solu-Medrol) followed by treatment with oral steroids is sometimes used. A trial of oral prednisone in patients with visual problems suggests that this steroid is not only ineffective in speeding recovery but may also increase patients' risk for future MS attacks. Curiously, prednisone injected directly into the veins—at ten times the oral dose—did seem to produce short-term recovery. Because of the link between optic neuritis and MS, the study's investigators believe these findings may hold true for the treatment of MS as well. A follow-up study of optic neuritis patients will address this and other questions.

Fatigue

Fatigue, especially in the legs, is a common symptom of MS and may be both physical and psychological. Avoiding excessive activity and heat are probably the most important measures patients can take to counter physiological fatigue. If psychological aspects of fatigue such as depression or apathy are evident, antidepressant medications may help. Other drugs that may reduce fatigue in some, but not all, patients include amantadine (Symmetrel), pemoline (Cylert), and the still-experimental drug aminopyridine.

Pain

People with MS may experience several types of pain. Muscle and back pain can be helped by aspirin or acetaminophen and physical therapy to correct faulty posture and strengthen and stretch muscles. The sharp, stabbing facial pain known as trigeminal neuralgia is commonly treated with carbamazepine or other anticonvulsant drugs or, occasionally, surgery. Intense tingling and burning sensations are harder to treat. Some people get relief with antidepressant drugs; others may respond to electrical stimulation of the nerves in the affected area. In some cases, the physician may recommend codeine.

Urinary and Sexual Malfunction

As the disease progresses, some patients develop bladder malfunctions. Urinary problems are often the result of infections that can be treated with antibiotics. The physician may recommend that patients take vitamin C supplements or drink cranberry juice, as these measures acidify urine and may reduce the risk of further infections. Several medications are also available. The most common bladder problems encountered by MS patients are urinary frequency, urgency, or incontinence. A small number of patients, however, retain large amounts of urine. In these patients, catheterization may be necessary. In this procedure, a catheter or drainage tube is temporarily inserted (by the patient or a caretaker) into the urethra several times a day to drain urine from the bladder. Surgery may be indicated in severe, intractable cases. Scientists have developed a "bladder pacemaker" that has helped people with urinary incontinence in preliminary trials. The pacemaker, which is surgically implanted, is controlled by a hand-held unit that allows the patient to electrically stimulate the nerves that control bladder function.

MS patients with urinary problems may be reluctant to drink enough fluids, leading to constipation. Drinking more water and adding fiber to the diet usually alleviates this condition. Sexual dysfunction

Table 14.1. Drugs Used to Treat Symptoms of Multiple Sclerosis

Symptom	Drug
Spasticity	Baclofen (Lioresal) Tizanidine (Zanaflex) Diazepam (Valium) Clonazepam (Klonopin) Dantrolene (Dantrium)
Optic neuritis	Methylprednisolone (Solu-Medrol) Oral steroids
Fatigue	Antidepressants Amantadine (Symmetrel) Pemoline (Cylert)
Pain	Aspirin or acetaminophen Antidepressants Codeine
Trigeminal neuralgia	Carbamazepine, other anticonvulsant
Sexual dysfunction	Papaverine injections (in men)

may also occur, especially in patients with urinary problems. Men may experience occasional failure to attain an erection. Penile implants, injection of the drug papaverine, and electrostimulation are techniques used to resolve the problem. Women may experience insufficient lubrication or have difficulty reaching orgasm; in these cases, vaginal gels and vibrating devices may be helpful. Counseling is also beneficial, especially in the absence of urinary problems, since psychological factors can also cause these symptoms. For instance, depression can intensify symptoms of fatigue, pain, and sexual dysfunction. In addition to counseling, the physician may prescribe antidepressant or antianxiety medications. Amitriptyline is used to treat laughing/weeping syndrome.

Tremors

Tremors are often resistant to therapy, but can sometimes be treated with drugs or, in extreme cases, surgery. Investigators are currently examining a number of experimental treatments for tremor.

Chapter 15

Movement Disorders

Chapter Contents

Section 15.1

Uncoordinated Movement

© 2007 A.D.A.M., Inc. Reprinted with permission.

Definition

Uncoordinated movement is an abnormality of muscle control or an inability to finely coordinate movements, resulting in a jerky, unsteady, to-and-fro motion of the trunk or the limbs.

Considerations

Smooth graceful movement results from a fine balance between opposing muscle groups. This balance is coordinated by a portion of the brain called the cerebellum.

Diseases that damage the cerebellum, spinal cord, and peripheral nerves (connecting the cerebellum to the muscle groups) can interfere with the fine tuning of muscular movement and result in coarse, jerky, uncoordinated movement. This condition is called ataxia, and is easily seen in the jerky, to-and-fro motion of the trunk and unsteady gait (walking style).

Ataxia may appear as a congenital defect, or follow a simple viral infection such as chickenpox. It may also appear following encephalitis, head trauma, and diseases affecting the central nervous system or spinal cord. Appearance as a genetic disorder, or as a toxic reaction to drugs, medications, alcohol or environmental toxins is also possible.

Common Causes

- transient ischemic attack (TIA)
- stroke
- multiple sclerosis
- vertebral abnormalities (such as compression fractures of the back)

172

- poisoning by heavy metals such as mercury, thallium, and lead, or solvents such as toluene or carbon tetrachloride

- alcohol or other drug intoxication

- drugs such as aminoglutethimide, anticholinergics, phenytoin (in high doses), carbamazepine, phenobarbital and tricyclic anti-depressants

- paraneoplastic syndromes (ataxia may appear months or years before cancer is diagnosed—an affected person produces anti-bodies against the neurons in the cerebellum)

- post-infectious condition (typically following chickenpox)

- hereditary condition (congenital cerebellar ataxia, Friedreich ataxia, ataxia telangiectasia, Wilson disease)

Home Care

Take safety measures around the home to compensate for difficulties in mobility that are inherent with this problem. For example, avoid clutter, leave wide walkways, and avoid throw rugs or other objects that might cause slipping or falling.

Other family members should encourage the affected person to participate in normal activities. Family members need to have extreme patience with people who suffer from poor coordination. Take time to demonstrate ways of performing tasks more simply, and take advantage of the afflicted person's strengths while avoiding weaknesses.

Call Your Health Care Provider If

- There is unexplained incoordination.

- Incoordination lasts longer than a few minutes.

What to Expect at Your Health Care Provider's Office

The medical history will be obtained, and a physical examination performed. In emergency situations, the patient will be stabilized first.

Medical history questions documenting uncoordinated movement in detail may include:

- When did it begin?

- Is it continuous or do episodes come and go?

- Is it getting worse?
- What medications are being taken?
- Is alcohol used?
- Are illegal/illicit drugs being used?
- Has there been any exposure to something that may have caused poisoning?
- What other symptoms are also present?
  - weakness or paralysis
  - numbness, tingling, or loss of sensation
  - confusion or disorientation
  - seizures

The physical examination may include detailed neurological and muscular examination.

Diagnostic tests that may be performed include:

- blood tests (such as a complete blood count [CBC] or blood differential);
- computed tomography (CT) scan of the head;
- magnetic resonance image (MRI) of the head;
- Romberg test—the patient is asked to stand erect with the feet together and the eyes closed. If the patient loses balance, this indicates a loss of the sense of position and the test is considered positive.

Referral to a specialist for counseling may be indicated.

References

Goetz, CG. *Textbook of Clinical Neurology. 2nd ed.* St. Louis, MO: WB Saunders; 2003: 713–736.

Goldman L, Ausiello D. Cecil *Textbook of Medicine, 22nd ed.* Philadelphia, PA: WB Saunders; 2004:2305–2306.

Section 15.2

Gait (Walking) Problems

Gait or Walking Problems: The Basic Facts

Many people with multiple sclerosis (MS) will experience difficulty with walking, which is more formally termed gait. Studies suggest that half the people with relapsing-remitting MS will need some assistance with walking within 15 years of their diagnosis. Gait problems in MS are caused by a variety of factors. MS frequently causes fatigue. MS damage to nerve pathways may hamper coordination and/or cause weakness, poor balance, numbness, or spasticity (abnormal increase in muscle tone). Concern about falling and the emotional impact of appearing impaired in public causes problems too.

"Gait problems in MS are all over the map," observes Sue Kushner, a physical therapist at Slippery Rock University in Pennsylvania, with long experience in multiple sclerosis. "This makes gait a difficult problem to address." Difficult, but not impossible.

Speak Up

If you are having difficulty walking or keeping your balance, if fatigue turns your legs to cement, don't despair, speak up. Many gait problems can be significantly improved with physical therapy, exercise, medication, or the right assistive device. You are not "giving in" when you seek treatment. Untreated gait problems can lead to emotional distress, injuries, added fatigue, and suspicion by other people that your gait problems stem from alcohol or drugs. Consulting your primary health-care provider and getting an accurate assessment of your ambulatory patterns are sensible things to do.

Diagnosis

You can expect to be referred to a physical therapist (PT). In order to analyze the biomechanics of your gait, a PT may ask you to walk across a room or down a hallway in order to observe coordination, positioning of feet, posture, and momentum. You may be asked to provide your medical history. You may be asked to perform tests that measure muscle strength, fatigue levels, range of motion, and spasticity. Some physical therapists use video cameras to record their observations. (Research labs specializing in gait analysis have a wide range of high-tech machines to calibrate body movement.)

Evaluation may be embarrassing, but it is not painful. Once the factors involved in your particular gait problems are identified, you, your physical therapist, and your physician will work together on a plan of action.

Your insurance may have tight limits on reimbursement for PT. Review your coverage to avoid nasty surprises. Your physician and the National MS Society may be able to help you battle for the coverage required by your problems. Or you may need to pay physical therapy costs yourself. It is wise to be frank and upfront with your PT about cost, payment plans, and the benefits you can expect from therapy.

Weakness

Muscle weakness clearly interferes with walking. Damage to neurons (nerve cells) can affect a particular muscle group or groups so they no longer respond to the nervous system input that normally guides the act of walking. Sue Kushner points out that, "Muscle weakness in MS isn't the same as the couch-potato syndrome that can be addressed by strength training." In fact, the wrong kind of exercise will do nothing to improve walking and can lead to fatigue and increased weakness.

Dr. Randall Schapiro of Fairview MS Center in Minneapolis is a strong advocate for exercise to keep people with MS fit, and he too warns, "What is good exercise for one person with MS may not be good for another." Working with an experienced PT, people can learn both appropriate exercises and ways to compensate for lost strength.

Muscle weakness that interferes with walking is not the same thing as MS fatigue. But MS fatigue can make walking problems worse. Since fatigue is so common in MS, an assessment will include exploration of these problems too—and you may be advised to use a mobility aid to manage fatigue and muscle weakness.

But, you say, you want to improve your walking, not give up on it. Using an aid is not an all or nothing choice. Many people continue to walk, and to work on improving their walking while using an aid. They find that assistive devices allow them to get where they want to go without exhausting all their energy reserves. Marie E., of Rhode Island, who lives with progressive MS, got a fold-up wheelchair for outings that involve long distances. Using it lets her focus on shopping or seeing the sights instead of concentrating all her energy on not tripping.

Balance

Impaired balance not only makes walking difficult, it can result in falls and injuries. A loss of balance and coordination can produce a swaying, uneven gait—called ataxia—that is often mistaken for drunkenness.

"Poor balance is not always an isolated symptom," observes Brian Hutchinson, a physical therapist at the Heuga Center for people with MS. "One leg may be weaker than the other or have spasticity, resulting in an uneven gait. Or, the source might be MS lesions in the parts of the central nervous system that control balance. It's important to identify what's causing the problem in order to find the best solution."

Therapeutic strategies that may help balance deficits include inner ear (or vestibular) exercises. Aerobic activity, stretching, and strengthening specific muscles can address some of the secondary reasons for balance difficulties, he said.

The right assistive device is often the most effective strategy. A brace called an ankle-foot orthotic, or AFO is often prescribed. An AFO is lightweight and designed to be hidden by socks or pant legs. A cane or walker is another solution to poor balance. An aid is far safer than "wall-walking" (holding onto a wall or nearby objects for support) and, Hutchinson notes, people who use them tend to move around more. Installing grab bars around the home can also make transfers easier and daily activities safer.

Numbness

Loss of feeling or tingling in the legs or feet means the brain is not receiving the full sensory input from the foot. As Marie E. describes it, "It's like I'm wearing thick heavy boots so I can't feel where I'm stepping." Foot numbness can also result in "foot drag," where the foot does not move forward in a smooth motion because the brain is not receiving input about where the foot is in space.

Solutions may involve using a cane, walker, or Canadian crutch (which has an arm cuff and grab handle). The aid relays missing information to the brain by carrying sensations from the ground through the device into the hand and arm. Visual cues may also work. People learn to watch where their feet are falling to compensate for the lack of sensation. Marie likes the convenience of collapsible canes, which can be easily stowed in a bag or under a chair.

Spasticity

Spasticity is abnormal muscle tone or tightness of muscles. As a person moves, the nervous system sends streams of signals to muscle groups to expand or contract in sequence. MS damage can interfere with these coordinated events, leaving certain muscles in a constricted or spastic state. Spasticity can cause uneven gait and more. In spastic limbs, muscles may atrophy from lack of use and joints may develop contractures—freezing in one painful position—if they remain rigid over time.

The right mix of medications, stretching, and exercise can control spasticity, improve gait, and prevent these serious complications. Baclofen and tizanidine are the most often used medications. A PT can recommend exercises to safely stretch spastic muscles. Good management calls for a team approach, with the individual, the physician or nurse, and the PT all contributing.

Sometimes spasticity actually helps gait problems. The increased stiffness allows some people who have weak legs to walk or stand more easily. However, Dr. Mindy Aisen, director of Rehabilitation Research and Development at Veteran's Administration Headquarters in Washington, DC, warns against relying on spasticity too much. "Excessive stress on joints or muscles can lead to unnecessary permanent damage," she said.

Fear of Falling

It is embarrassing as well as frightening to fall down in public. People have been known to stop going out at all to avoid the possibility of a fall. But staying put at home is not much of a solution. In fact, it may have unintended consequences.

Kathy Dieruf, assistant professor in the Physical Therapy Program at the University of New Mexico in Albuquerque, explained, "The painful consequences of a prior fall or current fear of falling may lead to a devastating downward spiral of decreased activity, decreased strength and endurance, diminished range of motion, and increased impairment that may actually add to the risk of falling."

It's Important to Be in the World

Janet L., of Philadelphia, pulled up to a neighborhood delicatessen and decided to leave her cane in the car. "It didn't seem that far to walk," she thought. As she threaded her way past some outdoor tables, she suddenly lost her balance—and fell across a stranger's lap. "I was so mortified I wanted to cry," she recalled. But she had the presence of mind to keep her sense of humor. "Come here often?" she asked. They both started laughing. She pulled herself up and explained that she sometimes looses her balance due to multiple sclerosis.

Janet works as a peer counselor at the Greater Delaware Valley Chapter. She knows that it's not always easy to keep a sense of humor in this kind of situation, but for her it's the best strategy. As she puts it, "MS is not something you have control over—but you do have control over how you choose to handle the problems." A former dancer, Janet is keenly aware of the ways in which her loss of balance and muscle weakness has changed her gait. Her advice: "Keep moving. It's important to be in the world."

Assistive Technology

We human beings are distinguished by our ability to develop technologies that make tasks easier. In a sense, all technology from safety pins to supersonic jets is assistive technology, helping us to accomplish feats we couldn't do otherwise. When physical disability develops, canes, braces, walkers, wheelchairs, and scooters assist. They help people move about easily.

The idea is not appealing initially. To many people, a cane represents feebleness; a wheelchair or scooter says that MS has taken over. The majority of people with MS who use the right assistive technology end up with a very different perspective. They recognize that a brace or cane allows them to walk with confidence; a wheelchair or scooter provides safety, speed, and saves energy for more important things.

But for some people, over-reliance on an aid can have an adverse effect on strength and stamina. As Dr. Aisen points out, "Being overly fatigued does nobody any good, but sometimes practicing walking makes walking better." A rehab professional with MS experience can help people improve their gait and manage fatigue, weakness, and balance problems. In other words, professionals look for individual solutions to individual gait problems.

The assistive technology industry offers options aplenty—from rolling walkers to weighted four-pronged canes and from ultra-light

179

power-assist wheelchairs to fully-powered multi-level wheelchairs. There are excellent web sites with information about such equipment. A good starting place is ABLEDATA (www.abledata.com), a federally funded project that offers product information, resources, and links. Their advice is worth noting: "To select devices most appropriate to your needs, we suggest combining ABLEDATA information with professional advice, product evaluations, and hands-on product trials." Do-it-yourselfers run the very real risk of using devices incorrectly and causing unnecessary damage to their muscles or joints.

Brian Hutchinson notes that physical and occupational therapists are often able to help people try out different devices before making a purchase. Sue Kushner encourages her clients to choose devices that are aesthetically pleasing. There are attractive choices available. Janet, the former dancer, used the internet to locate designer cane makers, and she now has a collection in different colors and styles, including a glittery Lucite cane that she used when she was a bridesmaid in a friend's wedding.

Reimbursement

Full or partial reimbursement for assistive technology (or durable medical equipment) may be available through private or public insurance, community organizations, social service agencies, or your state's vocational rehabilitation agency. Remember to explore veterans' benefits if you have done military service. Reimbursement programs require a prescription from a physician or a rehabilitation professional, and a statement that explains the medical necessity of the purchase. The statement may take some preparation.

People with MS often fail to fit standard disability categories because gait problems (like other MS symptoms) can come and go, and vary in intensity.

- Take some time to understand what your policy or program requires for reimbursement.

- Clearly communicate these requirements to your physician or therapist, as reimbursement will depend on supporting material from your health-care providers.

- Contact your National MS Society chapter for assistance if your health-care provider is unfamiliar with the procedures.

"It is important to have a strong advocate to explain why a device is justified," said Dr. Aisen.

Future Gait Research and Technology

At present, people with MS gait problems remain mobile and independent through physical therapy, exercise, medication, and assistive technology. New ways to prevent permanent losses and to improve the technology that compensates for losses are in development.

Dr. Aisen, for one, is optimistic that research being done in other conditions, such as spinal cord injury and stroke, will eventually prove useful in MS. There is some evidence that intensive, repetitive physical therapy can improve damaged neural function, perhaps by stimulating the brain to create new neural pathways.

Researchers are testing the compensatory effects of electrical stimulus for symptoms such as foot-drop or spasticity, and studies on the biomechanics of gait are underway that may give the health-care community a better basic understanding of gait problems.

Innovations in assistive technology are also expected to continue at a brisk pace—in part to keep up with aging baby-boomers. Lighter, more flexible mobility aids with sporty styling and cheerful colors are already available. "Sick" is out and "active" is in for people who compensate for disabilities with assistive devices.

Chapter 16

Tremor

Tremor is an unintentional, somewhat rhythmic, muscle movement involving to-and-fro movements (oscillations) of one or more parts of the body. It is the most common of all involuntary movements and can affect the hands, arms, head, face, vocal cords, trunk, and legs. Most tremors occur in the hands. In some people, tremor is a symptom of another neurological disorder. The most common form of tremor, however, occurs in otherwise healthy people. Although tremor is not life-threatening, it can be embarrassing to some people, and make it harder to perform daily tasks.

Causes of Tremor

Tremor is generally caused by problems in parts of the brain that control muscles throughout the body or in particular areas, such as the hands. Neurological disorders or conditions that can produce tremor include multiple sclerosis, stroke, traumatic brain injury, and neurodegenerative diseases that damage or destroy parts of the brainstem or the cerebellum. Other causes include the use of some drugs (such as amphetamines, corticosteroids, and drugs used for certain psychiatric disorders), alcohol abuse or withdrawal, mercury poisoning, overactive thyroid, or liver failure. Some forms of tremor are inherited and run in families, while others have no known cause.

"Tremor Fact Sheet," National Institute of Neurological Disorders and Stroke (NINDS), NIH Publication No. 06-4734, updated March 19, 2007.

Characteristics of Tremor

Characteristics may include a rhythmic shaking in the hands, arms, head, legs, or trunk; shaky voice; difficulty writing or drawing; or problems holding and controlling utensils, such as a fork. Some tremors may be triggered by or become exaggerated during times of stress or strong emotion, when the individual is physically exhausted, or during certain postures or movements.

Tremor may occur at any age but is most common in middle-aged and older persons. It may be occasional, temporary, or occur intermittently. Tremor affects men and women equally.

A useful way to understand and describe tremors is to define them according to the following types.

- **Resting or static tremor** occurs when the muscle is relaxed and the limb is fully supported against gravity, such as when the hands are lying on the lap. It may be seen as a shaking of the limb, even when the person is at rest. This type of tremor is often seen in patients with Parkinson disease.

- **Action tremor** occurs during any type of movement of an affected body part. There are several subclassifications of action tremor.

  - Postural tremor occurs when the person maintains a position against gravity, such as holding the arms outstretched.

  - Kinetic (or intention) tremor occurs during purposeful voluntary movement, such as touching a finger to one's nose during a medical exam.

  - Task-specific tremor appears when performing highly skilled, goal-oriented tasks such as handwriting or speaking.

  - Isometric tremor occurs during a voluntary muscle contraction that is not accompanied by any movement.

Categories of Tremor

Tremor is most commonly classified by clinical features and cause or origin. Some of the better known forms of tremor, with their symptoms, include the following.

Essential tremor (sometimes called benign essential tremor) is the most common of the more than 20 types of tremor. Although the tremor may be mild and nonprogressive in some people, in others, the tremor is slowly progressive, starting on one side of the body but affecting both sides within three years. The hands are most often affected but the head, voice, tongue, legs, and trunk may also be involved. Head tremor may be seen as a "yes-yes" or "no-no" motion. Essential tremor may be accompanied by mild gait disturbance. Tremor frequency may decrease as the person ages, but the severity may increase, affecting the person's ability to perform certain tasks or activities of daily living. Heightened emotion, stress, fever, physical exhaustion, or low blood sugar may trigger tremors and/or increase their severity. Onset is most common after age 40, although symptoms can appear at any age. It may occur in more than one family member. Children of a parent who has essential tremor have a 50 percent chance of inheriting the condition. Essential tremor is not associated with any known pathology.

Parkinsonian tremor is caused by damage to structures within the brain that control movement. This resting tremor, which can occur as an isolated symptom or be seen in other disorders, is often a precursor to Parkinson disease (more than 25 percent of patients with Parkinson disease have an associated action tremor). The tremor, which is classically seen as a pill-rolling action of the hands that may also affect the chin, lips, legs, and trunk, can be markedly increased by stress or emotions. Onset of parkinsonian tremor is generally after age 60. Movement starts in one limb or on one side of the body and usually progresses to include the other side.

Dystonic tremor occurs in individuals of all ages who are affected by dystonia, a movement disorder in which sustained involuntary muscle contractions cause twisting and repetitive motions and/or painful and abnormal postures or positions. Dystonic tremor may affect any muscle in the body and is seen most often when the patient is in a certain position or moves a certain way. The pattern of dystonic tremor may differ from essential tremor. Dystonic tremors occur irregularly and often can be relieved by complete rest. Touching the affected body part or muscle may reduce tremor severity. The tremor may be the initial sign of dystonia localized to a particular part of the body.

Cerebellar tremor is a slow, broad tremor of the extremities that occurs at the end of a purposeful movement, such as trying to press a button or touching a finger to the tip of one's nose. Cerebellar tremor is caused by lesions in or damage to the cerebellum resulting from stroke, tumor, or disease such as multiple sclerosis or some inherited degenerative disorder. It can also result from chronic alcoholism or overuse of some medicines. In classic cerebellar tremor, a lesion on one side of the brain produces a tremor in that same side of the body that worsens with directed movement. Cerebellar damage can also produce a "wing-beating" type of tremor called rubral or Holmes tremor—a combination of rest, action, and postural tremors. The tremor is often most prominent when the affected person is active or is maintaining a particular posture. Cerebellar tremor may be accompanied by dysarthria (speech problems), nystagmus (rapid, involuntary rolling of the eyes), gait problems, and postural tremor of the trunk and neck.

Psychogenic tremor (also called hysterical tremor) can occur at rest or during postural or kinetic movement. The characteristics of this kind of tremor may vary but generally include sudden onset and remission, increased incidence with stress, change in tremor direction and/or body part affected, and greatly decreased or disappearing tremor activity when the patient is distracted. Many patients with psychogenic tremor have a conversion disorder (defined as a psychological disorder that produces physical symptoms) or another psychiatric disease.

Orthostatic tremor is characterized by rhythmic muscle contractions that occur in the legs and trunk immediately after standing. Cramps are felt in the thighs and legs and the patient shakes uncontrollably when asked to stand in one spot. No other clinical signs or symptoms are present and the shaking ceases when the patient sits or is lifted off the ground. Orthostatic tremor may also occur in patients who have essential tremor.

Physiologic tremor occurs in every normal individual and has no clinical significance. It is rarely visible to the eye and may be heightened by strong emotion (such as anxiety or fear), physical exhaustion, hypoglycemia, hyperthyroidism, heavy metal poisoning, stimulants, alcohol withdrawal, or fever. It can be seen in all voluntary muscle groups and can be detected by extending the arms and placing a piece of paper on top of the hands. Enhanced physiologic tremor is a strengthening of physiologic tremor to more visible levels. It is generally not caused by a neurological disease but by reaction to certain drugs, alcohol withdrawal, or medical conditions including an overactive thyroid and hypoglycemia. It is usually reversible once the cause is corrected.

Other tremors. Tremor can result from other conditions as well. Alcoholism, excessive alcohol consumption, or alcohol withdrawal can kill certain nerve cells, resulting in tremor, especially in the hand. (Conversely, small amounts of alcohol may help to decrease familial and essential tremor, but the mechanism behind this is unknown. Doctors may use small amounts of alcohol to aid in the diagnosis of certain forms of tremor but not as a regular treatment for the condition.) Tremor in peripheral neuropathy may occur when the nerves that supply the body's muscles are traumatized by injury, disease, abnormality in the central nervous system, or as the result of systemic illnesses. Peripheral neuropathy can affect the whole body or certain areas, such as the hands, and may be progressive. Resulting sensory loss may be seen as a tremor or ataxia (inability to coordinate voluntary muscle movement) of the affected limbs and problems with gait and balance. Clinical characteristics may be similar to those seen in patients with essential tremor.

Diagnosis

During a physical exam a doctor can determine whether the tremor occurs primarily during action or at rest. The doctor will also check for tremor symmetry, any sensory loss, weakness or muscle atrophy, or decreased reflexes. A detailed family history may indicate if the tremor is inherited. Blood or urine tests can detect thyroid malfunction, other metabolic causes, and abnormal levels of certain chemicals that can cause tremor. These tests may also help to identify contributing causes, such as drug interaction, chronic alcoholism, or another condition or disease. Diagnostic imaging using computerized tomography or magnetic resonance imaging may help determine if the tremor is the result of a structural defect or degeneration of the brain.

The doctor will perform a neurological exam to assess nerve function and motor and sensory skills. The tests are designed to determine any functional limitations, such as difficulty with handwriting or the ability to hold a utensil or cup. The patient may be asked to place a finger on the tip of her or his nose, draw a spiral, or perform other tasks or exercises.

The doctor may order an electromyogram to diagnose muscle or nerve problems. This test measures involuntary muscle activity and muscle response to nerve stimulation.

Treatments

There is no cure for most tremors. The appropriate treatment depends on accurate diagnosis of the cause. Some tremors respond to treatment of the underlying condition. For example, in some cases of psychogenic tremor, treating the patient's underlying psychological problem may cause the tremor to disappear. Eliminating tremor triggers such as caffeine and other stimulants from the diet is often recommended.

Symptomatic drug therapy is available for several forms of tremor.

• Drug treatment for parkinsonian tremor involves levodopa and/or dopamine-like drugs such as pergolide mesylate, bromocriptine mesylate, and ropinirole. Other drugs used to lessen parkinsonian tremor include amantadine hydrochloride and anticholinergic drugs.

• Essential tremor may be treated with propranolol or other beta blockers (such as nadolol) and primidone, an anticonvulsant drug.

• Cerebellar tremor typically does not respond to medical treatment. Patients with rubral tremor may receive some relief using levodopa or anticholinergic drugs.

• Dystonic tremor may respond to clonazepam, anticholinergic drugs, and intramuscular injections of botulinum toxin. Botulinum toxin is also prescribed to treat voice and head tremors and several movement disorders.

• Clonazepam and primidone may be prescribed for primary orthostatic tremor.

• Enhanced physiologic tremor is usually reversible once the cause is corrected. If symptomatic treatment is needed, beta blockers can be used.

Physical therapy may help to reduce tremor and improve coordination and muscle control for some patients. A physical therapist will evaluate the patient for tremor positioning, muscle control, muscle strength, and functional skills. Teaching the patient to brace the affected limb during the tremor or to hold an affected arm close to the body is sometimes useful in gaining motion control. Coordination and balancing exercises may help some patients. Some therapists recommend the use of weights, splints, other adaptive equipment, and special plates and utensils for eating.

Surgical intervention such as thalamotomy and deep brain stimulation may ease certain tremors. These surgeries are usually performed only when the tremor is severe and does not respond to drugs.

- **Thalamotomy**, involving the creation of lesions in the brain region called the thalamus, is quite effective in treating patients with essential, cerebellar, or parkinsonian tremor. This in-hospital procedure is performed under local anesthesia, with the patient awake. After the patient's head is secured in a metal frame, the surgeon maps the patient's brain to locate the thalamus. A small hole is drilled through the skull and a temperature-controlled electrode is inserted into the thalamus. A low-frequency current is passed through the electrode to activate the tremor and to confirm proper placement. Once the site has been confirmed, the electrode is heated to create a temporary lesion. Testing is done to examine speech, language, coordination, and tremor activation, if any. If no problems occur, the probe is again heated to create a three-millimeter permanent lesion. The probe, when cooled to body temperature, is withdrawn and the skull hole is covered. The lesion causes the tremor to permanently disappear without disrupting sensory or motor control.

- **Deep brain stimulation (DBS)** uses implantable electrodes to send high-frequency electrical signals to the thalamus. The electrodes are implanted with procedures used for thalamotomy. The patient uses a hand-held magnet to turn on and turn off a pulse generator that is surgically implanted under the skin. The electrical stimulation temporarily disables the tremor and can be reversed, if necessary, by turning off the implanted electrode. Batteries in the generator last about five years and can be replaced surgically. DBS is currently used to treat parkinsonian tremor and essential tremor.

The most common side effects of tremor surgery include dysarthria (problems with motor control of speech), temporary or permanent cognitive impairment (including visual and learning difficulties), and problems with balance.

Research

The National Institute of Neurological Disorders and Stroke, a unit of the National Institutes of Health (NIH) within the U.S. Department of Health and Human Services, is the nation's leading federal fund provider of research on disorders of the brain and nervous system. The NINDS sponsors research on tremor both at its facilities at the NIH and through grants to medical centers.

Scientists at the NINDS are evaluating the effectiveness of 1-octanol, a substance similar to alcohol but less intoxicating, for treating essential tremor. Results of two previous NIH studies have shown this agent to be promising as a potential new treatment.

Other NINDS-funded grantees are studying two antidepressant medications, paroxetine and venlafaxine, to see if they can help control depression in Parkinson disease and affect motor symptoms such as tremor, stiffness, slowness, and loss of balance.

An additional NINDS study will examine how dextromethorphan, a drug that alters reflexes of the larynx (voice box), might reduce voice symptoms in people with voice disorders, including vocal tremor. This study will compare the effects of dextromethorphan, lorazepam (a tranquilizer), and a placebo in patients with four types of voice disorders.

Additional Information

Brain Resources and Information Network (BRAIN)
P.O. Box 5801
Bethesda, MD 20824
Toll-Free: 800-352-9424
Website: http://www.ninds.nih.gov
E-mail: braininfo@ninds.nih.gov

International Essential Tremor Foundation
P.O. Box 14005
Lenexa, KS 66285-4005
Toll-Free: 888-387-3667
Phone: 913-341-3880
Fax: 913-341-1296
http://www.essentialtremor.org
E-mail: staff@essentialtremor.org

WE MOVE (Worldwide Education and Awareness for Movement Disorders)
204 West 84th Street
New York, NY 10024
Phone: 212-875-8312
Fax: 212-875-8389
Website: http://www.wemove.org
E-mail: wemove@wemove.org

Tremor Action Network
P.O. Box 5013
Pleasanton, CA 94566-5013
Phone: 925-462-0111
Fax: 925-369-0485
Website: http://www.tremoraction.org
E-mail: tremor@tremoraction.org

National Ataxia Foundation (NAF)
2600 Fernbrook Lane N., Suite 119
Minneapolis, MN 55447-4752
Phone: 763-553-0020
Fax: 763-553-0167
Website: http://www.ataxia.org
E-mail: naf@ataxia.org

Chapter 17

Pain in MS Patients

Pain is a recognized symptom of multiple sclerosis (MS), affecting as many as seventy-five percent of people at some time during the course of their disease. However, only twenty-five percent of those who suffer with MS pain are being treated for it—presumably because pain is more difficult to manage than other MS symptoms. Pain is a subjective sensory experience: "Pain is whatever the experiencing person says it is, existing whenever he/she says it does.[1]" The subjective nature of pain, coupled with the different causal mechanisms seen in MS, contribute to the treatment challenge.

The most commonly reported pain syndromes in MS are burning dysesthesias in the lower extremities, headache, lower back pain, and painful spasms. People with MS describe their pain as having varying levels of severity and intensity, and characterize it as sharp, shooting, dull, or nagging pain that is either continuous or intermittent. Compared to the various types of pain described by the general population, the pain experienced by people with MS is reported as more intense, having greater impact on activities of daily living, and requiring greater use of analgesia.

The symptom of pain in MS demands attention, as it impacts activities of daily living and is associated with anxiety, depression, and fatigue. Pain in MS is also, but not exclusively, associated with longer disease duration, advancing age, higher disability scores, and secondary progressive disease course.

Classification of MS Pain

The etiology of MS pain is mixed. MS pain can be classified as either neurogenic (central) in origin or nociceptive (secondary to other factors). Whereas neurogenic pain is a consequence of lesions in the central nervous system (CNS), nociceptive pain is associated with noxious thermal, mechanical, electrical, or chemical stimuli that are generally a consequence of disease-related disability rather than the disease process itself. Differentiating types of MS-related pain according to the causal mechanism involved facilitates mechanism-tailored treatment strategies.

Neurogenic Pain

Neurogenic pain results from lesions in the CNS. The neurogenic pain syndromes described in MS include: trigeminal neuralgia; glossopharyngeal neuralgia; painful tonic seizures or spasms; dysesthesias of the extremities; thoracic and abdominal band-like sensations; certain types of headache; episodic facial pain; Lhermitte sign; and paroxysmal limb pain.

Neurogenic pain is further described by the character, duration, and intensity of symptoms that are experienced. Neurogenic pain often occurs spontaneously—for example, independent of any stimulus—and may be either paroxysmal or continuous. Spontaneous paroxysmal pain is typically characterized as shooting, stabbing, shock-like, lancinating, crushing, or searing. The most common forms of spontaneous continuous pain are dysesthesias—abnormal sensations that are characterized as burning, aching, prickling, tingling, nagging, dull and/or band-like. Dysesthesias are typically less intense than paroxysmal episodes of pain.

Stimulus-dependent forms of neuropathic pain (for example, occurring in reaction to a stimulus) include painful spasms and allodynia. Allodynia refers to pain in response to a stimulus that does not normally cause pain, such as gentle touch, massage, the feeling of clothing against the skin, or the weight of bed covers. Stimulus-dependent pain is usually of short duration and normally lasts only for the period of the stimulus.

The following is a review of the most common neuropathic pain syndromes seen in MS.

Paroxysmal Pain Syndromes

Trigeminal neuralgia (TN) is a spontaneous neurogenic pain experienced by approximately 4% of the MS population (a prevalence 400 times greater than in the general population). It affects one or more branches of the trigeminal nerve that innervates the eye, cheek, and jaw. TN is an intense, severe, sharp, electric-shock like pain, which is generally unilateral but may occasionally present bilaterally. Attacks can be spontaneous, or may be triggered or worsened by touching, chewing, smiling, or any facial movement. Periods in which sharp, shock-like attacks lasting 2–3 seconds to several minutes occur at varying frequency are typically interspersed with periods of remission. In rare instances the individual experiences episodes of longer duration (45–60 minutes) or continuous pain. TN rarely occurs during sleep. The onset of TN in MS occurs at an earlier age than in the general population. Presentation of TN pain in young adults may be diagnostic of MS.

TN in MS is thought to be associated with a lesion at the trigeminal root entry zone of the pons. Interrupting the pain pathway is the mechanism-tailored treatment strategy for trigeminal neuralgia in MS. Anticonvulsant medications, known to stabilize cell membranes—thereby decreasing the hyperexcitability of sensory neurons via sodium and calcium channel regulation—are the first-line treatment for the pain of trigeminal neuralgia. The second generation anticonvulsant agents have gentler side effect profiles; sustained-release, long-acting formulas minimize side effects.

When pain relief is not obtained through drug intervention, surgical gamma knife, radiofrequency, or nerve block procedures that interrupt the pain pathway may become an option. Percutaneous radiofrequency or glycerol rhizotomy is a safe and effective treatment, with lower reported risk of facial sensory loss than other invasive therapies.

Headache is more common in MS than in the general population, with 58% of patients experiencing episodic headache pain. Although the relationship between MS and headache is not clear, MS lesions in the midbrain have been associated with migraine-type headache. The headaches in MS are usually characterized as migraine-like, cluster, or tension-type. Migraine headache is more commonly reported in patients with relapsing-remitting disease. There is some evidence that migraine headaches are associated with exacerbation of MS symptoms.

Headaches should be treated following existing clinical guidelines for headache type. Mechanism-based treatment strategies include increasing the availability of the neurotransmitters serotonin and norepinephrine. The tricyclic antidepressants and the serotonin and norepinephrine reuptake inhibitors have been used with success in some patients. Increasing the availability of serotonin and norepinephrine may be an effective ongoing therapy for MS patients experiencing headache, as migraine is linked to changes in serotonin function and MS patients may have low serotonin levels.

Continuous Pain Syndromes

Dysesthetic Pain: The most common type of continuous pain experienced in MS is dysesthetic pain, which is defined as an unpleasant, abnormal sensation that is either spontaneous or evoked. Dysesthetic pain occurs more commonly in people with minimal disability and is characterized by sensations described as burning, prickling, or tingling, nagging, dull, or band-like. This persistent pain—often symmetric—typically affects the legs and feet but may also involve the arms, trunk, and perineum (called vulvodynia). Although dysesthetic pain is usually of moderate intensity, its nagging, persistent nature makes it difficult to tolerate. It is typically worse at night, and tends to be aggravated by changes in temperature. Dysesthetic pain can be associated with feelings of warmth or cold in the extremities that are unrelated to actual temperature. Allodynia is considered the hallmark of stimulus-induced dysesthetic pain. The use of a bed cradle and lambskin pads or booties may offer relief.

Dysesthetic pain is difficult to treat fully. Mechanism-based strategies include neuromodulation and interruption of pain pathways, with tricyclic antidepressants considered the first-line treatment. There is recent evidence that combination therapy (anticonvulsants plus antidepressants) provides greater effect with lower doses and fewer side effects. Topical agents such as capsaicin (Zostrix®), applications of heat and cold, and transdermal agents such as clonidine gel or patch (Catapres-TTS®) and the lidocaine patch (Lidoderm®) are effective management strategies. In the absence of allodynia, stimulation with fitted prescription pressure stockings at night, massage, acupuncture, or transcutaneous electric nerve stimulation (TENS), can also offer relief.

Nociceptive Pain

While nociceptive pain can be acute or chronic, the most common experiences in MS are chronic. This type of pain tends to be associated with greater disability and specifically described as low back pain and pain resulting from severe spasticity. Nociceptive pain can be intermittent or continuous, provoked or spontaneous. Some nociceptive pain can be easily localized—often described as aching, squeezing, stabbing, or throbbing. Other nociceptive pain is more variable in intensity and not as well-localized—generally described as gnawing or cramping, although sometimes described as sharp.

Musculoskeletal Pain

Common nociceptive pain experiences in MS, including back pain and painful spasms, involve the musculoskeletal system. MS musculoskeletal pain is a result of weakness, deconditioning, immobility, and stress on bones, muscles, and joints. Steroid use contributes to osteoporosis and possible compromise of the blood supply to large joints (avascular necrosis), with associated pain. Any pain of a musculoskeletal nature requires a thorough assessment for lumbar disc disease, avascular necrosis, or other condition.

Prevention is critical to the management of musculoskeletal pain. Bone antiresorptive therapies (for example, calcitonin [Miacalcin®], alendronate ([Fosamax®], raloxifene [Evista®], teriparatide [Forteo®]), smoking cessation, and calcium and vitamin D supplementation are preventive for pain associated with osteoporosis.

Physical therapy is essential for assessment and management of safety, gait, positioning, seating, and effective use of mobility aids, and ankle-foot-orthoses. Exercise and weight control are effective in preventing and treating musculoskeletal pain. Frequent position change and proper support relieve stress on muscles, bones, and joints.

Acetaminophen (Tylenol®), salicylates (aspirin), and nonsteroidal anti-inflammatory agents (NSAIDs) such as ibuprofen (Motrin®), naproxen (Aleve®), and celecoxib (Celebrex®) are first line medical treatments for musculoskeletal pain. All types of NSAIDs can cause gastrointestinal (GI) irritation and bleeding, They can also decrease renal blood flow, causing fluid retention and hypertension. NSAID labeling includes a black box warning for the potential risk of cardiovascular events and life-threatening GI bleeding. The U.S. Federal Drug Administration (FDA) recommends that NSAIDs be dosed exactly as prescribed or listed on the label. The lowest possible dose should be given for the shortest possible time.

Spasticity

Flexor and extensor muscle cramping, pulling, and subsequent pain occurs as spasticity in MS. Spasticity is evoked by noxious stimulation such as a decubitus ulcer, urinary tract infection, full bowel or bladder, or can result spontaneously from a CNS lesion. Management of spastic pain in MS follows standard spasticity medication management with baclofen (Lioresal®), tizanidine (Zanaflex®), diazepam (Valium®), dantrolene (Dantrium®), or botulinum toxin (Botox®).

Reference

1. McCaffery M. Two myths about pain. *Nursing Life* 2006;4(2):30.

Additional Information

National Multiple Sclerosis Society
733 Third Ave., 6th Fl.
New York, NY 10017-3288
Toll-Free: 800-344-4867 (FIGHTMS)
Phone: 212-986-3240
Fax: 212-986-7981
Website: http://www.nationalmssociety.org
E-mail: nat@nmss.org

Chapter 18

Fatigue in People with MS

MS and Fatigue

Fatigue is the most common symptom of multiple sclerosis (MS). As many as 75% to 95% of all people with MS have fatigue; 50% to 60% say that it's one of their worst problems. In fact, fatigue is one of the major reasons for unemployment among people with MS.

No one knows what really causes MS-related fatigue, but we do know some things that can help. If lack of energy is interfering with your regular activities or quality of life, tell your doctor. You could have a non-MS problem that can be treated. Even if it's related to MS, there are things you can do to improve the way you feel. Together, you and your doctor can select the best options for you.

One Size Doesn't Fit All

Everyone's circumstances are different: family situation, finances, support network, community resources, work flexibility, personal preferences, and physical function. Some options may not be practical for you. The more your health care team knows about these details, the better they'll be able to help.

What is MS-related fatigue?

Fatigue is a lack of physical energy, mental energy, or both. Everyone has low-energy days. And everyone knows what it's like to be down in the dumps and not feel like doing much of anything.

MS-related fatigue is different, and it's not always easy to spot. With MS fatigue, people have more off days than on days. Before it can be identified, other possible causes need to be crossed off the list of suspects.

If you have MS, ask yourself this question: Is fatigue interfering with my everyday activities or quality of life? If the answer is yes, your doctor needs to know.

Are there different types of fatigue?

Yes. The next step is to find out what type you have. This chapter refers to two general types of fatigue. Either type may, or may not, have a direct association with MS:

- *Chronic Persistent Fatigue*: Activity-limiting sluggishness or lassitude that goes on for more than six weeks, more than 50% of the days, during some part of the day.

- *Acute Fatigue*: Activity-limiting sluggishness that has either appeared (new) or become noticeably worse during the previous six weeks. Acute fatigue can be an early warning that other MS symptoms are about to flare up or become worse.

Think about your energy levels over the past several weeks. You may want to track how you feel for a couple of weeks, simply by making notes on a calendar. Then review the two descriptions of fatigue. Which one best fits you? Tell your doctor which type of fatigue you think you have, and why.

Each type of fatigue has different potential causes and treatments. All other possible causes need to be explored before MS-related fatigue is considered.

Important: Pay special attention to your MS after an episode of unusual fatigue. If your other MS symptoms seem to be getting worse, let your doctor know.

What are the types of MS-related fatigue?

Here again, there are broad categories:

- *Fatigue related to mobility problems*: With MS, sometimes ordinary activities take so much physical effort that they're exhausting. This is especially true for people who have leg weakness.

- *Fatigue related to respiratory problems*: MS can sometimes affect breathing, and when it does, even simple activities can be tiring. This is especially true for people who have the most serious physical symptoms of MS.

- *Primary MS fatigue*: This is a diagnosis of elimination. After all other causes of fatigue have been ruled out or treated successfully, primary MS fatigue is what's left.

Important: Pay special attention to your MS after an episode of unusual fatigue. If your other MS symptoms seem to be getting worse, let your doctor know.

Chapter 19

Speech Problems Associated with MS

Studies of dysarthria in multiple sclerosis (MS) indicate a prevalence ranging from 41% to 51%. Self-reporting of speech and other communication disorders has varied widely: 23% in a study in the United States (number in sample [N]= 656); 44% in a Swedish study (N= 200); and 57% in a preliminary South African study (N= 30). The range in prevalence figures reflects inconsistencies in study design, including the size and characteristics of the study samples, and the terminology and assessment tools used. In addition, a lack of congruence between evaluation results by a speech and language pathologist and self-report by individuals with MS has been proposed, and needs further study.

Speech and voice problems may be identified by the person with MS, a family member, or a healthcare professional. Common complaints include difficulty with precision of articulation, speech intelligibility, ease of conversational flow, speaking rate, loudness, and voice quality. When these problems interfere with a person's quality of life—particularly the ability to communicate daily needs—a referral for evaluation and treatment by a speech/language pathologist is recommended.

"Dysarthria in Multiple Sclerosis," by Pamela H. Miller. Reprinted in part with permission of the National Multiple Sclerosis Society. Copyright © 2007 National Multiple Sclerosis Society. All rights reserved. Material on the National Multiple Sclerosis Society website is regularly updated. For the latest version of this information, including references, please visit: www.national MSsociety.org.

Normal Speech Production

The normal processes of speech and voice production are overlapping and require the following five processes to work together smoothly and rapidly:

1. **Respiration:** Using the diaphragm to quickly fill the lungs fully, followed by slow, controlled exhalation for speech.

2. **Phonation:** Using the vocal cords and air flow to produce voice of varying pitch, loudness, and quality.

3. **Resonance:** Raising and lowering the soft palate to direct the voice to resonate in the oral and/or nasal cavities to further affect voice quality.

4. **Articulation:** Coordinating quick, precise movements of the lips, tongue, mandible, and soft palate for clarity of speech.

5. **Prosody:** Combining all elements for a natural flow of conversational speech, with adequate loudness, emphasis, and melodic line to enhance meaning.

Definition of Dysarthria and Dysphonia

Dysarthria refers to a speech disorder, caused by neuromuscular impairment, which results in disturbances in motor control of the speech mechanism. The demyelinating lesions caused by multiple sclerosis may result in spasticity, weakness, slowness, and/or ataxic incoordination of the lips, tongue, mandible, soft palate, vocal cords, and diaphragm. Therefore, articulation, speaking rate, intelligibility, and natural flow of speech in conversation are the areas most likely to be affected in those with multiple sclerosis.

Dysphonia, which refers to a voice disorder, often accompanies dysarthria because the same muscles, structures, and neural pathways are used for both speech and voice production. Therefore, voice quality, nasal resonance, pitch control, loudness, and emphasis may also be affected in those with MS.

Common Features of Dysarthria in MS

Dysarthria is considered the most common communication disorder in those with MS. It is typically mild, with severity of dysarthria symptoms related to neurological involvement.

Darley and colleagues published the first comprehensive, scientific study identifying common features of dysarthria in 168 people with MS. Analyses of speech characteristics and description of deviations in the five processes of respiration, phonation, resonance, articulation and prosody were rank ordered (see Table 19.1).

Since then, three replication studies have reported insufficient reliability of clinicians' judgments in the more specific areas, yet high agreement in such overall speech dimensions as intelligibility and naturalness.

A cross-linguistic analysis of dysarthria in Australian (N= 56) and Swedish (N= 77) speakers with MS, using a 33-point protocol identified six deviant features: harsh voice, imprecise articulation, impaired stress patterns, rate, breath support, and pitch variations. Even though different rank orders and problem frequencies were seen, agreement with Darley's list of seven most common features was noted, with the exception of loudness and hypernasality.

Table 19.1. Rank Order of Deviations in Speech and Voice in Multiple Sclerosis

Percent (N = 168)	Deviation	Description
77%	Loudness control	Reduced, mono, excess, or variable
72%	Harsh voice quality	Strained, excess tone in vocal cords
46%	Imprecise articulation	Distorted, prolonged, irregular
39%	Impaired emphasis	Phrasing, rate, stress, intonation
37%	Impaired pitch control	Monopitch, pitch breaks, high, low
35%	Decreased vital capacity	Reduced breath support and control
24%	Hypernasality	Excessive nasal resonance

Differential Diagnosis

There are three types of dysarthria associated with MS (see Table 19.2): spastic, ataxic, or mixed. Differential diagnosis depends on the extent and location of MS lesions, and the specific speech, voice, and accompanying physical signs that result. Mixed dysarthria is most common in MS because multiple neurological systems are typically involved.

Symptom Management of Contributing Factors

Differential diagnosis of the type of dysarthria has important implications for treatment planning by the speech and language pathologist as well as decision-making by the physician regarding pharmacologic management. Dysarthria and dysphonia in MS may be accompanied by the underlying symptoms of spasticity, weakness, tremor, and ataxia; and complicated by fatigue. Therefore, evaluation of medication trials to treat these symptoms, and ongoing communication with the patient and physician about the impact on speech and voice, is recommended during therapy.

Assessment of Dysarthria

Evaluation of dysarthria and dysphonia in MS typically involves three main aspects:

1. Assessment of oral-motor function of the peripheral speech mechanism by:

    *   Examining the structure and function of the articulators (lips, teeth, tongue, mandible, hard and soft palates) for symmetry, strength, speed, and coordination.
    *   Evaluating respiratory support and control for speech.
    *   Analyzing laryngeal control of loudness, pitch and voice quality during phonation.

2. Perceptual analysis to describe the various dimensions of respiration, phonation, articulation, resonance, and prosody. To classify type and severity of dysarthria.

3. Rating of speech intelligibility and naturalness in conversation.

Dysarthria evaluation in MS has traditionally included both informal and formal measures of a variety of oral-motor, speech, and voice functions, with comparison to referenced norms. Formal articulation tests are not commonly used because MS-related dysarthria tends to have an irregular pattern of breakdown that is not necessarily based on misarticulation of specific speech sounds. Rather, measures of oral reading rate in phonetically balanced passages (for example, *My Grandfather*—one of many standardized, phonetically-balanced oral reading passages) and analysis of a brief, recorded spontaneous speech sample (for example, describe job, family, interests, etc.) are standard procedures. Speaking rate, articulation precision, number of words per breath unit, pauses within and between words, intelligibility, and naturalness of conversational flow are then measured and described. Speaking rate varies according to the task: oral reading sentences—190 words per minute; oral reading of paragraphs—160–170 words per minute; speaking rate in conversation—150–250 words per minute. The wide range in conversation is due to a variety of cognitive-language factors, including the complex verbal formulations that are used, word retrieval/fluency abilities, turn-taking, and lack of concrete cues for pauses (such as the commas and periods in reading materials).

Some formal, published measures used in dysarthria evaluation in MS include:

- *Assessment of Intelligibility in Dysarthric Speech* (word and sentence levels), in which a judge, unfamiliar with the material, transcribes the recorded responses.

- *Dysarti-test*, which includes 54 test items, scored on a five-point interval scale. Items measured in each speech parameter include: respiration, phonation, oral-motor performance (divided into lips, jaw, tongue, and soft palate, plus a diadochokinesis rating), articulation, prosody and intelligibility.

- *Queensland Protocol*, an adapted version of the perceptual analysis/dysarthria classification procedure introduced by Darley and colleagues. This protocol includes 33 items relating to the five speech dimensions of respiration, phonation, resonance, articulation and prosody, and uses a four-point descriptive equal-interval scale to measure rate, intelligibility, articulation precision of consonants and vowels, and phoneme length.

Table 19.2. Comparing the Three Types of Dysarthria

Speech and Voice Signs	Related Neuromuscular/Physical Signs
Spastic dysarthria: Due to bilateral lesions of corticobulbar tracts	
Harsh, strained voice quality	Hypertonicity (excess muscle tone)
Pitch breaks	Bilateral spasticity
Imprecise articulation	Restricted range of motion (jaw)
Slow rate of speech	Reduced speed of movement
Reduced breath support and/or control	Bilateral hyperreflexia
Reduced or mono-loudness	Sucking and jaw jerk reflexes
Short phrases, reduced stress	Cortical disinhibition
Hypernasality	
Ataxic Dysarthria: Due to bilateral or generalized lesions of the cerebellum	
Vocal tremor	Intention tremor: head, trunk, arms, hands
Irregular articulation breakdown	
Dysrhythmic rapid alternating movements of the tongue, lips, and mandible	Broad-based, ataxic gait
	Nystagmus and irregular eye movements
Excess and equal stress (scanning speech)	Balance or equilibrium problems
	Hypertonicity
Excess and variable loudness	Overshooting; slow, voluntary movements
Prolonged phonemes and intervals	
Mixed dysarthria: Due to bilateral, generalized lesions of multiple areas in the cerebral white matter, brainstem, cerebellum, and/or spinal cord	
Impaired loudness control (reduced, mono-loudness, or excess and variable)	Any combination of spastic and ataxic features as previously mentioned
Harsh or hypernasal voice quality	
Impaired articulation (imprecise, distorted, prolonged, or irregular breakdowns)	
Impaired emphasis (slow, prolonged intervals or sounds, reduced, or excess and equal stress)	
Impaired pitch control (monopitch or pitch breaks, too low or too high)	

New Directions in Assessment

There has been a trend in recent years, to supplement perceptual analyses of dysarthria with acoustic analyses of speech parameters. Advancement in physiological instrumentation for assessment is aimed at improving objectivity in measurement, refining our understanding of dysarthria features specific to MS, and ultimately aiding clinical decision-making and treatment planning.

- Spectrographic displays have been used to obtain specific measures of acoustic distinctiveness during speech samples. For example, Tjaden and Wilding used a sound-treated booth, head-mounted microphone, and recording software (such as the CSpeechSP 4.0 or windows-based version TF32, Turbo Pascal 5.5) to objectively measure variations in sound/syllable duration, rate of articulation, vocal intensity, and size of working space for vowel and consonant production.

- Lip and tongue transducers have been used to objectively measure range, force, and diadochokinesis (or rapid alternating movements) of their function. Results of a recent study by Hartelius and Lillvik using this technique found that tongue function is more severely affected than lip function in MS, that tongue dysfunction can be detected subclinically (in non-dysarthric subjects), and that there was a moderate correlation to severity of neurological deficit and years in disease progression. Based on their findings, the importance of targeting improvement in tongue functioning early in articulation therapy was suggested.

Despite advances in the development of instrumental assessment techniques in recent years, perceptual analysis of recorded speech remains a primary tool for differential diagnosis and treatment planning.

Treatment

Evaluation of evidence-based research and expert opinion to support the treatment of dysarthria and to develop practice guidelines has been a project of the American Speech/Language Hearing Association (ASHA) and Academy of Neurologic Communication Disorders and Sciences (ANCDS) since 1997. A series of four practice guideline reports were published in the *Journal of Medical Speech / Language*

Pathology (2001–2004) and are available at www.ancds.org. Guidelines for improving speech intelligibility and naturalness are forthcoming. The World Health Organization's 2002 international classification of function, disability, and health has had a significant impact in the field of rehabilitation. The goal of addressing physical function and structure within the broader context of a person's ability to participate actively in his or her world, has influenced both assessment protocols and treatment planning. In dysarthria therapy, the trend has been away from a focus on specific impairments (for example, oral exercises to normalize movement patterns), toward the acquisition of specific skills to facilitate participation in functional real-world activities (for example, speaking with adequate loudness and intelligibility for telephone activities at work or home).

Clinical decision-making in treatment planning is individualized according to the person's specific problems and communication needs. Improving speech intelligibility and naturalness should be the ultimate goal of therapy. Selection of appropriate treatment approaches, and where to begin therapy, depend on which deviant speech dimension(s) are most disabling in these two areas. Work on one target behavior can have overlapping, indirect effects on other physiological and acoustic variables. For example, improving breath support/control can increase loudness and indirectly reduce rate, thus allowing more precise articulation and improving overall speech intelligibility. Measuring impact on participation and quality of life are recommended, to assess functional outcomes of dysarthria therapy.

Traditional dysarthric compensations taught to MS speakers include: improving breath support and control; reducing the rate of speech; using strategic pauses within and between words; exaggerating articulation; and actively self-monitoring/self-correcting speech.

In a recent review of the intervention literature on respiratory/phonatory dysfunction in dysarthria, evidence was found to support the following:

1. Improving breath support by using biofeedback to gauge respiration (and loudness or phrase length) during speech tasks; and when learning a new breath pattern with deeper inhalation, increased force at exhalation, and use of abdomen. Physiological and acoustic biofeedback methods, such as a Visipitch™, Computer software, volume/unit (VU) meter, recorder, Respitrace™, water manometer, velocity/air pressure transducer, oscilloscope, and electromyogram (EMG) were mentioned.

2. Improving respiratory/phonatory coordination by increasing awareness of the irregular speech-respiratory pattern, determining optimal words/breath groups, gradually increasing them, and practicing flexibility in cued and non-cued conversational scripts.

3. Improving phonatory functioning

   a. Hyperadduction (harsh voice quality, typical of MS): Often not directly treated because it is difficult to modify, with negligible impact on intelligibility.

   b. Hypoadduction (soft, breathy, whispered voice quality): Significant improvement has been demonstrated using the *Lee Silverman Voice Treatment* (LSVT™) in those with Parkinson disease and hypokinetic dysarthria. The LSVT seeks to increase vocal loudness, by increasing phonatory effort, which has been shown to improve speech intelligibility. Variable results with the LSVT technique have been noted in MS speakers and their spastic, ataxic, and mixed types of dysarthria.

A review of the literature on evidence-based practices in dysarthria therapy also found the technique of managing speaking rate to be effective in improving speech intelligibility. However, with rate control techniques there can be a negative impact on naturalness of conversational flow, which must be considered in treatment. Slowing rate can be accomplished by changing either the speech time (stretching out the word), or the increasing the pause time (within or between words). The two types of rate control include:

1. **Rigid:** Use of external aids—such as finger tapping, a pacing board, or a metronome—to slow speaking rate and allow more precise articulation of each word or syllable. Although this technique provides the fastest and greatest improvement in intelligibility, naturalness in flow of speech can suffer. It can be a motivating starting point, when combined with rhythmic rate control.

2. **Rhythmic:** Rate control techniques that also attempt to preserve naturalness by using biofeedback systems—including the Pacer/Tally software, Visipitch™, and delayed auditory feedback (DAF)—during speech tasks. The direct magnitude production technique (DMP), which uses no external device,

can also be effective. The DMP is self-devised and asks the individual to speak at half his habitual pitch. Whereas the rhythmic techniques take more time to learn, both speech intelligibility and naturalness may be improved.

Imprecise articulation of consonants has been noted as the greatest contributor to reduced overall speech intelligibility. In two studies specific to dysarthria treatment in MS speakers, the combined or overlapping effects of multiple techniques (increasing loudness, reducing rate, and exaggerating articulation) showed a positive impact on preciseness and speech intelligibility. Hartelius found tongue function to be more severely affected than lip function in dysarthric and non-dysarthric speakers with MS (N = 77). Therefore, increasing articulatory excursions while reducing rate is recommended.

Increasing loudness and reducing rate have also been associated with increasing the size of the articulatory-acoustic working space, and thus improving articulation precision and acoustic distinctiveness. Tjaden and Wilding performed acoustic and perceptual analyses of 15 mild to moderate spastic, ataxic, and mixed dysarthric speakers with MS and found that acoustic distinctiveness of vowels, as indexed by vowel space, was maximized in the slow condition, whereas distinctiveness of stop consonants was maximized in the loud condition. These findings are important for treatment planning.

Augmentative and Alternative Communication

The need for augmentative and alternative communication (AAC) devices in individuals with MS is relatively uncommon. However, when severe dysarthria interferes with the individual's well-being, safety, and functional communication of daily needs, evaluation for an appropriate speech generating device (SGD) is indicated. Speech supplementation devices (such as voice amplifiers) and nonspeech alternatives are also available. There are low-tech alternatives, such as: alphabet, picture, or eye gaze boards, as well as bells, buzzers, and yes-no systems—any of which offer manual, optical, or partner-assisted selection. And there are high-tech alternatives with dedicated devices such as Link™ or Lightwriter™, or multi-purpose integrated devices such as Mercury or Dynavox that use special personal computer (PC) software such as a keyboard with word-prediction software, EZ keys, touch screen, joystick, mouse, optical or switch scan as input, and text to digitized or synthesized speech output. Information about AAC devices, vendors, materials, and tutorials can be found at http://aac.unl.edu.

Yorkston and Beukelman (2000) developed a functional staging system for AAC intervention to aid in clinical decision-making. It rates five areas—speech, cognition, literacy, vision, and upper and lower extremity functioning—on a five-point scale. A team approach to AAC evaluation (including a physical therapist, occupational therapist, and speech/language pathologist) that takes into account the full range of a person's symptoms is recommended. Once assessment and training on the appropriate device has been completed, routine re-evaluation and update is essential.

In 2001, Medicare began providing reimbursement for evaluation, treatment, and appropriately-prescribed SGD devices. Medicare's assessment protocol and guidelines set the standard for state, federal, and private health plans. For example, prior to a speech language pathologist recommendation and physician prescription, an assessment trial of at least three systems that incorporate the necessary features is required before Medicare will provide authorization. Information about Medicare funding is available at http://aac-rerc.com.

Conclusion

In a preliminary MS study in South Africa, 62% of the respondents experiencing speech and language problems reported that these difficulties had a negative impact on their quality of life (QOL). Although the prevalence of dysarthria in MS has been reported to be at least 41%, referral rate is low—a significant gap that needs to be addressed.

Assessment protocols and treatment procedures for dysarthria in MS have shown recent advances. Trends have included the refinement of perceptual and acoustic analyses, and incorporation of the World Health Organization's international classification of function, disability and health, which aids functional goal-setting. Specific treatments are being studied with the MS population and controls, to add evidence-based research to the expert opinion of clinicians.

More MS research is needed in the international community in the areas of prevalence, acoustic and physiological dimensions and they relate to perceptual analysis, treatment outcomes as they relate to quality of life, and cross-linguistic perceptual ratings.

213

Chapter 20

Swallowing Disorders Associated with MS

Introduction

Permanent and transitory swallowing disorders (dysphagia) occur with high frequency in patients with multiple sclerosis (MS) (Abrahams and Yun, 2002; Calcagno et al., 2002; De Pauw et al., 2002; Prosiegel et al., 2004; Wiesner et al., 2002). In fact, swallowing disorders may be present long before the person with MS experiences any related symptoms.

In 1987, Dr. Angie Fabiszak studied three groups of individuals: healthy controls with no diagnosis of multiple sclerosis or other medical problems; patients with MS but no complaints of swallowing problems; and patients with multiple sclerosis who were complaining of a swallowing disorder. Results of x-ray studies (modified barium swallow) on these patients revealed that both of the groups of patients with multiple sclerosis exhibited similar abnormalities in swallowing, whereas the normal control group exhibited no swallowing disorders. In recent years, several other investigators have corroborated the fact patients with multiple sclerosis frequently exhibit swallowing disorders, even if they have no such complaints.

It is, therefore, important for the MS patient's primary care physician to refer the patient with multiple sclerosis—with or without a complaint of swallowing problems—for a full workup of his or her oropharyngeal and esophageal swallowing function as soon as the patient has a diagnosis of multiple sclerosis, in order to establish a baseline swallow physiology against which to compare any future changes.

Normal Swallowing

Normal swallowing involves cortical control of the facial muscles and tongue in placing food in the mouth, manipulating and tasting the food, chewing it, and forming it into a ball or bolus to be swallowed. Once the bolus is formed, the tongue begins to propel the food, or part of it, into the pharynx (throat), where control of the process is taken. The movements of the tongue and bolus stimulate sensory nerve endings which, in turn, trigger contractions in the pharynx, initiating the pharyngeal stage of the swallow. When the pharyngeal swallow is triggered, a number of motor components are initiated:

1. The soft palate closes to prevent food or liquid from going into the nose.

2. The larynx (entrance to the airway) lifts and closes to prevent food or liquid from entering the trachea.

3. The base of the tongue and walls of the throat converge to create pressure at the back of the bolus, propelling it throughout the pharynx into the esophagus.

4. The upper esophageal sphincter (located at the top of the esophagus) opens to enable the food to enter the esophagus.

Once in the esophagus, sequential esophageal motor contraction (peristalsis) propels the bolus through the esophagus to the stomach. The lower esophageal sphincter opens to allow the bolus to enter the stomach. The entire swallow, from placement of food in the mouth through entrance to the stomach, occurs rapidly (one second in the oral cavity, one second in the pharynx, and 8–10 seconds in the esophagus), safely (with no aspiration), and efficiently (with minimal residue).

The normal swallow depends upon a well-functioning central nervous system, including cortical and subcortical areas, the brainstem, and peripheral nerves—particularly cranial nerves. If the patient's MS lesions affect any of these areas, swallowing may be challenged. Many patients with MS will cough if food enters their airway or will require multiple swallows to clear food that has been left behind in the pharynx. Keep in mind, however, that patients who are experiencing reduced sensation may be unaware that food particles have entered the airway or that residual food particles have been left in the pharynx; they will not cough or repeat their swallows in spite of the need to do so.

Baseline Swallow Assessment: The Modified Barium Swallow and Esophagram

The patient with multiple sclerosis should receive a modified barium swallow to examine oral and pharyngeal swallow physiology, followed by an esophagram to examine esophageal function. The modified barium swallow is preferred because the MS patient may aspirate when given the usual large-volume swallows, including cup drinking, which are used for a standard barium swallow. In contrast to the standard barium swallow, the modified barium swallow is designed to introduce calibrated, measured volumes of thin liquids first, beginning with one milliliter (ml), which is similar to a saliva swallow, and building to three ml, five ml, and ten ml as tolerated by the patient without aspiration. Then, the patient is given a cup to drink from, followed by several swallows of three ml of pudding, and then two pieces of Lorna Doone cookie (1/4 of a cookie) coated with barium pudding (Logemann, 1993). This procedure, which involves a total of 14 swallows, allows the clinician to identify any abnormalities in the swallow as it progresses from small to large volumes of thin liquids, and thin to thicker viscosities. In healthy individuals, both volume and viscosity sequentially change the physiology of the swallow; it is important to determine whether the person with MS exhibits a similar systematic change in his or her swallow physiology in response to changing volume and viscosity (Logemann, 1998).

In addition to demonstrating the individual patient's swallow physiology, the modified barium swallow makes it possible to introduce and evaluate management strategies should they be needed. Strategies for management are introduced and evaluated on x-ray when the patient aspirates or has significant residual food left in the pharynx after the swallow. By the time the patient has completed the modified barium swallow procedure, the clinician should have an outline of recommendations for: 1) effective management strategies, including any swallowing therapy procedures that are needed; and 2) optimal, safe diet consistencies. The radiographic study should involve a speech-language pathologist who is familiar with the various management strategies and can introduce and evaluate the immediate effectiveness of the therapies during the radiographic study.

Common Swallowing Disorders in MS

The most common MS-related swallowing disorders in the oral and pharyngeal areas are:

- **Delay in triggering the pharyngeal swallow:** The delay in triggering the pharyngeal swallow, which is the most common problem seen in MS patients, can cause particular difficulties with liquid swallowing, including aspiration (Logemann, 2000). When the pharyngeal swallow is delayed, liquid may splash from the mouth into the pharynx. Because motor control of the pharynx has not been activated by the brainstem, the airway remains open and the upper esophageal sphincter remains closed, causing liquid that enters the pharynx to splash into the open airway and be aspirated.

- **Reduction in laryngeal elevation:** Reduced laryngeal elevation can contribute to weakened closure of the airway during the swallow and to reduced clearance of material from the pharynx, thereby causing residue after the swallow and possible aspiration.

- **Reduction in tongue base retraction:** Reduction in tongue base activity reduces the pressure generated during the swallow, allowing residual food to remain in the pharynx and be aspirated when the patient resumes breathing. These disorders can be mild, without causing any significant difficulties such as aspiration or inefficient swallow; or, they can be more severe and require therapeutic (behavioral) management.

The Barium Swallow Evaluation

Esophageal disorders require a standard barium swallow evaluation in which the patient is given a cup of barium and asked to swallow sequentially. A typical swallow from a cup or glass includes approximately 15 to 20 ml per swallow, a large volume that can cause difficulty if the patient has any significant abnormality. For this reason, the modified barium swallow should always precede the barium swallow to identify the locus of oropharyngeal swallow difficulty prior to giving the patient a large volume of liquid in a barium swallow or esophagram.

Dysphagia Management

The goal of dysphagia management is to maintain the patient on a normal diet as much as possible. Generally, two management plans are devised for each patient—one to promote safe and efficient swallowing for oral intake and one focused on exercise/therapy (Logemann, 2006). There are various kinds of strategies that can be introduced, including:

- postural change—which helps to redirect food along the correct pathway (for example, away from the airway);

- heightened oral sensation prior to the swallow—which enables the patient to get a faster pharyngeal swallow;

- voluntary control over swallows, such as holding one's breath to protect the airway, or increasing effort, if possible, to clear a greater amount of bolus;

- exercises to improve range of motion or coordination of the movement in the oral and pharyngeal structures as well as techniques to improve strength in the tongue.

One factor that can play a role in the selection of strategies for swallowing therapy is the patient's level of fatigue. If the patient is extremely fatigued, some swallow therapy strategies are not appropriate.

If the patient experiences significant exacerbations and/or the disease progresses, the nature or severity of his or her swallowing disorder could be expected to change as well. A re-assessment of the person's swallowing problems and a revised treatment plan are appropriate at that time.

Recommendations for Non-Oral Versus Oral Feeding

After the videofluoroscopic study of oropharyngeal swallow, the clinician will recommend continued oral feeding, or partial or complete non-oral feeding—depending upon the patient's safety and efficiency of swallow. If the patient is regularly aspirating on all foods, no matter what food viscosity is presented or therapy is used, non-oral feeding may be recommended for two reasons: First, regular aspiration can cause pneumonia; second, whatever the patient aspirates will not provide nutrition or hydration. Several studies have shown that patients who aspirate during the x-ray study have a significantly increased risk of pneumonia in the next six months than patients who do not aspirate during the study (Pikus et al., 2003; Schmidt et al., 1994). Non-oral supplements to ensure adequate nutrition and hydration may also be recommended for patients who have been exhibiting weight loss and fatigue when taking food orally. Whether or not the patient exhibits chronic aspiration or fatigue, partial non-oral feeding may be helpful. For example, the patient who aspirates may do so only on certain foods and be able to eat other foods orally. Or, the patient who fatigues easily may eat some foods orally and initiate non-oral nutrition when fatigue sets in.

The two basic types of non-oral feeding that allow food and liquids to be taken into the body without being swallowed are the nasogastric tube that goes through the nose and throat into the esophagus and stomach (generally used only on a very temporary basis because of the irritation it can cause to the nose and throat), and the percutaneous endoscopic gastrostomy (PEG) that involves inserting a feeding tube through the abdominal wall directly into the stomach. Both of these options for non-oral feeding are temporary and can be removed or not used when desired. Often patients and their significant others think that a decision to introduce partial or full non-oral feeding means that the patient will never eat by mouth again. This, however, is not the case. Non-oral feeding can serve as a temporary bridge while the patient improves and returns to oral feeding. Thus, at the end of the radiographic study, the recommendation for continued oral feeding, partial non-oral, or full non-oral feeding will be made. This is a recommendation to be carefully considered by the patient's physician, the patient, and their significant others.

Patient and Family Counseling Regarding Swallowing Management

The speech-language pathologist can also provide counseling to the patient and their family regarding the importance of completing the exercises given in therapy and ways in which the family can facilitate the patient's practice of exercise and application of techniques for swallowing improvement during mealtime.

Follow-Up

It is important for MS patients and their family members to contact both their physician and their speech-language pathologist if the swallow appears to worsen. It is common for dysphagia in patients with multiple sclerosis to wax and wane. This does not mean that swallowing management cannot be done, but rather that the therapy procedures used may need to be changed. The goal of swallowing management is to keep the MS patient from getting pneumonia or losing weight because of a swallowing difficulty.

References

Abraham SS, Yun PT. (2002 Winter). Laryngopharyngeal dysmotility in multiple sclerosis. *Dysphagia* 17(1): 69–74.

Calcagno P, Ruoppolo G, Grass MG, et al. (2002 Jan). Dysphagia in multiple sclerosis—Prevalence and prognostic factors. *Acta Neurol Scand* 105(1): 40–43.

De Pauw A, Dejaeger E, D'hooghe B, et al. (2002 Sep). Dysphagia in multiple sclerosis. *Clin Neurol Neurosurg* 104(4): 345–351.

Fabiszak A. (1987). *Swallowing patterns in neurologically normal subjects and two subgroups of multiple sclerosis patients.* Doctoral dissertation, Northwestern University.

Logemann JA. (1993). *A manual for videofluoroscopic evaluation of swallowing, 2nd ed.* Austin, TX: Pro-Ed.

Logemann JA. (1998). *Evaluation and treatment of swallowing disorders, 2nd ed.* Austin, TX: Pro-Ed.

Logemann JA. (2000). Dysphagia in multiple sclerosis. In Burks J, ed. *Multiple sclerosis: Diagnosis, medical management, and rehabilitation.* New York: Demos Medical Publishing. Pp. 485–490.

Logemann JA. (2004). Swallowing. In Kalb R, ed. *Multiple sclerosis: The questions you have—The answers you need, 3rd ed.* New York: Demos Vermande. Pp. 87–203.

Logemann JA. (2006). Speech and swallowing. *MS in Focus* 7: 9–10.

Pikus L, Levine MS, Yang YX, et al. (2003 Jun). Videofluoroscopic studies of swallowing dysfunction and the relative risk of pneumonia. *AJR Am J Roentgenol* 180(6): 1613–1616.

Prosiegel M, Schelling A, Wagner-Sonntag E. (2004). Dysphagia and multiple sclerosis. *Intl MS J* 11(1): 22–31.

Schmidt J, Holas M, Halvorson K, Reding J. (1994 Winter). Videofluoroscopic evidence of aspiration predicts pneumonia and death but not dehydration following stroke. *Dysphagia* 9(1): 7–11.

Wiesner W, Wetzel SG, Kappos L, et al. (2002 Apr). Swallowing abnormalities in multiple sclerosis: Correlation between videofluoroscopy and subjective symptoms. *Eur Radiol* 12(4): 789–792.

Additional Information

National Multiple Sclerosis Society
733 Third Ave., 6th Fl.
New York, NY 10017-3288
Toll-Free: 800-344-4867 (FIGHTMS)
Phone: 212-986-3240
Fax: 212-986-7981
Website: http://www.nationalmssociety.org
E-mail: nat@nmss.org

Chapter 21

Vision Problems and MS

Chapter Contents

Section 21.1

Optic Neuritis

Definition

Optic neuritis is inflammation of the optic nerve. It may cause sudden, reduced vision in the affected eye.

Causes, Incidence, and Risk Factors

The cause of optic neuritis is unknown. Sudden inflammation of the optic nerve (the nerve connecting the eye and the brain) leads to swelling and destruction of its outer shell, called the myelin sheath. The inflammation may occasionally be the result of a viral infection, or it may be caused by autoimmune diseases such as multiple sclerosis. Risk factors are related to the possible causes.

Symptoms

- acute loss of vision in one eye
- loss of color vision
- pain on movement of the eye
- decreased constriction of the pupil of the affected eye in bright light

Signs and Tests

A complete medical examination is usually used to rule out associated diseases. Tests may include the following:

- visual acuity testing
- color vision testing
- visualization of the optic disc by indirect ophthalmoscopy
- magnetic resonance imaging (MRI) of the brain to test for multiple sclerosis

Treatment

Visual acuity often returns to normal within 2–3 weeks with no treatment.

Intravenous corticosteroid therapy may accelerate visual recovery but may be associated with systemic side effects. Oral corticosteroid therapy may increase the risk of recurrence, and is seldom used for initial therapy. It may be used after initial intravenous corticosteroid therapy.

Further tests may be needed to determine the cause of the neuritis, and the condition causing the problem would then be treated.

Expectations (Prognosis)

Optic neuritis without underlying disease such as multiple sclerosis has a good prognosis for recovery. Optic neuritis resulting from multiple sclerosis, or other autoimmune disease such as systemic lupus erythematosus, is associated with a poorer prognosis.

Complications

* systemic side effects of therapy
* vision loss

About 20% of patients with a first episode of optic neuritis will develop multiple sclerosis.

Calling Your Health Care Provider

Call your health care provider immediately if sudden loss of vision in one eye occurs.

If you have optic neuritis, call your health care provider if vision decreases, pain in the eye develops, or if symptoms do not improve with treatment.

Section 21.2

Nystagmus (Uncontrollable Eye Movement)

© 2007 A.D.A.M., Inc. Reprinted with permission.

Definition

Uncontrollable eye movements are involuntary, rapid, and repetitive movement of the eyes.

Considerations

Nystagmus refers to rapid involuntary movements of the eyes that may be from side to side (horizontal nystagmus), up and down (vertical nystagmus), or rotary. Depending on the cause, these movements may be in both eyes or in just one eye. The term "dancing eyes" has been used in regional dialect to describe nystagmus.

The involuntary eye movements of nystagmus are caused by abnormal function in the areas of the brain that control eye movements. The exact nature of these disorders is poorly understood. Nystagmus may be either congenital (present at birth) or may be acquired (caused by disease or injury later in life).

Congenital Nystagmus

Congenital nystagmus is more common than acquired nystagmus. It is usually mild, does not change in severity, and is not associated with any other disorder.

Affected people are not aware of the eye movements, although they may be noticed by a careful observer. If the movements are of large magnitude, visual acuity (sharpness of vision) may be less than 20/20. Surgery may improve visual acuity.

Rarely, nystagmus occurs as a result of congenital diseases of the eye that cause poor vision. Although this is rare, an ophthalmologist should evaluate any child with nystagmus to check for this.

Acquired Nystagmus

A less-common cause of nystagmus is disease or injury of the central nervous system.

In young people the most common cause of acquired nystagmus is head injury from motor vehicle accidents. In older people the most common cause is stroke (blood vessel blockage in the brain). Any disease of the brain (such as multiple sclerosis or brain tumors) can cause nystagmus if the areas controlling eye movements are damaged.

Because control of eye movements is affected by input from the labyrinth (the part of the inner ear that senses movement and position), inner ear disorders such as Ménière disease can also lead to acquired nystagmus. Other causes may include Dilantin (an antiseizure medication) or alcohol intoxication.

Nystagmus may be observed through the following procedure: If the affected person spins around for about 30 seconds, stops, and tries to stare at an object, the eyes will first move slowly in one direction, then move rapidly in the opposite direction. The orientation of these alternating movements (side-to-side, up-and-down, or in a circular pattern) depends on the type of nystagmus.

Common Causes

Nystagmus is a symptom of many different disorders. Your health care provider will take a careful history and perform a thorough physical examination, which will emphasize the nervous system and inner ear.

Questions asked in a medical history may cover the following areas:

- When was it first noticed?
- How often does it occur?
- Has it ever happened before?
- Is it getting better, worse, or staying the same?
- Are there side-to-side eye movements?
- Are there up-and-down eye movements?
- What medications are being taken?
- What other symptoms are present?

Diagnostic tests that may be performed include:

- computed tomography (CT) scan of the head or magnetic resonance imaging (MRI) of the head

- electrooculography—an electrical method of measuring eye movements using tiny electrodes

Home Care

There is no therapy for most cases of congenital nystagmus. Availability of treatment for acquired nystagmus will vary with the cause. In most cases, except for those caused by Dilantin or alcohol intoxication, nystagmus is irreversible.

Call Your Health Care Provider If

Nystagmus is detected or suspected.

Chapter 22

Pulmonary and Respiratory Complications in MS Patients

Pneumonia and upper respiratory conditions are common causes of morbidity and mortality in patients with multiple sclerosis (MS), said Jodie K. Haselkorn, M.D., MPH, who chaired the Pulmonary Rehabilitation program at the Spring 2006 Consortium of Multiple Sclerosis Centers (CMSC) meeting. However, the medical literature provides the MS specialist little guidance in appropriate monitoring of deficits or treatment strategies. Dr. Haselkorn is an Associate Professor of Rehabilitation Medicine at the University of Washington and Director of the Multiple Sclerosis Center of Excellence at the West Veterans Affairs (VA) Puget Sound Health Care System.

"Pulmonary muscle strength and endurance is reduced in a large portion of our patients with MS, including those who are less disabled," agreed Donna Fry, PT, Ph.D., Associate Professor and Interim Director of Physical Therapy at the University of Michigan–Flint. "Yet, pulmonary muscle weakness often isn't considered in the MS population, and is not even listed as a symptom on the National Multiple Sclerosis Society website,"[1] she added.

Causes of Pulmonary Impairment in MS

Richard B. Goodman, M.D., Associate Professor of Pulmonary and Critical Care Medicine at the University of Washington in Seattle, also

"Pulmonary Complications in the MS Patient," by Barbara Merchant, *MS Exchange*, August 2006. © 2006 Consortium of Multiple Sclerosis Centers. Reprinted with permission.

229

presented at the symposium and has been collaborating with Dr. Haselkorn's MS Center of Excellence to screen patients with clinical respiratory symptoms by measuring their pulmonary function. According to Dr. Goodman, "it is clear that many MS patients have measurable pulmonary impairment."

Dr. Goodman reported on the work of Joshua Benditt, M.D., Professor of Medicine at the University of Washington, who has been studying respiratory function in general muscular diseases.[2] "Dr. Benditt has broken respiratory complications into three mechanistic categories: 1) bulbar weakness (glottic and pharyngeal muscles), which manifests as aspiration complications and impaired cough coordination; 2) inspiratory muscle weakness (diaphragm muscle), which presents with dyspnea and ventilatory insufficiency symptoms; and 3) expiratory muscle weakness (abdominal muscles), with resultant cough force impairment," reported Dr. Goodman. He added that, in MS, "impairments in any of these categories can result from plaques in the brain stem or spinal cord, from disease impairment, or from complications related to the treatment of MS-related spasticity."

Appropriate Screening Tools

Dr. Goodman uses spirometry to screen symptomatic patients who present to the pulmonary function laboratory. He evaluates forced vital capacity (FVC), forced expiratory volume in one second, maximal inspiratory pressure, and maximal expiratory pressure. He also monitors serum bicarbonate levels, because they serve "as a marker of ventilatory insufficiency in patients with measurable impairment of FVC, particularly in patients with diaphragm dysfunction."

Spirometers are portable and simple to operate, added co-presenter Toni Chiara, Ph.D., PT, a researcher at the Malcom Randall VA Medical Center in Gainesville, Florida and adjunct faculty member at the University of Florida. Their use is not limited to the respiratory therapist, she stressed.

Another useful tool for pulmonary assessment is the manometer, which Dr. Chiara said is helpful for getting "serial measurements of your patients in the clinic." The Index of Pulmonary Dysfunction (IPD) is an MS-specific tool for pulmonary function assessment, Dr. Chiara explained. The higher the patient's score (which ranges from 4–11), the greater the level of pulmonary impairment. The IPD consists of four questions:

1. Does the patient report a history of choking when he or she swallows?

2. Does the patient report his or her cough is normal or weak?

3. Does the evaluator perceive the cough as normal, weak, or absent?

4. On a maximal inhalation, how long can the patient count on one breath?

The impulse oscillometry system, previously a research tool now available for clinical use, measures airway resistance.

Improving Pulmonary Function

A number of trainers on the market boost inspiratory or expiratory muscle strength, or both. Dr. Chiara cited several studies that examined expiratory muscle strength training in MS patients. Some used trainers, but one study[3] performed by nurses, used music therapy. All studies reported that training helped MS patients to some degree.

The Role of the MS Specialist

Dr. Haselkorn stressed that MS specialists should effectively monitor their patients for decreases in respiratory function. In addition, MS clinicians should have knowledge of the role of exercise in strengthening inspiratory and expiratory muscles and prevention strategies for upper respiratory infections and pneumonia, such as the influenza vaccination, which has been proven not to exacerbate MS.

The goals in managing pulmonary complications in MS patients, added Dr. Goodman, are to "improve and stabilize gas exchange, ameliorate symptoms, improve sleep quality, extend survival, and improve quality of life."

References

1. The National Multiple Sclerosis Society website. Available at: www.nationalmssociety.org. Accessed July 25, 2006.

2. Benditt JO. Respiratory care and neuromuscular disease. *Respir Care*. 2006;51:828.

3. Wiens, M.E., Reimer, M.A., and Guyn, H.L. Music therapy as a treatment method for improving respiratory muscle strength in patients with advanced multiple sclerosis: a pilot study. *Rehabil Nurse*. 1999;24:74–80.

Chapter 23

Nerve Disease and Bladder Control Problems

For the urinary system to do its job, muscles and nerves must work together to hold urine in the bladder, and then release it at the right time. Nerves carry messages from the bladder to the brain to let it know when the bladder is full. They also carry messages from the brain to the bladder, telling muscles either to tighten or release. A nerve problem might affect your bladder control if the nerves that are supposed to carry messages between the brain and the bladder do not work properly.

What bladder control problems does nerve damage cause?

Nerves that work poorly can lead to three different kinds of bladder control problems.

Overactive bladder: Damaged nerves may send signals to the bladder at the wrong time, causing its muscles to squeeze without warning. The symptoms of overactive bladder include:

- urinary frequency—defined as urination eight or more times a day or two or more times at night;

- urinary urgency—the sudden, strong need to urinate immediately; and,

---

"Nerve Disease and Bladder Control," National Institute of Diabetes and Digestive and Kidney Diseases (NIDDK), NIH Publication No. 05–4560, January 2005.

- urge incontinence—leakage of urine that follows a sudden, strong urge.

Poor control of sphincter muscles: Sphincter muscles surround the urethra and keep it closed to hold urine in the bladder. If the nerves to the sphincter muscles are damaged, the muscles may become loose and allow leakage or stay tight when you are trying to release urine.

Urine retention: For some people, nerve damage means that their bladder muscles do not get the message that it is time to release urine or are too weak to completely empty the bladder. If the bladder becomes too full, urine may back up and the increasing pressure may damage the kidneys. Or, urine that stays too long may lead to an infection in the kidneys or bladder. Urine retention may also lead to overflow incontinence.

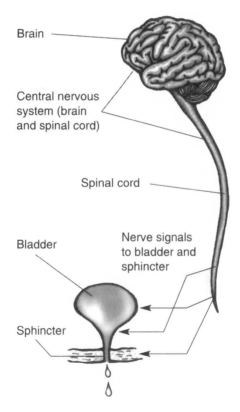

Figure 23.1. Nerves carry signals from the brain to the bladder and sphincter.

What causes nerve damage?

Many events or conditions can damage nerves and nerve pathways. Some of the most common causes are:

- vaginal childbirth
- infections of the brain or spinal cord
- diabetes
- stroke
- accidents that injure the brain or spinal cord
- multiple sclerosis
- heavy metal poisoning

In addition, some children are born with nerve problems that can keep the bladder from releasing urine, leading to urinary infections or kidney damage.

How will the doctor test for nerve damage and bladder control problems?

Any evaluation for a health problem begins with a medical history and a general physical examination. Your doctor can use this information to narrow down the possible causes for your bladder problem.

If nerve damage is suspected, the doctor may need to test both the bladder itself and the nervous system (including the brain). Three different kinds of tests might be used:

Urodynamics: These tests involve measuring pressure in the bladder while it is being filled to see how much it can hold and then checking to see whether the bladder empties completely and efficiently.

Imaging: The doctor may use different types of equipment—x rays, magnetic resonance imaging (MRI), and computed tomography (CT)—to take pictures of the urinary tract and nervous system, including the brain.

EEG and EMG: An electroencephalograph (EEG) is a test in which wires are taped to the forehead to sense any dysfunction in the brain. The doctor may also use an electromyograph (EMG) to test the nerves and muscles of the bladder.

What are the treatments for overactive bladder?

The treatment for a bladder control problem depends on the cause of the nerve damage and the type of voiding dysfunction that results.

In the case of overactive bladder, your doctor may suggest a number of strategies, including bladder training, electrical stimulation, drug therapy, and, in severe cases where all other treatments have failed, surgery.

Bladder training: Your doctor may ask you to keep a bladder diary—a record of your fluid intake, trips to the bathroom, and episodes of urine leakage. This record may indicate a pattern and suggest ways to avoid accidents by making a point of using the bathroom at certain times of the day—a practice called timed voiding. As you gain control, you can extend the time between trips to the bathroom. Bladder training also includes Kegel exercises to strengthen the muscles that hold in urine.

Electrical stimulation: Mild electrical pulses can be used to stimulate the nerves that control the bladder and sphincter muscles. Depending on which nerves the doctor plans to treat, these pulses can be given through the vagina or anus, or by using patches on the skin. Another method is a minor surgical procedure to place the electric wire near the tailbone. If you have this procedure, it will involve two steps. In the first step, the wire will be placed and connected to a temporary stimulator, which you carry with you for several days. If your condition improves during this trial period, then you go on to the second step. The wire is placed next to the tailbone and attached to a permanent stimulator under your skin. The Food and Drug Administration (FDA) has approved this device, marketed as the InterStim system, to treat urge incontinence, urgency-frequency syndrome, and urinary retention in patients for whom other treatments have not worked.

Drug therapy: Different drugs can affect the nerves and muscles of the urinary tract in different ways.

- Drugs that relax bladder muscles and prevent bladder spasms include oxybutynin chloride (Ditropan), tolterodine (Detrol), hyoscyamine (Levsin), and propantheline bromide (Pro-Banthine), which belong to the class of drugs called anticholinergics. Their most common side effect is dry mouth, although larger doses may cause blurred vision, constipation, a faster heartbeat, and flushing. A new patch delivery system for oxybutynin (Oxytrol) may decrease side effects. Ditropan XL and Detrol LA are time-release formulations that deliver a low level of the drug continuously in the body. These drugs have the advantage of once-a-day administration. In 2004, the FDA approved trospium chloride (Sanctura), darifenacin (Enablex), and solifenacin succinate (Vesicare) for the treatment of overactive bladder.

• Drugs for depression that also relax bladder muscle include imipramine hydrochloride (Tofranil), a tricyclic antidepressant. Side effects may include fatigue, dry mouth, dizziness, blurred vision, nausea, and insomnia.

Additional drugs are being evaluated for the treatment of overactive bladder and may soon receive FDA approval.

Surgery: In extreme cases, when incontinence is severe and other treatments have failed, surgery may be considered. The bladder may be made larger through an operation known as augmentation cystoplasty, in which a part of the diseased bladder is replaced with a section taken from the patient's bowel. This operation may improve the ability to store urine but may make the bladder more difficult to empty so that regular catheterization is needed. There is also a risk that the bladder may break open and leak urine into the body. Other risks include bladder stones, mucus in the bladder, and infection.

How do you do Kegel exercises?

The first step is to find the right muscles. Imagine that you are trying to stop yourself from passing gas. Squeeze the muscles you would use. If you sense a pulling feeling, those are the right muscles for pelvic exercises.

Try not to squeeze other muscles at the same time. Be careful not to tighten your stomach, legs, or buttocks. Squeezing the wrong muscles can put more pressure on your bladder control muscles. Just squeeze the pelvic muscles. Do not hold your breath.

Repeat, but do not overdo it. At first, find a quiet spot to practice—your bathroom or bedroom—so you can concentrate. Pull in the pelvic muscles and hold for a count of three. Then relax for a count of three. Work up to three sets of ten repeats. Start doing your pelvic muscle exercises lying down. This is the easiest position to do them because the muscles do not need to work against gravity. When your muscles get stronger, do your exercises sitting or standing. Working against gravity is like adding more weight.

Be patient. Don't give up. It takes just five minutes a day. You may not feel your bladder control improve for 3–6 weeks. Still, most people do notice an improvement after a few weeks.

Some people with nerve damage cannot tell whether they are doing Kegel exercises correctly or not. If you are not sure, ask your doctor or nurse to examine you while you try to do them. If it turns out that you are not squeezing the right muscles, you may still be able to learn proper Kegel exercises by doing special training with biofeedback, electrical stimulation, or both.

What are the treatments for lack of coordination between the bladder and urethra?

The job of the sphincter muscles is to hold urine in the bladder by squeezing the urethra shut. If the urethral sphincter fails to stay closed, urine may leak out of the bladder. When nerve signals are coordinated properly, the sphincter muscle relaxes to allow urine to pass through the urethra as the bladder contracts to push out urine. If the signals are not coordinated, the bladder and the sphincter may contract at the same time, so urine cannot pass easily.

Drug therapy for an uncoordinated bladder and urethra: Scientists have not yet found a drug that works selectively on the urethral sphincter muscle, but drugs used to reduce muscle spasms or tremors are sometimes used to help the sphincter relax. Baclofen (Lioresal) is prescribed for muscle spasms or cramping in patients with multiple sclerosis and spinal injuries. Diazepam (Valium) can be taken as a muscle relaxant or to reduce anxiety. Drugs called alpha-adrenergic blockers can also be used to relax the sphincter. Examples of these drugs are alfuzosin (Uroxatral), tamsulosin (Flomax), terazosin (Hytrin), and doxazosin (Cardura). The main side effects are low blood pressure, dizziness, fainting, or nasal congestion. All of these drugs have been used to relax the urethral sphincter in patients where the sphincter does not relax well.

Botox injection: Botulinum toxin type A (Botox) is best known as a cosmetic treatment for facial wrinkles. Doctors have also found that botulinum toxin is useful in blocking spasms like eye ticks or relaxing muscles in patients with multiple sclerosis. Urologists have found that injecting botulinum toxin into the tissue surrounding the sphincter can help the sphincter to relax. Although the FDA has approved botulinum toxin only for facial cosmetic purposes, researchers are studying the safety and effectiveness of botulinum toxin injection into the sphincter for possible FDA approval in the future.

What are the treatments for urine retention?

Urine retention may occur either because the bladder wall muscle cannot contract or because the sphincter muscle cannot relax.

Catheter: A catheter is a thin tube that can be slid through the urethra into the bladder to let urine flow out into a collection bag. If you are able to place the catheter yourself, you can learn to carry out the procedure at regular intervals, a practice called clean intermittent catheterization (CIC). Some patients cannot place their own catheters because nerve damage affects their hand coordination as well as their voiding function. These patients need to have a caregiver place the catheter for them at regular intervals. If this is not feasible, the patients may need to have an indwelling catheter that can be changed less often. Indwelling catheters have several risks, including infection, bladder stones, and bladder tumors. However, if the bladder cannot be emptied any other way, then the catheter is the only way to stop the buildup of urine in the bladder that can damage the kidneys.

Urethral stent: Stents are small tube-like devices inserted into the urethra and allowed to expand, like a spring, widening the opening for urine to flow out. Stents can help prevent urine backup when the bladder wall and sphincter contract at the same time because of improper nerve signals. However, stents can cause problems if they move or lead to infection.

Surgery: Men may consider a surgery that removes the external sphincter (sphincterotomy) or a piece of it (sphincter resection) to prevent urinary retention. The surgeon will pass a thin instrument through the urethra to deliver electrical or laser energy that burns away sphincter tissue. Possible complications include bleeding that requires a transfusion and rarely problems with erections. This procedure causes loss of urine control and requires the patient to collect urine by wearing an external catheter that fits over the penis like a condom. No external collection device is available for women.

Urinary diversion: If other treatments fail and urine regularly backs up and damages the kidneys, the doctor may recommend a urinary diversion, a procedure that may require an outside collection bag attached to a stoma, a surgically created opening where urine passes out of the body. Another form of urinary diversion replaces the bladder with a continent urinary reservoir, an internal pouch made from sections of the bowel or other tissue. This method allows the person to store urine inside the body until a catheter is used to empty it through a stoma.

Hope through Research

The National Institute of Diabetes and Digestive and Kidney Diseases (NIDDK) has many research programs aimed at finding treatments for urinary disorders, including bladder control problems caused by nerve damage. NIDDK-supported researchers have narrowed the search for a gene that causes neurological problems in bladder, bowel, and facial muscles. Finding the gene may lead to greater understanding of how nerves and muscles work together and how nerve damage can cause urination problems.

NIDDK is supporting another team of researchers that is testing an injectable form of oxybutynin, a drug for overactive bladder currently available in pill form. Injections may deliver a more effective and efficient dose of oxybutynin because the drug would not be broken down by the digestive system as the oral form is.

For More Information

American Urological Association Foundation
1000 Corporate Boulevard
Linthicum, MD 21090
Toll-Free: 866-RING-AUA (746-4282)
Phone: 410-689-3990
Fax: 410-689-3800
Website: http://www.urologyhealth.org

National Association for Continence
P.O. Box 1019
Charleston, SC 29402–1019
Toll-Free: 800-BLADDER (252-3337)
Phone: 843-377-0900
Fax: 843-377-0905
Website: http://www.nafc.org
E-mail: memberservices@nafc.org

National Kidney and Urologic Diseases Information Clearinghouse
3 Information Way
Bethesda, MD 20892-3580
Toll-Free: 800-891-5390
Fax: 703-738-4929
Website: http://kidney.niddk.nih.gov
E-mail: nkudic@info.niddk.nih.gov

Chapter 24

Cognitive Deficits in People with MS

Cognition means knowing or perceiving. No matter what you are doing, your nervous system is always trying to provide you with the most complete and accurate picture of reality. Your cognitive processes create and refine this picture, and make it possible for you to use it. Your adjustment in every area of your life depends upon your cognitive abilities because they are what enables you to recognize and understand what is going on around you. You use these adjustments to come up with plans for dealing with changes, and you can come up with ways to put your plans into effect. Judging whether or not your approaches and adaptations worked, remembering them if they did, and then modifying them if they didn't, are all cognitive processes. Every aspect of dealing with MS (as with everything else in your daily life) is based upon the use of your cognitive abilities, therefore it can benefit you to be aware of them.

There is another important benefit to becoming familiar with your cognitive symptoms. These symptoms tend to be extremely sensitive to changes in your level of stress, so they may serve as effective warning signals. Changes in the ways that your cognitive abilities are working may provide some useful clues that you are approaching your limits. Subtle changes in aspects of your cognitive functioning can alert you that you are in danger of exceeding your capacities. Armed with these

---

"Cognitive Deficits in Multiple Sclerosis," by Jennie Q. Lou, M.D., Carolyn Tischenkel, and Lindsey DeLange, reviewed 2005. © Multiple Sclerosis Foundation (www.msfacts.org). Reprinted with permission.

warning signals, you may be able to slow down and readjust, before your established symptoms begin to appear and/or intensify.

The most common cognitive difficulty in people with MS is mild to moderate impairment of short-term and working memory. People who usually have good memories may find themselves forgetting things, such as appointments. Their attention span and ability to concentrate may be diminished. Sometimes they find it hard to keep track of what they were doing before they were interrupted. For example, they may have difficulty getting back on track if the phone rings while they were sorting mail. While these problems can be quite subtle, they can be extremely frustrating and upsetting.

Some people with MS experience more serious cognitive problems. They have difficulty with planning and problem-solving and tend to become overwhelmed and inflexible when a task is too complex. They may lack the flexibility to generate alternative solutions. They may even be unaware of their difficulties and have problems monitoring their own behavior. Comprehension of the impact of their behavior on others may also be overlooked.

Difficulties with the self-regulation of behavior can create problems in many different ways. Some people with MS may be unable to plan and organize purposeful activity. Sometimes the problem is in the area of initiating action. Difficulties with getting started may appear to others as depression or lack of motivation. Other people who have MS may have the opposite problem of being unable to stop themselves. They may be very talkative and uninhibited, blurting out comments they would have kept to themselves in the past. Because they are unresponsive to the normal social clues that let them know their behavior is inappropriate, they seem very impulsive and oblivious to the reactions of others. Furthermore, they may have a short fuse and experience unpredictable angry outbursts.

Cognition involves the coordinated activity of your entire brain. Your cognitive symptoms can result from problems in any part of it. Following is a list of some of the changes in areas of cognitive functioning that people with MS commonly report. Remember, few people have all of these symptoms, and the symptoms come and go.

Simply put, take advantage of the times when your cognitive abilities are working at their best to prepare for the times when they're not. Remember that the pattern of cognitive decline is not uniform. The more frequently impaired areas are recent memory, sustained attention, verbal fluency, conceptual reasoning, and visual-spatial perception. The less frequently impaired areas include language, immediate memory, and remote memory.

Cognitive Difficulties Observed in People with MS

- problems with memory
- excessive drowsiness
- low levels of initiative or motivation
- emotional numbness
- poor mental acuity (fuzzy thinking)
- problems with balance, body awareness, or coordination
- indecisiveness
- problems with planning or organization
- problems with abstract thinking, judgment, or reasoning
- problems understanding what you read or hear
- poor concentration
- distractibility
- tangentiality (your mind wanders, you can't stay on task)
- impulsivity or disinhibition (you can't control or restrain your impulses)
- preservation (you get stuck on a thought, or a behavior)
- problems processing intense, complex, or fast moving sensory input
- problems with recognition (for instance, you can see it, but it doesn't register)
- processing delays (afterimages, trails, ringing in your ears)
- spatial disorientation (you get lost on the way to a familiar place)
- poor reflective awareness (you are not aware, or conscious of yourself)
- poor selective attention (you cannot choose what you want to think about, look at, or listen to)

Furthermore, many of these changes in your cognitive functioning may be evidence of depression. Emotional numbness, excessive drowsiness, poor initiative and motivation, and/or problems with mental acuity can be especially significant signs that someone is

245

depressed. As in most cases of the onset of an illness, depression is a frequent reaction to MS. MS-related lethargy and fatigue may also be confused with depression. You should talk to your doctor or counselor if you feel that your cognitive problems may be indicative of depression. Be assured that medical and alternative treatment options are available to help cope with some difficult feelings. Counseling services are often very accessible.

It is important to remember that when your cognitive abilities are not working well, flare-ups in any of your other symptoms may be more likely. However, you can learn to manage, and reduce disruptive effects on your cognitive abilities.

As with all of your other established symptoms, stress and demand can increase the intensity and frequency of your established cognitive symptoms. You can learn how this process works and how to manage it most effectively. The goal of stress management, and of symptom management, is not to eliminate stress, but to find and maintain the right level of stress that allows you to function at your best. This will allow you to keep your established symptoms at their lowest possible levels of frequency and intensity. The ultimate goal is to prevent them from appearing in the first place.

The majority of people with MS experience intermittent cognitive symptoms and so if you are among this majority, you may be able to achieve the goal of prevention. Even if your cognitive symptoms are present all or most of the time, with the proper approaches to symptom management, you may still be able to control the intensity, and reduce the disruptive effects. The benefits of managing your cognitive symptoms can accumulate over time.

Cognitive symptoms are complex and hard to understand, and they sometimes seem to threaten your grasp of reality. But they are not fundamentally different from any of your other symptoms. Many of these symptoms can be treated very effectively once they are identified. The MS Foundation is available to provide further referrals and information.

Strategies to Maximize Your Function in Your Daily Living

Strategy I: Respect the Complexity of Everyday Tasks

When you look closely at the cognitive demands of any of the tasks that you perform regularly, you may notice that things are more complicated than they appear to be.

There may be a lot of separate steps, or smaller tasks, involved in performing a particular task. Each one of these steps may place demands upon several different aspects of your cognitive functioning. For example, you may have a problem with auditory comprehension. There may be times when you cannot understand what people are saying to you. This could stem from problems with some of the most basic aspects of your cognitive functioning. You may not be able to focus on what the person is saying, or you might be dozing off while they are talking.

By the same token, difficulties with comprehension could be due to problems with aspects of sensory processing abilities, or memory. This would be evident when a person is talking too fast for you, or you cannot remember what they have already said. Problems with higher cognitive processes could also be involved. Maybe the other person is using a lot of complicated statements, or maybe they are talking in very abstract terms.

Remember, efficient cognitive functioning depends upon the coordinated activity of your entire brain, and many, if not most, tasks place demands upon several cognitive abilities at the same time. Even everyday tasks such as cooking can present incredibly complex cognitive demands.

This suggests one of the most important general strategies for dealing with your cognitive deficits: Recognize and respect the cognitive demands of the tasks that you are trying to perform. Often, people with MS say things like: "This is so simple. I never used to have any trouble figuring this out. I must really be stupid." But it is not so simple. Even everyday tasks can make many complicated cognitive demands, and you have to recognize and respect these demands before you can begin to look at the effects of your cognitive symptoms accurately, and begin to compensate for them.

One of the basic principles of managing all of your symptoms is that you cannot take things for granted anymore. You cannot look at the things you do in the old unconscious way that you used to. If you do, chances are you will feel stupid or inadequate. Having cognitive symptoms does not mean that you are stupid, but you may feel as if you are. This is especially true if you underestimate the demands of the tasks that you want to perform.

Strategy II: Stay Conscious of How Well or Poorly You Are Functioning

If you are going to perform a task successfully, you have to be aware not only of the demands of the task, but of your capacity to meet these demands. Those basic aspects of symptom management—observing and rating your abilities—may be even more essential with regard to your cognitive symptoms than in any other area of your functioning. The abilities that are declining are precisely the ones that you need to recognize. Their effectiveness can change very quickly. Noticing the beginnings of decline in your functioning should emphasize the importance of observing warning signals.

In order to effectively adapt activities, you have to develop effective ways of assessing your cognitive abilities. If you wait until your cognitive abilities (the control of your thoughts and behavior, or your ability to think things through) are very weak, it may be too late to do anything about it.

Many of the unnecessary, or preventable, symptom flare-ups that people with MS experience are due to lapses in their cognitive abilities. When the abilities that allow you to recognize that you are reaching your limits are not working well, and you have difficulty making decisions about how you should perform tasks or even if you should perform them at all, it is easy to keep going past your limits.

If you can learn to assess your cognitive abilities, you may be able to recognize when they are starting to fade, and do something to restore them to an effective level. This will allow you to keep any negative effects to a minimum.

Strategy III: Developing Your Survival Tactics

When you cannot prevent your cognitive symptoms from appearing, you have to develop ways to counter their effects. It is possible to develop techniques for enhancing your cognitive abilities, and these techniques may allow you to keep on functioning even during those periods when your cognitive symptoms are affecting you.

Strategy IV: Make the Most of Your Good Periods

A brief look at the list of general strategies and techniques which follow suggests why it is so important to make the most of your good periods. There are a lot of things you can do to deal with your cognitive symptoms and to enhance your cognitive functioning.

Remember, it takes some thought to come up with these things, and it is an effort to put them into effect. But in doing so, your approaches in dealing with your cognitive symptoms will be there for you when you need them, and they are going to be more effective if you've worked on them in advance.

Managing your symptoms presents a number of intense intellectual challenges, so you need to do most of the work during the periods when your cognitive abilities are at their best. Analyzing your experiences and developing and rehearsing your strategies has to take place during your periods of peak functioning. This concept cannot be overemphasized.

When you are in the middle of a demanding situation, and your cognitive symptoms are actually appearing or intensifying in response to it, it is usually pretty hard to keep up with everything that is happening to you. Coming up with new and creative ways to deal with this can be difficult. It is precisely these times when you usually have more urgent priorities like damage control.

If your symptoms catch you off guard, the demands of your efforts to figure out what to do about them can actually make them more intense. This can be a vicious circle. Again, take advantage of your good periods so that you can respond to your symptoms in ways that really can help.

Tips on Enhancing Your Cognitive Function for Daily Living

Externalize Your Cognitive Abilities

- Use post-it notes in areas where you are likely to see them, such as mirrors, television sets, telephones, or the refrigerator.
- Use pocket calendars, palm computers, and timers.

Arrange the Environment Where You Perform Tasks

- Always put things back where they belong.
- Keep items of importance within reach.

Develop and Use Task-Performance Routines

- Make a daily list and write down things that come to mind, and refer to the list frequently during the day.
- Keep a monthly calendar so that you can remember important events such as birthdays.

Adapt or Modify the Ways That You Perform Tasks

- Combine activities that you need to remember with tasks that you already perform everyday (for example, take your medication directly after you finish brushing your teeth).

- Do activities that require going outdoors during the early morning or evening to avoid extremely warm temperatures.

Simplify or Reduce Task Demands

- Prioritize and plan your week.
- Ask friends and family members to assist you.
- Use your inner dialogue.
- Talk to yourself while you are performing the task.
- Say things aloud several times to help you remember things.

Use Feedback from Other People

- Adjust your behavior according to the feedback from your family members or friends.
- Re-evaluate the effects that your productivity has on your work and make changes as needed.

Use Focusing Techniques to Create an Artificial Zone of Good Cognitive Functioning

- Practice yoga.
- Rest and relax before you start a new task.

Chapter 25

Depression in People with MS

"I have had MS for seven years. I think that I have been depressed on and off much of that time. My doctor never asked me about my mood and I never thought I needed any treatment. Recently, at my wife's urging, I saw a social worker who referred me to a psychiatrist. I have been taking an antidepressant for about two months now and seeing the social worker once a week. I feel like a new person." ~ Passage from *Multiple Sclerosis: The Questions You Have—the Answers You Need.*

Why is it that some people suffer from depression and others do not? Is one person a pessimist and the other an optimist? According to researchers and scientists, these oversimplifications are a far cry from the truth.

Does MS cause depression?

Depression can be a reaction to a difficult life situation, such as losing a job, going through a divorce, losing a loved one, or being diagnosed with an incurable disease. It is common among the general population, but even more so among those who have been diagnosed with MS. Some researchers believe that the effect of MS on the central nervous system, and the demyelination in certain parts of the brain contribute to depression. Other evidence suggests that some

"Hope for Depression," © 2005 Multiple Sclerosis Foundation (www.msfacts.org). Reprinted with permission.

people with MS show a dysfunction in the brain mechanisms that help to regulate the hormones involved in mood. Medications often used to treat MS and its symptoms, such as steroids and interferon drugs can contribute to depression. Sleep disturbances and fatigue, both common symptoms of MS, can contribute to depression as well.

When coping with MS, some people find themselves in a perpetual period of adjustment, grieving repeatedly with the onset of each new disability. All of the uncertainty and unpredictability associated with MS can lead to dramatic mood swings. "Adjustment to MS is as complex as it is slow," write Doctors Nicholas LaRocca and Jill Fischer in the book *Multiple Sclerosis: The Questions You Have - the Answers You Need*. "Many factors may influence how a person copes with the illness, including disease course, personality and coping style, the availability of social supports and financial resources, and other concurrent life stresses. A very important factor influencing adjustment is one's self-appraisal. People who view themselves as ineffectual and powerless are likely to adjust differently than those who view themselves as effective and able to manage what life brings them."

"It has been estimated that one out of every seven people with MS is experiencing a major depression," LaRocca and Fischer explain. "Approximately 50 percent of people with MS will experience a major depressive episode during the course of their illness, compared to five percent to fifteen percent in the general population."

Unfortunately, depression in individuals with MS goes undetected and untreated far too often. According to the National Institute of Mental Health (NIMH), half of all Americans still view depression as a character flaw or a personal weakness. As a result, thousands of people suffer needlessly for months or even years, trying to tough it out or shake it off.

Recognizing the Symptoms

Pessimism about the future, loss of self-esteem, shock, disbelief, sadness, anger, fear, and grief are all common reactions to a diagnosis of MS. So how do you know if you are responding "normally" or if you are suffering from depression?

"People who are depressed may lose interest in most of the things that used to be enjoyable, such as hobbies, visiting friends, reading, work-related projects, and sexual activity," writes LaRocca and Fisher. "They may experience loss of appetite or gradually begin eating much more than usual. Sleep may be disturbed by early morning awakening or they may begin wanting to sleep longer or more frequently.

Depression can include feelings of worthlessness and self-blame for everything that seems to be going wrong. Individuals who are depressed may also feel guilty without knowing why, as if they had done something horrible that must be punished. A depressed person's thoughts and actions may be slowed, and behavior may appear listless. However, unlike those who are simply suffering from MS fatigue," the doctors explain, "People who are depressed do not really care about feeling listless because they are not interested in doing anything. The person who is depressed may also be plagued by thoughts of death and even suicide." If you are clinically depressed, the feeling of sadness will be constant, with little or no relief.

There Is Good News

The good news is that depression is treatable. According to the American Psychiatric Association, at least 85 percent of all people with depression can be helped to a significant degree, and early diagnosis and treatment can dramatically reduce the length and intensity of depression.

Sadly, seeking help from a mental health professional still conjures images of Jack Nicholson in *One Flew Over the Cuckoo's Nest*. Seeking psychiatric help doesn't mean you're weak or crazy. In fact, it is a sign of strength and determination, two precious assets in the emotional battle against MS.

Assert Yourself

If you are depressed, don't wait for your neurologist to inquire about your mental health. Take the initiative and bring the subject up yourself. Remember that your neurologist's primary focus is on the physical aspects of your disease. One study found that in a sample of people moderately disabled by MS, 80 percent had experienced some type of psychiatric disorder during the past year. Of those, only 60 percent sought psychiatric treatment. Don't suffer needlessly. Assert yourself and ask for the help you need.

Treatment Options

Psychotherapy and medication, used separately or together, are highly effective in fighting depression. Psychotherapy is usually conducted one-on-one with a qualified psychiatrist, psychologist, or social worker. Finding the right person to talk to is essential. Ask yourself, do I feel comfortable with this person? Do I feel a sense of safety and trust? Is this someone who understands MS? Talk to your doctor, and decide together what course of treatment would be most conducive to your recovery. Research shows that psychotherapy may improve depression in just a few weeks. Substantial, long-lasting results, however, generally take several months. Support groups and peer counseling can be helpful but should be used in addition to private counseling and/or medication.

A variety of antidepressant medications are used successfully to treat depression. Each of these medications can produce slightly different side effects. Prozac, for example, provides a stimulant effect that could improve fatigue. Trazodone, on the other hand, is usually taken at night and often alleviates insomnia. It may take time to establish your ideal treatment plan. If side effects are bothersome after the initial adjustment period, let your doctor know. Changing medications is not uncommon. Be aware that it may take several weeks of medication before you feel any improvement. Then again, you could begin feeling better within a week.

There is hope for depression. Recognize its symptoms in yourself and in others. Assert yourself. Seek treatment. Then you, too, can say, I feel like a new person.

If you are experiencing at least five of the following symptoms, and they have persisted for at least two weeks, you are most likely suffering from depression.

- sadness, nearly all day, nearly every day

- loss of interest or pleasure in everyday activities

- loss of appetite or increased appetite

- sleep disturbances (insomnia, excessive sleeping, or nightmares)

- feelings of worthlessness or guilt

- persistent thoughts of death or suicide

- hopelessness

- violence or outbursts of rage

- inability to think or concentrate

Chapter 26

Pregnancy Concerns for Women with MS

The Decision

The decision to start a family is a life-changing one. For any couple, it is difficult to speculate how their relationship, employment, and financial status might change over the years. Speculation is a gamble and there are no guarantees. For those couples that must factor in the additional uncertainties of MS, both speculation and decision-making grow more complex. Nevertheless, there are steps that you and your partner can take that will enable you to make intelligent and realistic decisions.

Ideally, the decision to start a family should be a team effort. Parenting is a lifetime commitment and thoughtful consideration must be given to the various challenges that could arise as a result of MS. Worsening disability could change your financial status. Fatigue could be troublesome, particularly when caring for a baby or toddler.

With a little flexibility and a creative, proactive approach on the part of both parents, solutions to these and similar problems are within reach. For example, if you were not well for a period of time, would your partner be willing to take over household chores and parenting responsibilities as needed? Do you have caring friends or family members nearby to offer support and assistance throughout your labor, delivery, and postpartum period? Having a support system in place can make a tremendous difference.

"Pregnancy for Women with Multiple Sclerosis," © 2005 Multiple Sclerosis Foundation (www.msfacts.org). Reprinted with permission.

Attend a local MS support group meeting. Talk and listen to others who are successfully parenting with MS. What are their challenges? How are they handling them? What have they learned?

Together with your partner, visit your neurologist and discuss current disease activity and possible progression. Ask questions. In her book, *Multiple Sclerosis: The Questions You Have - The Answers You Need*, Rosalind Kalb, Ph.D. writes, "Historically (and occasionally even now), couples have found that some members of the medical profession discourage pregnancy, and even parenting for a woman who has MS. We now know that there is no medical reason for women with MS to avoid pregnancy." If you decide to start a family and your neurologist is not supportive, find another one. A supportive obstetrician is also important. As a team, these professionals can provide the care and encouragement that you and your baby deserve.

Will my baby develop MS?

The risk of your child developing MS, although higher than the general population, still remains low. "While there is some increase in the risk to children with a family history of the disease, the actual risk is small (95 percent chance that MS will not occur). At the present time there is no way to diagnose MS or assess the MS risk in a particular infant before or after birth," asserts Dr. Kalb.

Will MS affect my pregnancy?

Statistics show that only ten percent of women experience relapses during their nine months of pregnancy. Research indicates that women with MS who give birth show no signs of increased disability over their lifetime than women with MS who never become pregnant. One study even suggests that women with MS who become pregnant may be less likely to develop a progressive course of the disease when compared to women with MS who choose to forego having children.

For reasons still not entirely understood, pregnancy allows the body to enter a mildly immunosuppressive state. This means that during pregnancy, a woman naturally achieves the immunosuppressive state that is usually achieved artificially with some medications. This could be the reason for reduced disease activity during pregnancy. Many women with MS feel exceptionally well, especially during their third trimester, when relapse rates are at an all-time low.

On the other hand, fatigue—especially during the first three months, constipation, and urinary tract infections may be bothersome for some women. Your obstetrician may suggest using a stool softener to alleviate constipation or having regular urine cultures to detect potential infections.

Can I take medication?

Generally, there are two categories of medication used to treat MS. There are those that are used to treat symptoms, such as bladder infections. These medications are often safe to continue during pregnancy, but always check with your doctor first. Then there are the immunomodulating agents that actually reduce disease activity. These include Avonex®, Betaseron®, Copaxone®, and Rebif®, commonly called the ABCR drugs. The safety of these drugs during pregnancy, as well as their affect on the unborn baby, has yet to be determined. Recent research in animals suggests that Copaxone may carry a reduced risk to the fetus. More research is needed, however, to determine the effects of these drugs on the unborn human child. There is also some concern that these drugs could increase the risk of miscarriage.

As soon as you begin trying to conceive, talk with your doctor about your medications. Unless you plan to breastfeed your baby, you may, with your doctor's consent, resume your medication immediately after delivery.

Will MS influence my labor and delivery?

MS does not appear to influence the course of pregnancy, labor, or delivery. In fact, there is no reason to expect your labor to be significantly different from that of a woman without MS. An injection of anesthetic into the lumbar area of the spine (an epidural) to alleviate pain during labor is common and usually safe. General anesthesia is also considered safe. Many couples enroll in prenatal classes, or practice the Lamaze technique. This breathing and relaxation method has been widely practiced since the early 1950s. Meet with your doctor or anesthesiologist to explore your options.

Women with substantial lack of sensation or paralysis may be closely monitored during the ninth month, just in case they are unable to recognize the onset of contractions or need labor to be induced after dilation of the cervix begins. Should muscle weakness or fatigue occur after several hours of pushing, the delivery may be assisted with forceps, a suction cup on the baby's head, or a Caesarian section. If leg control or spasticity is a problem, an epidural can be beneficial.

Inform your obstetrician of any steroid use, particularly over the past twelve months. If you have taken steroids on a regular basis during that time, you will need steroid medication during labor.

What about the postpartum period?

Careful planning for the postpartum period can minimize stress, fatigue, and your risk of having an exacerbation. Exhaustion is typical for new mothers, but a new mother with MS must not ignore this fatigue. It is important to focus only on caring for yourself, resting, and feeding your new baby. Other household tasks, shopping, social events, and even some of the infant care should be delegated to others.

During the initial six months after delivery, 29 percent of women will experience a relapse. Due to this heightened risk, you may choose to start or restart one of the immunomodulating drugs right after your baby is born. If you are employed outside the home, you may require a longer maternity leave than the average six- to eight-week period that is customary in the U.S., because relapses occur most frequently between the fourth and eighth week of the postpartum period.

In the book, *Mother To Be: A Guide to Pregnancy and Birth For Women with Disabilities*, Judith Rogers and Molleen Matsumura interviewed Margie, a 27 year-old woman with MS, to discover the changes she experienced throughout her pregnancy, labor, delivery, and postpartum period.

"Margie had MS before she became pregnant. Her symptoms before pregnancy were weakness in the arm and leg on one side, and occasional bladder problems. About her first pregnancy Margie said, 'I felt great while I was pregnant. I enjoyed feeling so healthy, and I had a positive outlook on life'."

The authors go on to explain that, "After her first pregnancy, Margie's MS worsened slightly. Her main problem was blurred vision. After her second pregnancy, she made sure she had extra help, and there was no exacerbation of MS."

Should I breastfeed my baby?

"Historically, neurologists have discouraged women with MS from nursing, feeling that it posed an additional physical burden to a woman already at increased risk for an exacerbation," writes Dr. Kalb. "However nursing is now widely encouraged if you have adequate dexterity, strength, and stamina."

Breast milk not only provides optimal nutrition, but also eliminates the nuisance of bottle preparation. If you do choose to breastfeed, be consistent with all feedings during the first two weeks. This should generate a steady and sufficient milk flow. After this initial period, you can pump and store your milk or use formula so that your partner can handle the nighttime feedings. This is the best way for you to get the sufficient, uninterrupted rest that is so crucial for a new mother with MS. According to current medical information, there is no elevated risk of exacerbation caused by breastfeeding.

It is important to realize, though, that breastfeeding can be tiring. For women whose symptoms are exacerbated by fatigue, this could be a deciding factor. On the other hand, some women feel that breastfeeding is less demanding than bottle-feeding. Talk it over with your partner, your obstetrician, your neurologist, or a lactation consultant at your local hospital.

A Final Word

Make sufficient rest top priority from conception through the postpartum period. Proper nutrition and some form of physical activity are also important. Strive to communicate openly and honestly with your partner. Establish a support network before the baby arrives. Be flexible in terms of parental and domestic responsibilities. Things may not always be done exactly the way you would do them yourself, but they will be done. Let that suffice. Your health and the health of your child are far more important than any domestic chore.

Rather than ignoring the existence of your disease, acknowledge it in all its unpredictability and plan accordingly. Many of the things you plan for may never come to pass. Nevertheless, preparedness now will reduce stress and fatigue later, granting you and your partner ample time to delight in your new baby.

Part Three

Diagnostic Tests, Treatments, and Therapies for Multiple Sclerosis

Chapter 27

Neurological Diagnostic Tests and Procedures

Diagnostic tests and procedures are vital tools that help physicians confirm or rule out the presence of a neurological disorder or other medical condition. A century ago, the only way to make a positive diagnosis for many neurological disorders was by performing an autopsy after a patient had died. But decades of basic research into the characteristics of disease, and the development of techniques that allow scientists to see inside the living brain and monitor nervous system activity as it occurs, have given doctors powerful and accurate tools to diagnose disease and to test how well a particular therapy may be working.

Perhaps the most significant changes in diagnostic imaging over the past 20 years are improvements in spatial resolution (size, intensity, and clarity) of anatomical images and reductions in the time needed to send signals to and receive data from the area being imaged. These advances allow physicians to simultaneously see the structure of the brain and the changes in brain activity as they occur. Scientists continue to improve methods that will provide sharper anatomical images and more detailed functional information.

Researchers and physicians use a variety of diagnostic imaging techniques and chemical and metabolic analyses to detect, manage, and treat neurological disease. Some procedures are performed in specialized settings, conducted to determine the presence of a particular

Excerpted from "Neurological Diagnostic Tests and Procedures," National Institute of Neurological Disorders and Stroke (NINDS), NIH Publication No. 05–5380, updated December 2006.

disorder or abnormality. Many tests that were previously conducted in a hospital are now performed in a physician's office or at an outpatient testing facility with little if any risk to the patient. Depending on the type of procedure, results are either immediate or may take several hours to process.

What are some of the more common screening tests?

Laboratory screening tests of blood, urine, or other substances are used to help diagnose disease, better understand the disease process, and monitor levels of therapeutic drugs. Certain tests, ordered by the physician as part of a regular check-up, provide general information, while others are used to identify specific health concerns. For example, blood and blood product tests can detect brain or spinal cord infection, bone marrow disease, hemorrhage, blood vessel damage, toxins that affect the nervous system, and the presence of antibodies that signal the presence of an autoimmune disease.

- Blood tests are also used to monitor levels of therapeutic drugs used to treat epilepsy and other neurological disorders.

- Genetic testing of deoxyribonucleic acid (DNA) extracted from white cells in the blood can help diagnose Huntington disease and other congenital diseases.

- Analysis of the fluid that surrounds the brain and spinal cord can detect meningitis, acute and chronic inflammation, rare infections, and some cases of multiple sclerosis.

- Chemical and metabolic testing of the blood can indicate protein disorders, some forms of muscular dystrophy and other muscle disorders, and diabetes.

- Urinalysis can reveal abnormal substances in the urine or the presence or absence of certain proteins that cause diseases including the mucopolysaccharidoses.

What is a neurological examination?

A neurological examination assesses motor and sensory skills, the functioning of one or more cranial nerves, hearing and speech, vision, coordination and balance, mental status, and changes in mood or behavior, among other abilities. Items including a tuning fork, flashlight, reflex hammer, ophthalmoscope, and needles are used to help diagnose brain tumors, infections such as encephalitis and meningitis, and

264

diseases such as Parkinson disease, Huntington disease, amyotrophic lateral sclerosis (ALS), and epilepsy. Some tests require the services of a specialist to perform and analyze results.

X-rays of the patient's chest and skull are often taken as part of a neurological work-up. X-rays can be used to view any part of the body, such as a joint or major organ system. In a conventional x-ray, also called a radiograph, a technician passes a concentrated burst of low-dose ionized radiation through the body and onto a photographic plate. Since calcium in bones absorbs x-rays more easily than soft tissue or muscle, the bony structure appears white on the film. Any vertebral misalignment or fractures can be seen within minutes. Tissue masses such as injured ligaments or a bulging disc are not visible on conventional x-rays. This fast, noninvasive, painless procedure is usually performed in a doctor's office or at a clinic.

Fluoroscopy is a type of x-ray that uses a continuous or pulsed beam of low-dose radiation to produce continuous images of a body part in motion. The fluoroscope (x-ray tube) is focused on the area of interest and pictures are either videotaped or sent to a monitor for viewing. A contrast medium may be used to highlight the images. Fluoroscopy can be used to evaluate the flow of blood through arteries.

What are some diagnostic tests used to diagnose neurological disorders?

Based on the result of a neurological exam, physical exam, patient history, x-rays of the patient's chest and skull, and any previous screening or testing, physicians may order one or more of the following diagnostic tests to determine the specific nature of a suspected neurological disorder or injury. These diagnostics generally involve either nuclear medicine imaging, in which very small amounts of radioactive materials are used to study organ function and structure, or diagnostic imaging, which uses magnets and electrical charges to study human anatomy.

The following list of available procedures—in alphabetical rather than sequential order—includes some of the more common tests used to help diagnose a neurological condition.

Angiography is a test used to detect blockages of the arteries or veins. A cerebral angiogram can detect the degree of narrowing or obstruction of an artery or blood vessel in the brain, head, or neck. It is used to diagnose stroke and to determine the location and size of a brain tumor, aneurysm, or vascular malformation. This test is usually performed in a hospital outpatient setting and takes up to three hours, followed by a 6- to 8-hour resting period.

Biopsy involves the removal and examination of a small piece of tissue from the body. Muscle or nerve biopsies are used to diagnose neuromuscular disorders and may also reveal if a person is a carrier of a defective gene that could be passed on to children. A small sample of muscle or nerve is removed under local anesthetic and studied under a microscope.

Brain scans are imaging techniques used to diagnose tumors, blood vessel malformations, or hemorrhage in the brain. These scans are used to study organ function or injury or disease to tissue or muscle. Types of brain scans include computed tomography, magnetic resonance imaging, and positron emission tomography.

Cerebrospinal fluid analysis involves the removal of a small amount of the fluid that protects the brain and spinal cord. The fluid is tested to detect any bleeding or brain hemorrhage, diagnose infection to the brain or spinal cord, identify some cases of multiple sclerosis and other neurological conditions, and measure intracranial pressure. The procedure is usually done in a hospital. The sample of fluid is commonly removed by a procedure known as a lumbar puncture, or spinal tap. A common after-effect of a lumbar puncture is headache, which can be lessened by having the patient lie flat. The entire procedure takes about 45 minutes.

Computed tomography, also known as a CT scan, is a noninvasive, painless process used to produce rapid, clear two-dimensional images of organs, bones, and tissues. Neurological CT scans are used to view the brain and spine. They can detect bone and vascular irregularities, certain brain tumors and cysts, herniated discs, epilepsy, encephalitis, spinal stenosis (narrowing of the spinal canal), a blood clot or intracranial bleeding in patients with stroke, brain damage from head injury, and other disorders. Many neurological disorders share certain characteristics and a CT scan can aid in proper diagnosis by differentiating the area of the brain affected by the disorder.

Intrathecal contrast-enhanced CT scan (also called cisternography) is used to detect problems with the spine and spinal nerve roots. This test is most often performed at an imaging center. The patient is asked to put on a hospital or imaging gown. Following application of a topical anesthetic, the physician removes a small sample of the spinal fluid via lumbar puncture. The sample is mixed with a contrast dye and injected into the spinal sac located at the base of the lower back. The patient is then asked to move to a position that will allow the contrast fluid to travel to the area to be studied. The dye allows the spinal canal and nerve roots to be seen more clearly on a CT scan. The scan may take up to an hour to complete. Following the test, patients may experience some discomfort and/or headache that may be caused by the removal of spinal fluid.

Electroencephalography, or EEG, monitors brain activity through the skull. EEG is used to help diagnose certain seizure disorders, brain tumors, brain damage from head injuries, inflammation of the brain or spinal cord, alcoholism, certain psychiatric disorders, and metabolic and degenerative disorders that affect the brain. EEG is also used to evaluate sleep disorders, monitor brain activity when a patient has been fully anesthetized or loses consciousness, and confirm brain death.

Electromyography, or EMG, is used to diagnose nerve and muscle dysfunction and spinal cord disease. It records the electrical activity from the brain and spinal cord to a peripheral nerve root (found in the arms and legs) that controls muscles during contraction and at rest.

An EMG is usually done in conjunction with a nerve conduction velocity (NCV) test, which measures electrical energy by assessing the nerve's ability to send a signal. This two-part test is conducted most often in a hospital.

Electronystagmography (ENG) describes a group of tests used to diagnose involuntary eye movement, dizziness, and balance disorders, and to evaluate some brain functions. The test is performed at an imaging center. Small electrodes are taped around the eyes to record eye movements. If infrared photography is used in place of electrodes, the patient wears special goggles that help record the information. Both versions of the test are painless and risk-free.

Evoked potentials (also called evoked response) measure the electrical signals to the brain generated by hearing, touch, or sight. These tests are used to assess sensory nerve problems and confirm neurological conditions including multiple sclerosis, brain tumor, acoustic neuroma (small tumors of the inner ear), and spinal cord injury. Evoked potentials are also used to test sight and hearing (especially in infants and young children), monitor brain activity among coma patients, and confirm brain death.

Testing may take place in a doctor's office or hospital setting. It is painless and risk-free. Two sets of needle electrodes are used to test for nerve damage. One set of electrodes, which will be used to measure the electrophysiological response to stimuli, is attached to the patient's scalp using conducting paste. The second set of electrodes is attached to the part of the body to be tested. The physician then records the amount of time it takes for the impulse generated by stimuli to reach the brain. Under normal circumstances, the process of signal transmission is instantaneous.

Visual evoked potentials detect loss of vision from optic nerve damage (in particular, damage caused by multiple sclerosis). The patient sits close to a screen and is asked to focus on the center of a shifting checkerboard pattern. Only one eye is tested at a time; the other eye is either kept closed or covered with a patch. Each eye is usually tested twice. Testing takes 30–45 minutes.

Somatosensory evoked potentials measure response from stimuli to the peripheral nerves and can detect nerve or spinal cord damage or nerve degeneration from multiple sclerosis and other degenerating diseases. Tiny electrical shocks are delivered by electrode to a nerve in an arm or leg. Responses to the shocks, which may be delivered for more than a minute at a time, are recorded. This test usually lasts less than an hour.

Magnetic resonance imaging (MRI) uses computer-generated radio waves and a powerful magnetic field to produce detailed images of body structures including tissues, organs, bones, and nerves. Neurological uses include the diagnosis of brain and spinal cord tumors, eye disease, inflammation, infection, and vascular irregularities that may lead to stroke. MRI can also detect and monitor degenerative disorders such as multiple sclerosis and can document brain injury from trauma.

Functional MRI (fMRI) uses the blood's magnetic properties to produce real-time images of blood flow to particular areas of the brain. An fMRI can pinpoint areas of the brain that become active and note how long they stay active. It can also tell if brain activity within a region occurs simultaneously or sequentially. This imaging process is used to assess brain damage from head injury or degenerative disorders such as Alzheimer's disease and to identify and monitor other neurological disorders, including multiple sclerosis, stroke, and brain tumors.

Positron emission tomography (PET) scans provide two- and three-dimensional pictures of brain activity by measuring radioactive isotopes that are injected into the bloodstream. PET scans of the brain are used to detect or highlight tumors and diseased tissue, measure cellular and tissue metabolism, show blood flow, evaluate patients who have seizure disorders that do not respond to medical therapy and patients with certain memory disorders, and determine brain changes following injury or drug abuse, among other uses. PET may be ordered as a follow-up to a CT or MRI scan to give the physician a greater understanding of specific areas of the brain that may be involved with certain problems.

Single photon emission computed tomography (SPECT), a nuclear imaging test involving blood flow to tissue, is used to evaluate certain brain functions. The test may be ordered as a follow-up to an MRI to diagnose tumors, infections, degenerative spinal disease, and stress fractures.

Thermography uses infrared sensing devices to measure small temperature changes between the two sides of the body or within a specific organ. Also known as digital infrared thermal imaging, thermography may be used to detect vascular disease of the head and neck, soft tissue injury, various neuromusculoskeletal disorders, and the presence or absence of nerve root compression. It is performed at an imaging center, using infrared light recorders to take thousands of pictures of the body from a distance of 5 to 8 feet. The information is converted into electrical signals which results in a computer-generated two-dimensional picture of abnormally cold or hot areas indicated by color or shades of black and white. Thermography does not use radiation and is safe, risk-free, and noninvasive.

Ultrasound imaging, also called ultrasound scanning or sonography, uses high-frequency sound waves to obtain images inside the body. Neurosonography (ultrasound of the brain and spinal column) analyzes blood flow in the brain and can diagnose stroke, brain tumors, hydrocephalus (build-up of cerebrospinal fluid in the brain), and vascular problems. It can also identify or rule out inflammatory processes causing pain. It is more effective than an x-ray in displaying soft tissue masses and can show tears in ligaments, muscles, tendons, and other soft tissue masses in the back. Transcranial Doppler ultrasound is used to view arteries and blood vessels in the neck and determine blood flow and risk of stroke.

Chapter 28

The MS Health Care Team

The multiple sclerosis (MS) team of caregivers generally consists of:

- neurologists,
- neuropsychologists,
- nurses,
- social workers,
- psychologists,
- occupational therapists,
- physical therapists,
- vocational rehabilitation specialists,
- registered dietitians,
- speech-language pathologists.

Neurologists

A neurologist is a medical specialist trained to evaluate problems of the nervous system, including the symptoms of MS. Neurologists have an in-depth understanding of the central nervous system and

"Multiple Sclerosis Caregiving Team," © 2007 The Cleveland Clinic Foundation, 9500 Euclid Avenue, Cleveland, OH 44195, www.clevelandclinic.org. Additional information is available from the Cleveland Clinic Health Information Center, 216-444-3771, toll-free 800-223-2273 extension 43771, or at http://www.clevelandclinic.org/health.

how it is affected by multiple sclerosis. Ideally, it is helpful if the neurologist is affiliated with an MS center, research facility, or a teaching hospital. Neurologists:

- diagnose MS;

- make recommendations for treatment, testing, and symptom management; and,

- are available to answer your medical questions, sign forms, fill prescriptions, and provide help with disability-related issues.

A consulting neurologist makes recommendations to your local doctor or neurologist for treatment, testing, and symptom management.

Neuropsychologists

Neuropsychologists specialize in memory, problem-solving, and other cognitive problems. They can evaluate and diagnose people with MS so they can seek the appropriate treatment. Neuropsychologists might offer cognitive rehabilitation exercises to improve memory, attention, information processing, and reasoning. All of these functions might become slowed due to the process of demyelination in the brain.

Nurses

Nurses possess a broad range of experience in advanced practice nursing, research, and treatment procedures. Advanced practice nurses (APN) are clinical nurse specialists, nurse practitioners, and registered nurses with additional education (certification or master's degree) and expertise in a specialty area or clinical practice.

Working independently and in collaboration with a doctor, advanced practice nurses are able to provide a wide variety of services. Advanced practice nurses who treat people with MS provide many health services including:

- patient and family education about MS and related problems;

- ongoing assessment and management of MS symptoms;

- counseling on general health maintenance and wellness;

- information about medicines and monitoring side effects;

- education in the management of bowel, bladder, or other personal care issues;

- guidance in determining when change might be needed in the treatment plan;

- administration and monitoring of medicines according to treatment and research protocol;

- coordination of outpatient care with home care services;

- consultation to health team members as well as outside providers; and,

- speaking at community programs about MS and related topics.

Social Workers

Social workers provide personal support to people with MS and their families by offering:

- short-term counseling and referrals for ongoing counseling;

- information about home care assistance services and assistive devices;

- recommendations of community resources, and local and national agencies that offer both information and support for people with MS and their families;

- financial resource information such as Social Security disability, supplemental security income, Medicaid, Waiver 4, and PASSPORT financial assistance programs;

- information about quality of life issues including living wills and durable power of attorney for health care.

Psychologists

Psychologists are available to help people with MS cope with the cognitive, emotional, and interpersonal aspects of the disease. They offer:

- psychological evaluation of emotional and interpersonal problems;

- individual psychological counseling sessions to reduce emotional distress and improve stress management skills;

- group psychological counseling to develop strategies for coping with the illness and the resulting life changes;

- neuropsychological testing to determine if MS is affecting cognitive functions such as attention or memory.

Occupational Therapists

Occupational therapists analyze how MS affects the way people perform their daily tasks, help them learn new ways to do familiar activities, and prescribe proper seating as needed. Occupational therapists assist individuals in maximizing their level of functional independence. They offer:

- Individualized treatment through appropriate exercise and adaptive equipment, following an accurate assessment of each patient's current level of functional performance.

- Ongoing evaluation and appropriate treatment strategies to optimize the range of motion and muscle strength of patients' upper extremities (arms and hands) to help them successfully complete activities of daily living such as dressing, eating, toileting, and bathing.

Physical Therapists

Physical therapists are available to assess muscle strength, flexibility, coordination, balance, endurance, walking ability, and mobility. They specialize in:

- improving function and providing instruction on managing physical disabilities;

- recommending appropriate exercises to maintain flexibility while preventing and reducing pain;

- providing instruction regarding the use of assistive devices, braces, or other mobility aids to maximize independence.

Vocational Rehabilitation Specialists

A satisfying work life is as important to the person with MS as to anyone. For people with MS, finding work that matches their skills, interests, and abilities can be especially challenging.

Vocational rehabilitation specialists assist individuals with:

- recognizing their skills and abilities;
- exploring new careers;
- locating jobs;
- preparing for interviews;
- developing safe work sites;

- coping with work-related issues; and,

- learning the many resources available for making career choices.

Assessing an individual's needs is the first step in vocational rehabilitation. Information from the assessment helps the patient and the counselor make the best use of vocational services. During the initial interview, a counselor reviews the person's educational, work, and medical histories and assesses any factors that might affect his or her ability to work. A vocational evaluation also measures the person's general abilities, and specific needs and interests. After the consultation, the individual might be referred to other services or community resources.

Registered Dietitians

Registered dietitians provide nutritional counseling through diet management to promote good nutrition while preventing malnutrition. They are available to:

- assess each patient's nutritional needs based upon the progression of the disease;

- recommend changes in each patient's diet to assist in the treatment of MS;

- develop individual care plans for each patient to promote a good nutritional status;

- if necessary, provide calorie and protein supplements to increase daily caloric and nutrient consumption; and,

- adapt the consistency of foods and liquids if swallowing becomes difficult.

Speech-Language Pathologists

Speech-language pathologists can help people with MS maintain as many verbal communication skills as possible. They also teach techniques that conserve energy, including non-verbal communication.
The speech-language pathologists are available to:

- evaluate and treat speech disorders and communication problems;

- assess swallowing problems to provide assistance with eating and drinking; and,

- recommend appropriate communication technologies to provide treatment that will aid in the success of daily activities.

Chapter 29

Benign MS Treatment: Taking a Wait-and-See Approach

One of the biggest challenges faced by clinicians who treat patients with multiple sclerosis (MS) is the variability and unpredictability of the disease course. Should all MS patients be treated with disease-modifying agents right away? Or are there some instances where a "wait-and-see" approach would be the best course to pursue?

The current trend among neurologists is to treat all cases of relapsing-remitting MS with immunomodulatory medications as early as possible. A National Multiple Sclerosis Society consensus statement[1] (updated in February of 2005) recommends initiation of a disease-modifying agent as soon as possible following a definite diagnosis of MS with a relapsing course, and in selected patients with a first attack who are at high risk for MS.

But what about patients whose disease appears to follow a benign course? Although various definitions of benign MS exist, it is generally described as disease that is present for ten or more years with little or no disability. Although patients may experience MS-related symptoms, the disease does not restrict their activities of daily living.[2]

The Olmsted County MS Prevalence Cohort

"Regardless of the definition used," said Sean J. Pittock, M.D. of the Department of Neurology, Mayo Clinic, in Rochester, Minnesota,

"To Treat or Not to Treat? The Controversy Over Benign MS," *MS Exchange*, May 2006. © 2006 Consortium of Multiple Sclerosis Centers. Reprinted with permission.

"the question remains as to whether these patients should be treated with immunomodulatory therapies."

In a 2004 article in the *Annals of Neurology*, [3] Dr. Pittock et al. reported the results of a natural history study of MS patients in Minnesota. In 2001, the researchers followed up all patients from the 1991 Olmsted County MS prevalence cohort. "We identified patients who had had MS for 10 years or more in 1991. At follow-up, they had had MS for at least 20 years," remarked Dr. Pittock.

Although many of the patients were still doing well, some had developed disability. "We wanted to determine whether there was a way to predict which patients with so-called benign MS would eventually reach a level of significant disability," he explained.

In an effort to develop a method for predicting future disability, Dr. Pittock and colleagues divided the patients into two groups: those with Expanded Disability Status Scale (EDSS) scores between 0 and 2 and those with EDSS scores of 2.5 to 4.0 in 1991. Among the key findings of the study:

- Patients with EDSS scores of two or lower and a disease duration of at least ten years had a 93% chance of continuing to have low disability in the second decade.

- Patients with EDSS scores of 2.5 to 4.0 for at least ten years had a 43% chance of continuing to have low disability in the second decade.

- Those with motor pathway deficit at onset were significantly less likely to be in the mild group after 20 years. (No other differences between groups were found.)

Based on these results, Dr. Pittock and colleagues proposed that benign MS be defined as "patients with MS for ten years or more who have EDSS score of two or less because they have a less than 10% likelihood of developing significant disability." According to this study, patients with benign MS make up 17% of all MS patients.

"There are currently about 211,000 MS patients in the United States," stated Dr. Pittock. "If 17% of those patients have benign MS, that would mean about 36,000 patients may not need to be taking an injectable drug every week for the rest of their lives."

Taking a Reasonable Approach?

How can neurologists identify which newly diagnosed patients are likely to follow a benign disease course? "When a patient is first diagnosed with MS, the duration of the disease from onset is often less than ten years. As a result, it is difficult for clinicians to predict long-term disability," explained Dr. Pittock. However, he added, it is not uncommon for a clinician taking the history of a patient presenting with a first MS attack to find that he or she had symptoms suggestive of an attack (visual blurring, hemisensory loss, etc.) several years earlier. "Thus, the clinician is provided information of the natural course and duration of disease for that particular patient.

"For example, a patient might present with symptoms suggestive of a spinal cord attack with weakness or sensory loss in the lower extremities that resolved after four weeks. The neurologist learns from the patient's history that he or she had a brief episode of left-sided facial numbness ten years prior to the current episode but never saw a clinician," said Dr. Pittock. "The neurologic examination reveals minimal abnormalities. A brain magnetic resonance image (MRI) shows several signal abnormalities consistent with MS but no enhancing lesions."

These are the kinds of patients for whom he would recommend a "wait and see" approach to treatment. "For some patients, the automatic commencement of medication may not be the best thing."

However, which treatment approach should be used for patients presenting with their first attack if the clinician has no clear knowledge of the disease course over time? A recent issue of *Archives of Neurology* contained two articles on the controversy over whether to begin early treatment of benign MS. In one article, Dr. Pittock elaborated on his suggested approach to treating such patients:[4] "Until it is clear that the patient has continuing disease activity clinically and/or radiographically, in which case the need for treatment is clear to the clinician and to the patient, it is advisable to observe a period of no treatment while monitoring for inflammatory disease activity."

MS Studies Advocating Early Treatment

Dr. Pittock also discussed the "Controlled High Risk Avonex® Multiple Sclerosis (CHAMPS)" trial and the "Early Treatment of MS" study. These studies demonstrated that treatment with interferon beta-1a reduces the likelihood of conversion to clinically definite MS within two years of a clinically isolated syndrome (CIS).[5, 6]

"However," he pointed out, "there is no evidence that delaying the second attack has any long-term effect on disability. Based on CHAMPS, seven patients need to be treated to prevent one person from developing clinically definite MS within three years." Additionally, more than half of placebo-treated patients in both studies did not have a second attack during the two- to three-year follow-up. Those who did convert to clinically definite MS usually did so during the first year, suggesting that a brief observation period could adequately identify those who most need treatment.

Dr. Pittock also noted that approximately 50% of interferon beta-1a–treated patients still demonstrated clinical or MRI evidence of active disease during the initial 18 months of the CHAMPS trial. "The incomplete benefit from early interferon treatment is shown by this finding," he stated.

"At the Mayo Clinic, we treat most, but not all, of our relapsing-remitting MS patients with disease-modifying therapy. Treating all patients with a diagnosis of MS or CIS immediately with disease-modifying drugs overlooks an important subset of MS patients who may not need to go through the monetary costs and side effects of injecting themselves with medicines for the rest of their lives," he explained. "The final decision about whether and when to initiate treatment should be shared by the patient and clinician after an unbiased review of the relevant information.

References

1. The National Multiple Sclerosis Society's Disease Management Consensus Statement Summary. Available at: www.nationalmssociety .org/Sourcebook-Early.asp. Accessed April 13, 2006.

2. McAlpine D. The benign form of multiple sclerosis. A study based on 241 cases seen within three years of onset and followed up until the tenth year or more of the disease. *Brain.* 1961;84:186–203.

3. Pittock SJ, McClelland RL, Mayr WT, et al. Clinical implications of benign multiple sclerosis: a 20-year population- based follow-up study. *Ann Neurol.* 2004; 56:303–306.

4. Pittock SJ, Weinshenker BG, Noseworthy JH, et al. Not every patient with multiple sclerosis should be treated at time of diagnosis. *Arch Neurol.* 2006;63:611–614.

5. Jacobs LD, Beck RW, Simon JH, et al. Intramuscular interferon beta-1a therapy initiated during a first demyelinating event in multiple sclerosis. CHAMPS Study Group. *N Engl J Med.* 2000;343:898–904.

6. Comi G, Filippi M, Barkhof F, et al. Effect of early interferon treatment on conversion to definite multiple sclerosis: a randomised study. *Lancet.* 2001;357:1576–1582.

Chapter 30

Drug Treatments and Therapies for MS

Chapter Contents

Section 30.1

Treating Exacerbations and Relapses

Excerpted from *Multiple Sclerosis: The Process and Medical Treatments, Fourth Edition*, © 2002 Multiple Sclerosis Association of America. All rights reserved. Reprinted with permission. Reviewed in June 2007 by Dr. David A. Cooke, M.D., Diplomate, American Board of Internal Medicine.

How Multiple Sclerosis (MS) Treatments Are Approached

Physicians and researchers approach the treatment of MS in three ways:

1. The first approach is to treat an exacerbation, usually with a high-dose, short-term, powerful drug such as a corticosteroid. The goals are to (1) reduce the severity and duration of the relapse by decreasing inflammation, and (2) potentially minimize any permanent damage resulting from the attack.

2. The second approach is an attempt to slow or stop disease activity and progression. Trials in this area are normally conducted with drugs that affect the immune system and may be tolerated for prolonged periods of time. Surgical techniques and even complex alterations to the blood are also under investigation.

3. The third approach uses drugs and therapies to manage MS symptoms.

The ultimate goal is to cure the disorder and repair any damage to the myelin and axons. Trials are presently underway to study the potential of transplanted remyelinating cells to grow new myelin within MS lesions.

Without a definitive cause or cure, finding the best treatment for MS is challenging. Drug therapies available today for MS have limited efficacy, but they do show positive results. For the first time, individuals with MS may now choose from five different approved drug therapies.

In the past, these drugs were only available to those with relapsing-remitting multiple sclerosis (RRMS), but now people with progressive disease forms have choices too. More options are anticipated in the near future, but trials for MS treatments require several years to test dosages, side effects, and overall success.

Administering Drugs

Drug treatments are usually administered either orally (by mouth) or by injection. Injections may be performed in one of four ways:

1. **Intrathecally (IT):** By making a lumbar puncture (inserting a needle into the base of the spine), the drug is injected directly into the cerebrospinal fluid. This method is used when the drug must act directly upon specific areas within the central nervous system (CNS) and physicians are uncertain if the drug is able to pass through the blood-brain barrier (BBB) to enter the CNS. Initial trials of MS treatments often begin with intrathecal injections for potentially optimum drug performance within the CNS. Intrathecal injections may be performed only by a medical professional.

2. **Intravenously (IV):** This method injects the drug into the vein, allowing the agent to enter the bloodstream directly. If desired, small amounts of a drug may be administered continuously or intermittently through intravenous injection. This type of injection must also be performed by a medical professional.

3. **Intramuscularly (IM):** This form of injection disperses the drug into the muscle. This allows for slower absorption of the drug, enabling it to enter the system gradually. Although this type of injection is typically performed by a nurse or doctor at a medical facility, patients may be taught to give themselves intramuscular injections and may do so in their own home.

4. **Subcutaneously (SC):** These injections are given under the skin. Following instruction from a medical professional, patients are able to administer these injections themselves in the convenience of their own homes. Drugs given this way are absorbed more quickly than those given intramuscularly. The biggest advantage to subcutaneous injection is the ease and comfort by which a person may administer a drug.

A new device for subcutaneous injection is now available for those who give themselves self-injections. The autoinjector is an enclosed needle and syringe that offers a number of benefits over the traditional style. Because it is fully enclosed, the needle is hidden and this helps to alleviate any discomfort one might have about needles. Additionally, the depth of the injection is controlled, the user may reach more difficult injection areas, and the drug is delivered with just a push of a button. Many drug companies now offer an autoinjector device for their medications that are injected subcutaneously.

Treating Exacerbations with Steroids

Most people with MS experience exacerbations, which often last from one to three months. Acute neurologic and physical symptoms must be present for at least 24 hours—without any signs of infection or fever—before the treating physician can consider that it is a true relapse.

Pseudoexacerbation is a temporary symptom flare-up that is brought on by external influences—such as infection, exhaustion, heat, or depression. Checking for a fever is important, since even a minor infection can cause old symptoms to reappear, or new ones to develop. Urinary tract infection (UTI) is the most common illness to cause a pseudoexacerbation. People with heat-sensitive MS should also avoid situations—such as hot tubs or saunas—which can raise the body's temperature. These too can cause a temporary flare-up.

During a relapse, gadolinium-enhanced magnetic resonance image (MRI) scans may show new active lesions. Sometimes older lesions become reactivated as well. Although most relapses remit without any drug intervention, most doctors will recommend treatment when the symptoms are severe enough to affect the person's ability to function normally.

Inflammation with damage to myelin appears to cause the exacerbation; conversely, reduction of the inflammation is thought to assist with recovery. By treating the inflammation, the exacerbation will hopefully be less severe, subside sooner, and possibly cause little or no permanent damage. Anti-inflammatory medications are used for this purpose.

Steroid (or corticosteroid) treatments are considered to be the most effective anti-inflammatory therapy at this time. Corticosteroids are natural or synthetic hormones associated with the adrenal glands. These include glucocorticoids. These drugs decrease the production of cytokines and antibodies which in turn reduces inflammation. Through chemical changes, steroids may also improve the conduction of nerve impulses along demyelinated areas.

In addition to its anti-inflammatory properties, corticosteroid treatment also acts as an immunomodulator (this is an agent that alters one or more functions of the immune system). Corticosteroids have been shown to reduce the duration and degree of an exacerbation while bringing about recovery sooner. These agents are also thought to reduce defects in the BBB, reduce edema (swelling), and possibly promote remyelination, which in turn improves the conduction of nerve impulses. Despite all of these benefits, their long-term effects on the course of the disease are not yet proven.

Corticosteroids tend to have more dramatic results for people with newer cases of MS (less than five years). These drugs are usually more effective in alleviating visual difficulties, facial weakness, and spasticity, while having less influence on tremor, coordination problems, and loss of balance.

High-dose corticosteroids are typically given for periods that vary from three to fourteen days. Following this high-dose course, a patient may need to be taken off the drug slowly to avoid withdrawal problems. Common side effects with short-term use (less than six weeks) include water retention, acne, increased appetite and weight gain, as well as anxiety and difficulty sleeping.

Less common side effects are associated with long-term use. These include excess hair growth, fragile bones and skin, severe acne, slower healing of wounds, joint problems, psychosis, convulsions, euphoria, cataracts, high blood pressure, peptic ulceration, and increased susceptibility to infections. "Cushingoid state" is an unusual condition which also may occur with long-term use. Symptoms of this condition include many of those mentioned, along with a reddening and swelling of the face and neck, raised blood sugar levels, and osteoporosis.

Synthetic adrenal glucocorticoids (betamethasone, cortisone, dexamethasone, methylprednisolone, prednisolone, and prednisone) are the most commonly used steroid treatments for acute exacerbations. In addition, adrenocorticotropic hormone (ACTH) is a protein hormone extracted from animal pituitary glands. It is given by intramuscular injection and has been used to treat MS for more than 30 years.

ACTH causes the release of glucocorticoid hormones by stimulating the adrenal gland. These hormones can now be made synthetically and appear to be stronger, have fewer side effects, and last longer than ACTH. Steroids work by restricting or arresting an enzyme that is required for inflammation after an injury. In addition to anti-inflammatory actions, these steroids display immunosuppressive properties (traits which suppress or weaken the immune system), and appear to affect the T-lymphocytes.

Often nerve flow is temporarily increased in affected areas. A rise in energy may be experienced by those taking these hormones, as well as a sense of well-being or possibly even an exaggerated feeling of happiness. Some individuals, however, may feel depressed while taking steroids.

High doses of methylprednisolone (Depo-Medrol®, Solu-Medrol®) given intravenously (IV) is now the treatment of choice among treating physicians. Compared to ACTH, methylprednisolone is more convenient and more consistent, while offering faster results with fewer side effects.

Preferred dose, duration, and even method of administration vary widely. Most prescribe 500 to 2000 milligrams (mg) given orally or via IV over two to 24 hours, for three to ten days. IV steroids can be administered as an outpatient procedure or at the person's home if a hospital stay is not necessary for other reasons. This therapy may be followed with a short, tapering course of oral corticosteroids. The benefits of adding this oral taper are mixed, and some doctors do not prescribe it for their patients.

A rapid reduction in active lesions, as seen through gadolinium-enhancement on an MRI, is associated with this type of high-dose corticosteroid therapy. Some studies suggest that taking high-dose steroids orally is as effective as IV administration. Steroids given orally are less expensive and more convenient than those given intravenously, but comparative results are not definitive.

Low-dose steroid treatment is controversial and believed to possibly shorten the time between relapses. While studies suggest that low-dose glucocorticoids may reduce symptoms, this therapy may also increase some patients' risk for subsequent relapses. Many doctors support the idea of keeping a close eye on a patient who is only experiencing mild symptoms, while immediately initiating a steroid treatment for a severe attack.

Although intravenous dexamethasone is not prescribed as often as methylprednisolone, it does have many of the same characteristics. Dexamethasone is typically less expensive than methylprednisolone, and when given in a brief course, may offer similar benefits. While no studies have been performed to compare the two drugs, dexamethasone may provide a less-expensive option.

The *Optic Neuritis Treatment Trial* has given doctors some new insights into prescribing steroids to those with MS. Individuals with optic neuritis were selected because it is often a presenting symptom for people who have yet to be diagnosed with MS, and related outcome measures (such as visual field, visual sharpness, and the ability to see color and contrast) are very sensitive.

A group of 457 patients experiencing optic neuritis were randomly selected to receive one of three treatments:

- Group 1: high-dose IV methylprednisolone daily for three days followed by low-dose oral prednisone for 11 days

- Group 2: low-dose oral prednisone for 14 days

- Group 3: oral placebo

Those in the first group had a significantly faster rate of recovery than those in the second two groups—whose rates of recovery were the same. Researchers were surprised to see that during the six-month to two-year follow-up analysis, those who were in the second group (and treated with the low-dose oral prednisone) had an increased risk of experiencing a reoccurrence of optic neuritis in either eye.

Those in the first group (who were treated with high-dose IV methylprednisolone), were 50 percent less likely to experience a new attack leading to the diagnosis of MS within the two-year follow-up period. This result was especially true for those with the most lesions at the beginning of the trial (and who had the greatest chance of having a relapse).

After three years, the treatment groups did not differ in terms of relapse rate. The result suggests that the group treated with high-dose IV methylprednisolone may have experienced a delay in the onset of MS, but ultimately, the treatment was unable to stop the development of the disease.

While most treating physicians have prescribed steroids for their patients who are experiencing a significant relapse, physicians do not all agree on the ideal treatment regimen. Research has yet to confirm the best type of steroid, the optimal route of administration (such as IM, IV, or oral), the most effective dosage, and the value of an oral steroid taper.

In the past, researchers thought that intrathecal injections of methylprednisolone directly into the cerebrospinal fluid would be beneficial by allowing the drug to reach MS lesions directly and at higher concentrations. After 20 years of use, results are questionable. For this reason, along with the risks involved, intrathecal injection of this drug is rarely used today.

Long-term use of steroids is not generally recommended. They can cause many side effects when given over a long period of time and appear to have no affect on the progression of MS.

Although MRI scans illustrate a rapid response to steroids—with a reduction in gadolinium-enhancing lesions—the results are brief. Within as little as a week's time following treatment, new enhancing lesions can begin to reappear. In addition, with each corticosteroid treatment an individual receives, the drug's effectiveness is reduced.

Non-Steroidal Treatment of Relapses

Plasmapheresis (plasma exchange or PE) is used for individuals who are experiencing a severe exacerbation, and are not responding to high-dose IV steroid treatment. With this procedure, blood is taken from the patient and cleansed of toxic elements. The cleansed blood is then returned to the patient. The long-term effectiveness of PE has not been proven. Side effects are mild—typically a transient drop in blood pressure for some, which may cause fainting during the process. A reduction in red blood cells and platelets may also occur. PE is not effective for those with progressive forms of MS, but it may be helpful in treating very severe relapses. PE can also be very expensive.

Anti-Inflammatory Drugs Not Used to Treat Exacerbations

Nonsteroidal anti-inflammatory drugs (NSAIDs) include fenoprofen (Nalfon®), ibuprofen (Advil®, Motrin®), indomethacin (Indocin®), ketoprofen (Orudis®), naproxen (Naprosyn®), phenylbutazone (Butazolidin®), sulindac (Clinoril®), and tolmetin (Tolectin®). Most of these synthetic drugs slow or stop the formation of prostaglandins. Produced by macrophages, certain prostaglandins promote inflammation and immune functions, while others suppress these same functions. These drugs are not used to treat exacerbations, but they may be helpful in treating the flu-like side effects of interferons. Indomethacin, however, may worsen MS in some individuals.

Aspirin and sodium salicylate are two moderately anti-inflammatory agents that affect the prostaglandin pathways. Peptic ulceration and gastrointestinal bleeding are two side effects common to these agents that appear to have no effect on MS. Aspirin may be beneficial for pain relief, but acetaminophen has fewer side effects and certain advantages over aspirin. Neither is used to treat MS.

Sulfasalazine is a drug similar to aspirin yet also contains an antibacterial component. Immunomodulating, anti-inflammatory, and analgesic, this drug has been prescribed for more than 50 years—typically to treat inflammatory diseases of the bowel. Following trials, results indicate that sulfasalazine provides no therapeutic benefit in the treatment of MS.

Treating Disease Progression

The drugs and other therapies used in an attempt to slow or stop the progression of MS are based upon research into possible causes and suspected cellular changes within a person with MS. For instance, evidence strongly suggests that MS is an autoimmune disease. With this in mind, agents affecting the immune system are often used. These include drugs which cause immunosuppression (the weakening of most or certain aspects of the immune system) and immune modulators (agents which alter the immune system). Most treatments in these categories affect the lymphocytes—either by destroying, redirecting, or removing those causing damage. Several anticancer drugs and therapies have been investigated for MS disease progression.

Autoimmune diseases fall under the category of allergy since this type of malfunction is a reaction to a substance—only this time the reaction is to the individual's own myelin. To treat an allergy, desensitization therapies (those that promote a tolerance) may be used.

Oral tolerization is based on the fact that the body naturally builds a tolerance to things that are ingested, and an immune response to such substances is rare. Actual cow (bovine) myelin taken orally was in clinical trials for MS (Myloral®), but failed to show an effect. Based on this theory, an oral form of glatiramer acetate (Copaxone®) was tried but did not prove effective.

Viruses are also suspects in the development and worsening of MS. For this reason, antiviral drugs have been investigated for many years in the treatment of MS. These include the interferon (IFN) drugs (drugs which "interfere" with viruses) and agents which prevent and treat viruses such as influenza type A and herpes viral infections. The advantage of such drugs is twofold. First, should a slow-acting virus be involved in the acquisition of MS, an antiviral drug may have an effect on the cause of the disease. Second, these drugs might theoretically prevent the cause of some attacks. For example, many relapses are preceded by a viral upper respiratory infection.

Some physicians will prescribe a combination of drugs or therapies to be used at one time. One possible advantage to this type of approach may be a reduction of side effects, since patients may be receiving a smaller dose of each agent. Another advantage is the potential for treating more than one aspect of MS at one time—and, as mentioned, MS could well be the result of a combination of factors. On the downside, no data is available on combination therapies, and such treatment could have negative results. Trials are presently being conducted to assess the potential of various combination treatments.

Section 30.2

Long-Term Treatment for Disease Progression

Excerpted from *Multiple Sclerosis: The Process and Medical Treatments, Fourth Edition,* © 2002 Multiple Sclerosis Association of America. All rights reserved. Reprinted with permission. Updated in June 2007 by Dr. David A. Cooke, M.D., Diplomate, American Board of Internal Medicine.

An Overview and Comparison of the "A-B-C" Drugs, Rebif®, Novantrone®, and Tysabri®

In the early-1990s, individuals with MS had no proven long-term disease treatment options. Treatments at that time were limited to steroids for relapses, and cytotoxic drugs (strong immunosuppressive drugs often used for cancer) to minimize relapses and disease progression. While these agents are still used to treat MS, six drug treatments for MS have since become available within a nine-year span. These drugs are well-tolerated and approved by the Food and Drug Administration (FDA) to reduce disease activity.

The first three long-term MS treatments to be approved were dubbed the "A-B-C" drugs because of their brand names: Avonex®, Betaseron®, and Copaxone®. These are interferon beta-1a, interferon beta-1b, and glatiramer acetate, respectively. All were approved for treating relapsing-remitting multiple sclerosis (RRMS).

The fourth drug to be approved was mitoxantrone (Novantrone®), and this was the first drug indicated for both worsening RRMS and secondary-progressive multiple sclerosis (SPMS). News then arrived of a fifth FDA-approved drug for RRMS: interferon beta-1a (Rebif®). This is the same drug as Avonex®, but is given subcutaneously (under the skin) in more frequent and higher doses. A sixth drug, Tysabri®, was subsequently approved, then withdrawn from the market, and then reintroduced under new prescribing restrictions.

This is a promising time for individuals who have been diagnosed with MS. In less than a decade, treatment options have gone from zero to six—and more therapeutic agents are on their way. Approximately 80 drugs and therapies are being investigated worldwide for the treatment of MS, the most in the history of MS research. And these include everything from antiviral medications, to vaccines, to procedures and agents that repair myelin.

Each of the approved treatments is well tolerated and side effects are mild. Novantrone® is the only drug that has a set limit of doses, which is necessary to avoid cardiotoxicity. The other drugs appear safe as long as the person taking the drug is not experiencing any adverse effects and blood tests continue to be normal. While no damage to the reproductive systems has been observed, none of these drugs may be taken if a patient is pregnant or considering pregnancy during her treatment period.

Treating Early

More experts are now recommending treatment as early as possible with one of these agents, possibly delaying time to the second relapse. Early treatment is also thought to possibly limit axonal injury, which may be irreversible, and later lead to progressive disease.

Two independent trials were conducted with Avonex® (known as the CHAPS study) and with Rebif® (known as the ETOMS study) to determine if early treatment could delay the second disease event leading to a confirmed MS diagnosis. Individuals whose symptoms indicated they were at high risk of developing CDMS (clinically definite multiple sclerosis), took part in these two trials.

In the Avonex® study, treated and placebo groups received IV methylprednisolone followed by oral prednisone. The treatment group then received the regular weekly dose of Avonex®. At 18 months, investigators found that compared to the placebo group, the rate of conversion to CDMS was decreased by 44 percent, and the MRI showed reductions in the number of new lesions, the number of enhancing lesions, and the percentage of change in T2 lesion volume.

Similar results were observed with the Rebif® study, although the dose used was one-sixth of the normal dose. At two years, a 24-percent reduction in the rate of conversion was realized, along with reductions in T2 active lesions and T2 disease burden.

Clearly the use of interferon beta-1a (Avonex® and Rebif®) has the ability to delay the time to the next disease episode, when an individual with possible or probable MS would be diagnosed with CDMS. Investigators do not know if delaying time between the first and second MS events will affect the long-term outcome of MS, nor do these results support the idea that such treatment could prevent the development of CDMS.

Some medical professionals delay treatment because they may want to see if the disease is taking a benign early course. They may feel that evidence does not support the long-term efficacy of the treatment, or they may be concerned with the development of neutralizing antibodies, which might prevent this treatment option later on in the disease course.

Neutralizing Antibodies

Neutralizing antibodies may occur with the interferons. Those produced with the interferons (Avonex®, Betaseron®, Rebif®), and Tysabri® may potentially neutralize the drug's effectiveness. The antibodies associated with Copaxone® do not appear to neutralize the drug's performance. Fewer antibodies are developed with Avonex® and Rebif® than Betaseron®.

The actual impact of neutralizing antibodies is not known. Most doctors would not switch treatments based on neutralizing antibodies. In most cases, if an individual is doing well but has neutralizing antibodies, the treating physician would not change this person's treatment. Conversely, if an individual is not responding optimally to treatment but hasn't developed neutralizing antibodies, many doctors would consider changing the treatment.

How the Approved Drugs Work

Interferons

Avonex®, Betaseron®, and Rebif® work to decrease inflammatory or damaging cells and increase those that suppress inflammation. Avonex® and Rebif® are derived from mammalian cells (specifically Chinese hamster ovaries), and their amino acid sequence is identical to that of naturally occurring interferon beta. Betaseron® comes from bacterial cells and its amino acid sequence is nearly identical to naturally occurring interferon beta.

The study of interferons is an intriguing component of antiviral treatment research. Interferons are produced by cells in the body as a response to certain substances, including viruses. Interferons are appropriately named as they are secreted by cells exposed to viruses and "interfere with" viral different lymphocytes that produce different interferons. For instance, natural killer lymphocytes (NK cells) create interferon alpha; fibroblast cells create interferon beta; and Th-2 lymphocytes create interferon gamma when "turned on" by an antigen or virus. Interferons are able to protect nearby cells from viral infection as well as affect immune regulation.

Natural interferons are difficult to produce in large numbers and most interferons used in treatments today are produced by recombinant deoxyribonucleic (DNA) techniques. This process allows researchers to synthetically produce interferons in cell cultures programmed with interferon genes. Recombinant interferons have greater "purity" than those produced by "natural" methods.

Trials with interferon alpha had slightly positive results, and studies with this agent are ongoing. Interferon gamma trials showed a rapid worsening of MS. It promotes human leukocyte antigen (HLA) expression on cell surfaces, a factor enabling sensitized T-lymphocytes and macrophages to target and destroy these cells. Interferon gamma along with interferon gamma producing drugs (such as tilorone and staphage lysate) should not be used in the treatment of MS.

Interferon betas have been shown to affect the immune system through several actions. Examples include:

- reducing the production of tumor necrosis factor alpha (TNF) and T-cells, known to induce damage to myelin;

- switching cytokine production from type 1 (pro-inflammatory) to type 2 (anti-inflammatory) cells, which reduce inflammation;

- decreasing antigen presentation, to reduce the attack on myelin;

- increasing levels of interleukin 10 (IL-10), also known to reduce inflammation;

- reducing the ability of immune cells to cross the BBB, by affecting adhesion molecules, chemokines, and proteases.

Copaxone®

Copaxone® is a synthetic chain of four amino acids that structurally resembles the myelin basic protein (MBP) molecule. Formerly known as copolymer 1 or COP 1, this drug is believed to block the immune system from attacking myelin. Copaxone® also switches the immune response from Th-1 cells (pro-inflammatory) to Th-2 cells (anti-inflammatory) which could reduce myelin damage.

Copaxone® is the first approved treatment for MS management which does not involve steroids or interferons. The antibodies produced by Copaxone® do not appear to affect the drug's performance, and unlike interferon treatments, Copaxone® does not cause certain side effects such as flu symptoms, fatigue, or depression.

Tysabri®

Tysabri® (natalizumab) is a monoclonal antibody approved for use in relapsing multiple sclerosis. A monoclonal antibody is a preparation of identical antibodies, all of which attack the same target. The exact manner in which Tysabri® helps multiple sclerosis is not known, but it is known to block white blood cells carrying alpha-4-beta 1-integrin from interacting with cells in the blood vessel lining and cells of the brain. This may help prevent the immune system attacks that occur in multiple sclerosis. It is given as monthly intravenous infusions.

Tysabri® appears to be moderately effective in patients with the relapsing subtype of multiple sclerosis. It is well-tolerated in most patients, but allergic reactions can occur, and about 6% of patients develop antibodies that inactivate the drug.

Nevertheless, Tysabri® is generally reserved for patients with severe disease in which other drugs have failed. A rare but devastating brain disease called progressive multifocal leukoencephalopathy (PML) has been observed in a small number of patients taking this drug. This is a result of reactivation of a latent virus in immunosuppressed patients; most reported cases occurred in patients who were taking other immunosuppressive drugs in combination with Tysabri®. While PML has been reported in only about 1/1000 patients taking Tysabri®, PML is untreatable, and may lead to severe neurologic damage or death. Due to this risk, it must not be used with other drugs that suppress the immune system, and is only available through a special and closely monitored prescribing program.

Novantrone®

Novantrone® is an antineoplastic agent, which means that it inhibits or prevents the development of any uncontrolled new or abnormal growth (such as a neoplasm or tumor). This drug has been identified as an immunosuppressant and specific immunomodulator. Its actions include suppressing B-cell as well as T-cell immunity.

Novantrone® is the first treatment approved in the U.S. specifically for SPMS (along with RRMS). This drug is indicated for reducing neurologic disability and/or frequency of clinical relapses in those with SPMS, or worsening RRMS.

Costs and Marketing

Avonex®, Betaseron®, and Copaxone® have each been extensively marketed to individuals with MS and medical professionals. All three cost approximately the same (about $16,000 per year) and all three appear to be the most effective for those with early RRMS. Rebif® has also been aggressively marketed, and costs approximately $19,000 per year.

Novantrone® costs less than the various interferon preparations, but requires periodic heart and blood tests. As noted, Tysabri® is suitable only for a relatively small number of patients and its use is under special restrictions. It currently costs about $28,000 per year.

Individual Study Results

Several large, double-blind, placebo-controlled, randomized clinical trials have been conducted to study each of these drugs separately for their effects on MS. Although differences exist in study design and specific findings, trials generally showed these common results:

- reduced the number of relapses;

- reduced the severity of relapses;

- reduced the development of new, gadolinium-enhancing lesions on MRI;

- showed some evidence of delaying short-term disease progression.

Following are the results of some of the individual trials conducted on the approved drugs for MS.

Avonex®

A two-year trial with 301 RRMS participants with mild to moderate neurologic disability ended early when the dropout rate was less than expected. Those who completed the two years experienced one-third fewer exacerbations, as well as a reduction in gadolinium-enhancing lesions and new or enlarging lesions on MRI. No differences were observed with total lesion load. Also, a significant percentage of people in the treated group did not progress to new levels of disability as measured by the EDSS.

Avonex® significantly delays the time to the second MS episode and diagnosis of clinically definite multiple sclerosis (CDMS). Additionally, the full benefit of Avonex® may be delayed for a year or more after beginning treatment.

At double the regular dose, according to a preliminary report, Avonex® was shown to be beneficial for treating individuals with SPMS over a two-year period.

Betaseron®

In a U.S. multicenter trial, 372 RRMS participants with mild to moderate disability were given a high dose of Betaseron®, low dose, or placebo. The higher dose group experienced a reduction in relapse rate by about one-third. Time to first relapse was increased, as well as the number of those who did not have a relapse. Also, the treated groups had a significant reduction in disease activity as measured by MRI. Progression of disease was not statistically different with Betaseron®.

In this study, Betaseron® was found to specifically reduce the number of relapses by 31 percent, and reduce the number of severe attacks by 51 percent. As a result, these patients had 20 percent fewer days on steroid treatment, and the need to stay in a hospital was reduced by 48 percent. MRI studies showed that 93 percent of these patients experienced a significant reduction in the amount of total or new enhancing lesions.

A group of participants from this original study have continued to be monitored. After 12 years, these patients have remained stable (according to MRI studies), with few side effects and minimal neutralizing antibodies.

A large study in Europe has shown that interferon beta-1b is effective in slowing the progression of disability in people with SPMS. The European study consisted of 718 patients with SPMS, ranging from moderate to severe stages of disability.

The study was conducted by the company that markets interferon beta-1b in Europe (known there as Betaferon®). Following two years of this three-year trial, the results were so impressive that the independent advisory board recommended all patients in the placebo group be switched to the active drug. Progression of disease, annual relapse rate, and MRI measures were used in determining the success of this treatment.

In the U.S., the marketers of Betaseron® conducted a trial with more than 800 individuals with SPMS in North America. While this trial did not show a reduction in rate of progression, it did have significant reductions in clinical attack rate, MRI attack rate, and volume of lesions on T2 MRI.

Why the results of the two SPMS trials differed is not known, however, this latter study had individuals with significantly fewer relapses than those in Europe. This suggests that interferon beta-1b might be more effective for people who are still experiencing relapses and are in an earlier phase of SPMS.

Rebif®

A major trial of Rebif® was conducted with 560 individuals who were diagnosed with RRMS and exhibited mild to moderate disability. They were given a low dose, high dose, or placebo three times a week for two years.

The results showed a significant decrease in the number and severity of relapses, as well as a delay in time to the second relapse, and a delay in the time to confirmed progression as measured by EDSS. The percentage of those in the treated groups who remained relapse-free was increased. MRI disease activity was also significantly reduced along with total T2 lesion load.

Similar to Avonex®, Rebif® also delays the time to the second MS episode and diagnosis of CDMS (clinically definite MS), according to the results of the ETOMS study. In a large SPMS study, disease progression was not significantly affected, however, positive results were similar to the Betaseron® SPMS study in North America.

Copaxone®

A two-year U.S. trial with 251 individuals with RRMS who had mild to moderate disability resulted in 29 percent fewer relapses per year. This study may have also shown a favorable effect on EDSS progression, although this is not confirmed. MRI studies were not included in this trial.

A nine-month study was conducted to determine the Copaxone® affect on disease activity as measured by MRI. Results included a reduction in enhancing lesions, clinical attack rate, and T2-weighted burden of disease.

EDSS change. A subgroup of the 251 individuals from the original two-year trial chose to continue in a follow-up study. At the six-year mark, the 152 participants have experienced a stabilization of

EDSS score and a substantial reduction in clinical attack rate. This study is one of the longest continuous follow-up of any MS treatment, but with 40 percent of the original participants dropping out, the robustness of the findings is reduced.

Novantrone®

A multisite study in France and London found a combination of Novantrone® and methylprednisolone (steroid) was effective for people with MS who have very active disease in improving both clinical and MRI indications of disease activity over a period of six months. Those taking the two drugs experienced a month-by-month decrease almost to zero in the number of new enhancing lesions as well as the total number of enhancing lesions.

Additionally, twice as many participants in the Novantrone®-steroid group remained free of exacerbations compared to the steroid-alone group. The steroid-alone group also experienced more than four times as many relapses as the combination-drug group. Those taking the two drugs exhibited a mean average EDSS improvement of more than one point.

In a two-year European multi-center phase III study of 194 individuals with SPMS, participants received two doses of either IV Novantrone® or placebo, every three months. Results showed a significant reduction in relapse rate and progression of disability for those in the treatment group.

Tysabri® (Natalizumab)

Two published studies examined the effects of Tysabri® in patients with relapsing multiple sclerosis. One study found that 17% of patients progressed on Tysabri® alone, as compared to 29% with placebo. The other study found 23% of patients on Tysabri® in combination with interferon progressed, as compared to 29% with interferon alone. However, Tysabri® is not recommended to be used with interferon, due to the findings of increased rates of progressive multifocal leukoencephalopathy (PML).

Three patients out of 3000 studied developed progressive multifocal leukoencephalopathy while on therapy with Tysabri®. Two of these patients were taking Tysabri® with interferon, and one was taking Tysabri® with azathioprine. While this represents a 1/1000 risk, this is a vastly higher rate of PML than what occurs in untreated patients, and this lead to the precautions and restrictions on the use of Tysabri®.

Section 30.3

Tysabri (Natalizumab) for Relapsing Forms of MS

"Patient Information Sheet for Natalizumab," U.S. Food and Drug Administration (FDA), June 2006; and excerpts from "Questions and Answers on Natalizumab," FDA, June 2006.

Natalizumab (marketed as Tysabri®)

Tysabri® is an intravenous (IV) medicine used to treat patients with relapsing forms of multiple sclerosis (MS) to reduce the number of relapses. A relapse is a time when new symptoms can appear and old symptoms come back or worsen. Relapses are followed by periods of time when no new symptoms occur (remission).

Tysabri® is indicated for use as monotherapy, meaning it should not be used in combination with other immune system modifying drugs, and is for patients who have not responded adequately to, or cannot tolerate, other treatments for MS.

What are the risks?

The following are the major potential risks and side effects of Tysabri® therapy. However, this list is not complete. Tysabri® increases the chance of patients getting a rare brain infection that usually causes death or severe disability. This infection is called progressive multifocal leukoencephalopathy (PML). PML usually happens in people with weakened immune systems. Because of the risk of PML, Tysabri® is available only through a special restricted distribution program.

Tysabri® may cause severe allergic reactions. These severe reactions usually happen within two hours of the start of the Tysabri® infusion. Symptoms of a severe allergic reaction include an itchy swelling on the skin (hives), dizziness, fever, rash, shaking, nausea, flushing, low blood pressure, breathing problems, and chest pain. People who have these severe reactions with Tysabri® must have their infusion stopped right away, be treated for the reaction, and should not be treated with Tysabri® again.

The serious side effects with Tysabri® include:

- serious infections, such as pneumonia; and,

- severe or life threatening allergic reactions.

Other side effects may include infections, such as in the urinary tract or upper respiratory tract, headache, tiredness, depression, joint pain, diarrhea, and stomach area pain.

What should I tell my health care professional?

Before being treated with Tysabri® tell your health care professional if you:

- have any new or worsening medical problems (such as a new or sudden change in your thinking, eyesight, balance, or strength or other problems) that have lasted several days;

- have a fever or infection (including shingles or any unusually long lasting infection); or,

- are pregnant, planning to become pregnant, or are breast-feeding.

During or after treatment with Tysabri® tell your health care professional if you experience itching or any of the symptoms of an allergic reaction (listed under risks) after receiving Tysabri®.

Are there any interactions with drugs or foods?

Tell your health care professional about all the medicines you take, including prescription and non-prescription medicines, vitamins, and herbal supplements. Especially tell your health care professional if you take:

- corticosteroid medicines; or

- any other medicines to treat multiple sclerosis, such as interferon beta-1a (Avonex®, Rebif®); interferon beta-1b (Betaseron®), or glatiramer acetate (Copaxone®).

These medicines and Tysabri® may interact causing side effects or affect how each other work.

Questions and Answers on Natalizumab (marketed as Tysabri®)

What action is the FDA taking with Tysabri®?

The Food and Drug Administration (FDA) approved an application for resumed marketing of Tysabri® (natalizumab) with a special restricted distribution program on June 6, 2006. Tysabri® is a monoclonal antibody, for the treatment of patients with relapsing forms of multiple sclerosis (MS). Tysabri® is indicated for use as monotherapy, because we don't know enough about how its use with other immune modifying drugs could impact risk. It is also meant for patients who have not responded adequately to, or cannot tolerate, other treatments for MS.

Why was marketing of Tysabri® previously halted?

Tysabri®, which was initially approved by the FDA in November, 2004, was withdrawn by the manufacturer in February 2005 after three patients in the drug's clinical trials developed progressive multifocal leukoencephalopathy (PML), a serious viral infection of the brain. In addition, FDA put clinical trials of the drug on hold in February, 2005 based on this information.

Why is this product being allowed to go on the market?

FDA allowed a clinical trial of Tysabri® to resume in February 2006, following a reexamination of the patients who had participated in the previous clinical trials, confirming that there were no additional cases of PML. In March 2006, FDA consulted with its Advisory Committee on drugs for peripheral and central nervous systems about the possibility of making Tysabri® available to appropriate MS patients while decreasing the possibility of patients developing PML. The Advisory Committee recommended a risk-minimization program with mandatory patient registration and periodic follow-up to identify as early as possible any cases of PML that do occur and to try to determine the reason the infection occurs. In response, the manufacturer, Biogen Idec submitted to the agency a Risk Management Plan, called the TOUCH Prescribing Program, to help ensure safe use of the product.

How can consumers get the product?

Tysabri® is available only through a Risk Management Plan, called the TOUCH Prescribing Program. In order to receive Tysabri®, patients must talk to their doctor and understand the risks and benefits of Tysabri® and agree to all of the instructions in the TOUCH Prescribing Program.

What are the main features of the Risk Management Plan?

- The drug will only be prescribed, distributed, and infused by prescribers, infusion centers, and pharmacies registered with the program.

- Tysabri® will only be administered to patients who are enrolled in the program.

- Prior to initiating the therapy, health care professionals are to obtain the patient's magnetic resonance imaging (MRI) scan to help differentiate potential future multiple sclerosis symptoms from PML.

- Patients on Tysabri® are to be evaluated at three and six months after the first infusion and every six months after that, and their status will be reported regularly to Biogen Idec.

Who will manage the program?

Biogen Idec Inc., the company that manufactures Tysabri®, and Elan Pharmaceuticals Inc., the company that distributes Tysabri®, will manage the program.

How will FDA evaluate the program?

Biogen Idec and Elan Pharmaceuticals will be monitoring the conduct of the program continuously. Periodically they will submit reports to FDA about the functioning of the program. Biogen Idec and Elan Pharmaceuticals will also submit to FDA proposals for any changes in the program to help ensure safe use of the product.

How can consumers get additional information?

Consumers who would like more information or have any questions can talk with their health care provider. Consumers can also call 1-800-456-2255 or visit www.tysabri.com.

Chapter 31

MS Pain Management

Management of pain in multiple sclerosis involves a combination of behavioral, physical, surgical, and medical interventions.

Behavioral Mechanisms

Cognitive and behavioral approaches to MS pain management include education, relaxation, behavior modification, distraction, psychotherapy, support groups, imagery, hypnosis, biofeedback, recreation, laugh therapy, music therapy, and, meditation.

Physical Mechanisms

Physical modalities include: physical therapy; stretching; application of heat, cold, and pressure; reconditioning to improve strength, endurance, and flexibility; counter irritation; massage; acupuncture; exercise; yoga and Tai Chi; attention to ergonomics and positioning; electroanalgesia such as transcutaneous electric nerve stimulation (TENS); and, sound nutrition and weight control.

"Pain in Multiple Sclerosis," by Heidi Maloni. Reprinted in part with permission of the National Multiple Sclerosis Society. Copyright © 2006 National Multiple Sclerosis Society. All rights reserved. Material on the National Multiple Society website is regularly updated. For the latest version of this information, including references, please visit: www.national MSsociety.org.

Medication Management

Neurogenic Pain

Neurogenic pain is often resistant to therapy, requiring an in-depth and ongoing assessment of pain indicators, sleep, mood, and quality of life. Medication management includes topical agents, anticonvulsants, antidepressants, antiarrhythmics, N-methyl D-aspartate (NMDA)-receptor antagonists, and nonnarcotic and narcotic opioids.

The use of opioids in neurogenic pain remains controversial as studies show equivocal results. A meta-analysis of several randomized controlled trials demonstrated significant efficacy of opioids over placebo for non-MS neurogenic pain. Rowbotham and colleagues (2003) randomized eight MS patients to either high-dose or low-dose levorphanol and found a significant effect of the high-dose opioid on pain intensity. Opioids should be considered when other agents become ineffective or are not well tolerated. Clearly, further studies are needed to confirm their long-term efficacy and safety for the treatment of neurogenic pain in MS.

In April 2005, Health Canada, the drug regulatory agency for Canada, approved the use of the cannabis-derived drug Sativex® (GW Pharmaceuticals) to treat MS-related pain. The approval was based on a four-week clinical trial conducted in the United Kingdom in 66 people with MS. Sativex contains extracts from the marijuana plant and is administered as a spray into the mouth. This drug is not approved in the United States. Studies of the herbal cannabis, delta-tetrahydrocannabinol, and the oral form dronabinol (Marinol®) indicate a modest analgesic effect on MS pain. Current studies have been short-term and the long-term adverse events of cannabinoid use in MS have not been determined. Modest therapeutic effect must be balanced with disruption in cognitive function, and increases in anxiety and depression.

The goal of pain management is to enhance comfort, function, mood, sleep, and quality of life. The benefits of the medications used must be weighed against their side effects. The use of combination therapy (low doses of different drug classes and different drugs within classes) may increase efficacy while minimizing the unwanted effects.

Nociceptive Pain

Medications commonly used to manage nociceptive pain include acetaminophen, salicylates, and nonsteroidal anti-inflammatory agents, and nonnarcotic and narcotic opioids. The section titled, "Pharmacological Treatment of Neurogenic or Neuropathic Pain in MS," provides information about the medications commonly used to manage neurogenic or neuropathic pain in MS, including dosage, adverse events, and indications for use. The indications for medication use are derived primarily from evidence-based trials in diabetic and post-herpetic neuropathy.

Invasive Interventions

Invasive procedures include intrathecal medication administration of either baclofen (Lioresal®) or morphine, or both in combination; botulinum toxin (Botox®) injection; phenol injection of trigger-points; epidural steroids; regional blocks; spinal cord stimulators; and various surgical procedures.

- Deep brain stimulation, which generates a pulse to relieve pain through electrodes planted in the brain, has the advantage of being reversible.

- Neurosurgical procedures include: cordotomy, rhizotomy, percutaneous balloon compression, percutaneous glycerol injection, radiofrequency rhizotomy, and Gamma knife radiosurgery. Microvascular decompression surgery (MVD) has not shown an effect that outweighs side effects for pain in MS.

- Neuroablative techniques are considered when medical therapy is not well tolerated or is ineffective in managing pain. Quality of life is balanced with possible adverse effects of localized numbness, pain recurrence, and possible worsening of the underlying pain.

Pharmacological Treatment of Neurogenic or Neuropathic Pain in MS

Following is information about the medications commonly used to manage neurogenic or neuropathic pain in MS, including dosage, adverse events, and indications for use. The indications for medication use are derived primarily from evidence-based trials in diabetic and post-herpetic neuropathy.

Antidepressants

Used in MS for chronic neurogenic pain (for example, dysesthetic extremity pain such as burning, tingling); often prescribed at night, but split dosing is recommended.

- Tricyclic antidepressants

  - amitriptyline (Elavil®)

  - imipramine (Tofranil®)

  - desipramine (Norpramin®)

  - nortriptyline (Pamelor®)

- Serotonin noradrenaline reuptake inhibitor (SNRI) antidepressants: Used in MS for migraine; episodic and continuous neurogenic pain (sharp, shooting, burning or dull sensations; nighttime pain).

  - duloxetine (Cymbalta®)

  - venlafaxine (Effexor®)

Antiepileptics

For MS use primarily in sharp, lancinating neurogenic pain (for example, trigeminal neuralgia); also used in dull or burning, continuous neurogenic pain.

- carbamazepine (Tegretol®; Carbatrol® extended release): trigeminal neuralgia; tonic painful seizures; pelvic pain; intense episodic, lancinating, burning pain.

- gabapentin (Neurontin®): Trigeminal neuralgia; pins or needles sensations; cramping; dysesthetic extremity pain; tonic spasms; nocturnal spasms; good combination drug with little drug-drug interaction; better tolerated than carbamazepine

- pregabalin (Lyrica®): same indications for MS use as gabapentin; better tolerated with lower effective doses

- lamotrigine (Lamictal®): trigeminal neuralgia; continuous and episodic dysesthetic extremity pain; burning; painful tonic spasms; better tolerated than carbamazepine

- levetiracetam (Keppra®): trigeminal neuralgia; painful spasms

- oxcarbazepine (Trileptal®): trigeminal neuralgia

- tiagabine (Gabitril®): painful tonic spasms

- topiramate (Topamax®): trigeminal neuralgia; sharp, episodic paroxysmal pain

- zonisamide (Zonegran®): neurogenic pain

Antiarrhythmic Agents

- mexiletine (Mexitil®): neurogenic pain; painful tonic seizures; trigeminal neuralgia; itching, or Lhermitte sign

- lidocaine: not well tolerated; use as add-on therapy

Transdermal Agents

In MS, used for moderate, continuous, dysesthetic neurogenic pain and to reduce oral medication load or side effects.

- clonidine (Catapres-TTS®): acts synergistically with morphine

- lidocaine patch (Lidoderm®): neurogenic, dysesthetic, continuous, burning, tingling pain of recent onset; less effective for long-term and severe dysesthetic pain

- capsaicin (Zostrix®): mild or moderate neurogenic or nociceptive pain

- fentanyl (Duragesic®): moderate neurogenic or nociceptive pain not responsive to non-opioid

Antispasmodic Agents

Used in multiple sclerosis for painful spasms.

- baclofen: painful spasticity; trigeminal neuralgia; glossopharyngeal neuralgia

- tizanidine (Zanaflex®): painful spasms

- botulinum-A: painful spasms

Nonsteroidal Antiinflammatories (NSAIDs) (Selective Representation)

In MS, used for nociceptive pain (ineffective for neurogenic pain).

- ibuprofen (Motrin®; Advil®)

- naproxen sodium (Naprosyn®; Aleve®)

- celecoxib (Celebrex®)

- aspirin (ASA)

Non-Opioid and Opioid Agents

Used in MS as add-on for moderate to severe neurogenic or nociceptive pain, or when non-opioids are ineffective—caution in combination with carbamazepine or tricyclic antidepressants (TCA).

- tramadol (Ultram®; Ultracet®): neurogenic pain

- methadone (Dolophine HCl®): neurogenic pain (continuous and touch-evoked); nociceptive pain

- oxycodone (OxyContin®), hydromorphone (Dilaudid®), hydrocodone (plus acetaminophen = Vicodin®, Lortab®), and levorphanol (Levo-Dromoran®): moderate to severe neurogenic pain; allodynia, tolerance not developed to side effect, constipation

- morphine sulfate (Kadian®; MS Contin®; Avinza®): nociceptive and neurogenic pain when other agents have failed

Summary

Pain control is an achievable goal that begins with a thorough assessment, including the identification of pain triggers. Recommendations for effective pain management include:

- Use preventive measures and non-drug strategies in conjunction with medications.

- Be familiar with the treatment options and side effects—and treat the side effects promptly.

- Use low doses of several different medications to achieve greater efficacy with fewer adverse effects.

- Begin with low doses and titrate slowly to an effective pain control. If pain free for three months, titrate back the dosage slowly.

Pain is a symptom that demands serious attention, as it has such pervasive impact on role, mood, capacity to work and rest, and interpersonal relationships. Untreated pain causes isolation, anger, and depression. Optimum therapeutic treatment involves a commitment to the goal of controlling pain and improving quality of life.

Chapter 32

Treating Involuntary Movement

Chapter Contents

Section 32.1

Controlling Spasticity in MS

Introduction

Spasticity is one of the most mysterious of all multiple sclerosis (MS) symptoms. It comes; it goes. It feels different to different people—and even to the same person at different times. There are even occasions when a physician finds spasticity but the person affected has no symptoms. There's also an inherent paradox. Spasticity is not all negative. The stiffness it may give the legs can be a real help to moving about or transferring from beds to chairs, to car seats, on and off a toilet, and more.

What is spasticity?

The word spasticity refers to involuntary muscle stiffness or spasms (sudden muscle contractions or movements). In any coordinated movement, some muscles relax while others contract. Spasticity occurs when this coordination is lost. Too many muscles contract at the same time. MS-related spasticity can cause a leg to lock up and refuse to bend.

Spasticity is not completely understood, but doctors believe that the problem is caused by increased sensitivity in the parts of muscles to tightening, relaxing, and stretching of the muscles. This may lead to excessive firing of the nerves that control muscles. In mild cases, the condition is noticeable only as a feeling of tight or stiff muscles. When the condition is severe, the person can experience painful spasms or twisted limbs, which can impede mobility and other physical functions.

There are two types of MS-related spasms: flexor and extensor. Flexor spasticity is defined as an involuntary bending of the hips or knees (mostly involving the hamstring muscles on the back of the upper leg). The hips and knees bend up toward the chest. Extensor spasticity is an involuntary straightening of the legs. Extensor spasticity involves the quadriceps (muscles on the front of the upper leg) and the adductors (inner thigh muscles). The hips and knees remain straight with the legs very close together or crossed over at the ankles. Spasticity may also occur in the arms, but in MS this is less common.

How common is spasticity?

Spasticity is one of the more common symptoms of MS. If all degrees of spasticity are taken together, it occurs in an estimated 80 percent of people with the disease. The question of degree is important. In one person, spasticity may cause a stiff leg, and in another, it makes it impossible to walk. For many people, the extra effort needed to move around when muscles are spastic contributes significantly to fatigue. On the other hand, sometimes spasticity can compensate for muscle weakness, making it easier to stand, walk, and move.

Treatment

The Treatment Partnership

Because the condition is so individual, successful treatment of spasticity demands a true partnership between you and your doctor, nurse, physical therapist, and occupational therapist. Your family also plays an important role. The first step in building a good treatment partnership is knowing that something can be done.

"Treating spasticity is not a matter of the doctor writing out a prescription for pills and saying come back in three months," said Charles R. Smith, M.D., Director of the Multiple Sclerosis Comprehensive Care Centers at White Plains Hospital in White Plains, New York, and at Bronx Lebanon Hospital in Bronx, New York.

A doctor can identify the presence and degree of spasticity by checking for involuntary resistance when the limbs are passively stretched. For example, if your leg is spastic, there is resistance when the leg is quickly bent at the knee by your doctor. When spasticity is mild, the resistance is barely felt. When it is severe, the leg may be so stiff it cannot be bent at all.

Treatment begins with the doctor recommending ways to relieve the symptoms. These may include medication, exercise, or changes in daily activities, singly or in combination. To individualize the plan, and to adjust the dosage of any medication to its most effective level, your doctor will need to follow your progress. She or he may also make referrals to other health care professionals, such as physical and occupational therapists.

The nurse is an important part of this process, since nurses normally have responsibility for health education and for learning in detail how patients' daily lives are affected by their symptoms. Take the time to ask your nurse questions and provide personal information. Both your doctor and nurse will guide you through the sometimes tricky process of medication adjustment.

Self-Help

Your spasticity, like other aspects of your MS, is in many ways unique to you. As with other MS symptoms, it tends to come and go and to be worse under specific conditions. Typical triggers include cold temperatures, high humidity, tight clothing, tight shoes, constipation, poor posture, and having a viral infection such as a cold or the flu, or a bacterial infection including skin sores or bladder infections. A sudden dramatic increase in spasticity, as a result of any of these conditions, can even suggest a pseudoexacerbation of the MS.

In time you will become aware of the triggers that affect you most. Some, like tight shoes, can be avoided. Others merit an intervention. Effective self-help means:

- Don't assume that nothing can be done. Spasticity does not have to be tolerated. Improvement is usually possible.

- Make sure an appropriate exercise program is a regular part of your routine. The National MS Society's illustrated booklets, "Stretching for People with MS" and "Stretching with a Helper for People with MS," which are available from local chapters of the Society, include exercises specifically for spasticity. Ask your physical therapist, nurse, or doctor for suggestions.

- Explore complementary relaxation techniques such as progressive muscle relaxation, yoga, meditation, or deep-breathing exercises. None of these is a cure, but they can make it easier to sleep at night and face the next day's problems with a clearer head.

- If your doctor agrees, explore massage. You may even receive a prescription, which might entitle you to some insurance reimbursement depending on your plan. Massage can help relax muscles and enhance range-of-motion exercises and may be helpful in preventing pressure sores. However, it should not be used if pressure sores or reddened areas of skin are present. The American Massage Therapy Association has a national locator service and can supply names of qualified therapists. Call 1-877-905-2700 or visit their website at http://www.amtamas sage.org/findamassage/locator.htm.

- Be patient but persistent through adjustments in daily activities, the types and doses of medication, the type and timing of exercise, and the use of devices, gadgets, and adaptations.

Treatment Goals

Spasticity interferes with daily activities—so the primary goal of treatment is to reduce the negative effects as much as possible. Sections of this chapter detail what can be accomplished by medication, physical therapy, orthotic devices (splints or braces), and occupational therapy. Some strategies seek to relieve the affected muscles; others involve learning to work around spasticity by adopting new ways to do things.

Treatment also aims at preventing the serious complications of spasticity. These include contractures (frozen or immobilized joints) and pressure sores. Since these complications also act as spasticity triggers, they can set off a dangerous escalation of symptoms. In fact, surgical measures are considered for those rare cases of spasticity that defy all other treatments.

Contractures are not only painful and disabling. If left untreated, they become permanent, leaving legs that can never be straightened and limiting joint mobility in such places as the shoulder. Treatment—and prevention—of contractures usually combines treatment of spasticity and physical therapy, prescribed and tailored to the individual by the physician.

Pressure Sores

Pressure sores, sometimes called bed sores, occur in people who spend much of their day sitting or lying down. The term bed sore is misleading. One does not need to be in bed all the time to be at risk for a pressure sore. MS reduces the thousands of small movements people ordinarily make both in sleep and while sitting down. MS can dull sensation in the buttocks or legs, eliminating the usual sensory cues for shifting position.

Spasticity contributes to pressure sores by making normal movement more difficult and by causing posture changes that create pressure points. Complicated infected pressure sores are contributing factors in some MS-related deaths.

Pressure sores begin innocently enough, as small reddened areas. The spot may not even feel painful or tender. However, there may already be significant damage to the soft tissues underneath reddened areas of skin. If pressure on the area is not relieved, the skin will break down, forming a sore. These sores can deepen quickly. They are prone to infection, and they can eventually destroy large areas of underlying tissue and even bone. Your nurse or doctor can provide instruction in prevention and early detection. Controlling spasticity is part of good pressure sore prevention.

Rehabilitation

Physical Therapy

A physical therapist recommends and teaches specific exercises and movements that can increase flexibility and relieve spasticity. First, you will have several tests that measure muscle tone, resistance, strength, and coordination. You'll also be asked about your general functioning in routine daily activities.

In addition to active exercises (ones you do yourself), physical therapists also relieve spasticity with passive exercises (done with the help of another person) to stretch and relax shortened muscle fibers, increase joint movement, extend contracted muscles, and improve circulation. Some of these techniques may be taught to a family member or helper so that they can be performed on a routine basis at home.

Physical therapists also use and teach hydrotherapy (therapy using water) and local application of cold packs or ice. Hydrotherapy is a very effective way to temporarily relax spastic limbs, especially when used in combination with gentle stretching.

Physical therapists usually require a written referral from a physician.

Orthotic Devices

Orthotic devices may make it easier to move around or get into a more comfortable position. These are braces and splints, and they should be fitted by professionals. A common example is the ankle-foot orthosis (AFO). Although many drugstores and catalogs offer them over-the-counter, ill-fitting devices can aggravate spasticity and cause pressure sores or pain.

Trained physical therapists can steer you to the best options and teach you how to use them. Physical therapy can help maintain range of motion to prevent contractures. Strengthening the muscles that oppose the spastic ones may be particularly beneficial.

Occupational Therapy

Occupational therapists are experts in modifications to make daily life with spasticity more comfortable. That might include replacing small drawer pulls with large knobs, spraying drawer tracks with silicone to make the drawers glide, or lowering the clothes bar in your closets. Occupational therapists will recommend devices and let you try out samples. You may be amazed at the ingenuity of the gadgets available. Here is a small sample:

- **Dressing aids:** These include sock pullers, long shoehorns, shoe and boot removers, and dressing sticks, all of which help you dress with a minimum of bending. There are stretchy elastic shoelaces that let you slip in and out of shoes without having to retie them, zipper pulls with long handles, buttoning gadgets, and more.

- **Toiletry and grooming aids:** In addition to electric shavers and electric toothbrushes, there are easy-grip handles for shaving cream cans, combs, or brushes, and palm or wrist cuffs to hold either regular bath brushes or bent-handled brushes. For people who use wheelchairs, occupational therapists may also suggest positioning changes that minimize spasticity. Sometimes simple adjustments in the height of a footrest or the width of a seat can make a world of difference. Occupational therapists can also develop exercise programs for your hands and arms.

Medications: Drug Therapy

There are two medications approved for the treatment of spasticity and other medications that can serve well in certain situations. The most effective dosage will depend on striking a balance between the drug's good and bad effects. An effective dosage tends to vary from time to time. An infection, cold weather, an ingrown toenail—whatever triggers your spasticity—will also influence the amount of medication needed to control it.

Typically, a prescription dose will be increased slowly until the full benefit is evident, and if side effects occur, the dose will be reduced. In addition, people on your health care team can suggest timing your medication in specific situations. For example, taking an antispasticity medication an hour before sexual activity can prevent painful spasms during orgasm.

Baclofen (Lioresal®) is a muscle relaxant that works in the spinal cord. It is most often taken three or four times a day, and common side effects are drowsiness and muscle weakness. Baclofen relaxes normal as well as spastic muscles. Nausea, a less common side effect, can usually be avoided by taking baclofen with food. The drug has a good safety record with long-term use. The side effects don't build up or become worse over time. But at high doses, this medication reduces concentration and contributes to fatigue.

Because it usually restores flexibility within a short period, baclofen may allow other treatment, such as physical therapy, to be more effective. Baclofen does not cure spasticity or improve coordination or strength. It should not be greatly reduced or stopped suddenly without consultation with your physician.

Intrathecal baclofen: Some people require a higher dose of baclofen but cannot tolerate higher side effects. A surgically implanted pump can administer very small amounts of the drug directly and continuously to the spinal cord (specifically, to an area called the intrathecal space).

The baclofen pump has been extremely successful. The pump can improve—or at least maintain—a person's level of functioning. It may even help some people remain ambulatory. And it permits people with very limited mobility to be positioned to minimize pain and the risk of skin breakdown.

The computer-controlled, battery-operated pump, which weighs about six ounces, is surgically implanted under the skin of the abdomen. A tube runs from the pump to the spinal canal. The pump is programmed to release a preset dose specific for the individual. People who use the pump return to their physician for a new drug supply and a check of the computer program every one to three months. New drug is injected into the pump through the skin. The little computer can be reprogrammed painlessly by radio signals. When the battery wears out—in three to seven years—the pump itself is surgically re-moved and replaced. The tube remains in place.

Tizanidine (Zanaflex®) is the first new medication for muscle spasticity to be approved by the FDA in over 20 years. It works quickly to calm spasms and relax tightened muscles. Although it doesn't pro-duce muscle weakness directly, it often causes greater sedation than other medications. Tizanidine is typically taken three times a day. In addition to drowsiness, dry mouth is a common and usually tempo-rary side effect. Hypotension (low blood pressure) is another poten-tial side effect although less frequent.

This drug also has a good safety record with long-term use. It does not cure spasticity or improve muscle coordination or strength. A com-bination of baclofen and tizanidine may give the best results.

Diazepam: Spasticity can also be treated with diazepam (Valium®), often in small doses. This drug is not as effective as those previously mentioned, but it has the benefit of relieving anxiety, making it easier for someone who is restless or has disturbing night time spasms to relax and get a good night's sleep.

Drowsiness and potential dependency with long-term use make diazepam a less desirable choice. However, in some circumstances, diaz-epam and another antispasticity drug may be prescribed together. People for whom this works say that they would rather be a bit slug-gish and fully flexible than wide awake and spastic. Another benzo-diazepine, clonazepam (Klonopin®), can also help control spasms, particularly at night.

Gabapentin (Neurontin®) is used to control some types of sei-zures in epilepsy. In MS it controls certain types of pain, and can re-duce spasticity. The most common side effects include blurred or double vision, dizziness, and drowsiness. Once you've started on it, gabapentin should not be stopped without consulting your physician.

Dantrolene (Dantrium®) is generally used only if other drugs—alone or in combination— have been ineffective. It works by partially paralyzing muscles, making it a poor choice for people who walk. Dantrolene can produce serious side effects, including liver damage and blood abnormalities. The longer a person takes this drug, the more these problems are likely to develop. People taking dantrolene must have periodic blood tests.

Botulinum toxin: Injection of botulinum toxin (Botox®) has been shown to help spasticity. However, the benefit is limited to the injected muscles, and the treatment must be repeated every three to six months. Only small amounts of the drug can be injected into the body at any one time. Otherwise, the immune system might create antibodies against it. For these reasons, Botox is not a good choice when many muscles are spastic or the spastic muscles are large. It is a very good choice when muscles of the arm are spastic, as these muscles are small and do not require a lot of medication. Side effects include weakness of the injected muscle and some nearby muscles, and a brief flu-like syndrome. Despite the drug's effectiveness, the FDA has not yet approved Botox for MS-related spasticity, and the drug is very expensive.

Phenol: Another older treatment is the injection of a nerve block called phenol. This treatment also needs to be repeated every three to six months, and is rarely used today as there are better choices.

Final Option

Severe Spasticity

Enormous progress has been made in controlling spasticity in the past two decades. But if none of the treatments discussed have helped, surgery will be recommended for relief. The relief is permanent but so is the resulting disability. The techniques include severing tendons (tenectomy) or nerve roots (rhizotomy) in order to relax cramped-up muscles. These measures are only undertaken after serious consideration and for the most difficult cases of spasticity.

Section 32.2

Deep Brain Stimulation for MS

What is deep brain stimulation?

Deep brain stimulation (DBS) is a variation of an old surgery. Surgery for tremor due to multiple sclerosis, Parkinson disease, and essential tremor has been available since the 1960s. Back then, surgery was used to destroy a small part of the brain called the thalamus (thalamotomy) or another part of the brain called the globus pallidus (pallidotomy).

These surgeries are still done today, although less frequently because of the availability of deep brain stimulation. These surgeries carry significant risks: both thalamotomy and pallidotomy require purposeful destruction of the brain. If the surgeon is off by even a fraction of an inch, the surgery may not be effective and severe complications such as paralysis, loss of vision, or loss of speech can result.

Deep brain stimulation is a way to inactivate the thalamus or globus pallidus without purposefully destroying the brain. Therefore, the risks are much lower. In deep brain stimulation, an electrode is placed with the tip of the electrode in the thalamus (for essential tremor and multiple sclerosis) or in the subthalamic nucleus or globus pallidus (for Parkinson disease). Rather than destroying the brain, small electrical shocks are given. This has the same effect as thalamotomy or pallidotomy, but with less destruction of the brain.

The electrode for deep brain stimulation is left in the brain. It is connected by a wire to a pacemaker-like device that is implanted under the skin over the chest. The pacemaker-like device generates the electrical shocks.

319

What are the advantages of deep brain stimulation?

Deep brain stimulation offers a number of advantages. The electrical stimulation is adjustable, whereas surgical destruction is not. The electrode has four metal contacts that can be used in many different combinations. Even if one electrode contact is not in the exact location, it is likely that one of the others or some combination of the electrical contacts will be closer to the proper target. As the patient's response to surgery changes over time, the stimulation can be adjusted without requiring a repeat operation.

Another significant advantage of deep brain stimulation relates to future treatments. Destructive surgery, such as thalamotomy or pallidotomy, may reduce the patient's potential to benefit from future therapies. With deep brain stimulation, the stimulator could be turned off if others were to be attempted.

What kinds of movement problems are helped by deep brain stimulation?

Because the right side of the brain controls the left side of the body, and the left side of the brain controls the right side of the body, a stimulator will help only on the opposite side of the body. Most patients will have the stimulator placed in only one side of the brain; a few will have stimulators placed on both sides, but not at the same time. The risks for complications increase when stimulators are placed in both sides of the brain.

The main purpose of deep brain stimulation for patients with essential tremor and tremor due to multiple sclerosis is to control the tremor of the arm. While tremor of the head and body may be helped, the decision to have surgery should be based on the goal of decreasing arm tremor. In the case of multiple sclerosis, other problems such as loss of vision, sensation, motor incoordination or strength are not helped by deep brain stimulation. Electrical stimulation does not cure multiple sclerosis, nor does it prevent the disease from getting worse.

What sort of benefit can be expected from deep brain stimulation?

The benefit of deep brain stimulation varies from one patient to another, so no specific results can be guaranteed. The main benefit seen in multiple sclerosis patients is with very severe tremors in the arm or leg. These severe tremors often involve the distal part of the arm or hand. Tremors can interfere with the most basic daily activities, such as eating, dressing, bathing, and toileting. Deep brain stimulation can improve severe tremors so that it is easier for multiple sclerosis patients to sustain these basic daily activities, or allow caregivers to more easily provide care. Deep brain stimulation in multiple sclerosis patients typically does not improve tremors to allow for writing, walking, or other fine coordination skills. It is important for multiple sclerosis patients to have appropriate expectations regarding the potential benefits of deep brain stimulation.

Is deep brain stimulation experimental?

Deep brain stimulation is not experimental. It has been approved by the U.S. Food and Drug Administration (FDA) for stimulation of the thalamus in patients with Parkinson disease and essential tremor.

Deep brain stimulation of the thalamus for patients with multiple sclerosis has not been approved specifically by the FDA. However, this does not mean that the treatment is experimental or that it would not be covered by insurance. There are many examples of treatments that are used every day and are standard and accepted but have not been approved by the FDA.

Who should consider deep brain stimulation?

There are many important issues to be addressed when considering deep brain stimulation. These issues should be discussed with a movement disorders expert or a specially trained neurologist. A movement disorders expert is someone who has trained specifically in movement disorders (such as through a fellowship) or who has done research in or published articles about movement disorders.

One of the most important criteria is that the patient has had an adequate trial of medications. It would be inappropriate to expose a person to the risks of surgery if medications could control the disease. However, surgery should be considered for people with severe tremors who do not achieve satisfactory control through medications. If there is any question whether surgery will help, the patient should consult a movement disorders expert or a neurologist who has experience with movement disorders.

Where should the operation be done?

The first and most important recommendation is that the patient has surgery where there is a team of experts. This means neurologists and neurosurgeons that have experience and specialized training in doing these types of surgeries.

The next most important question is how the surgery is done. Different centers may perform the surgeries in different ways. It is very important to ask how the target (that is, the thalamus or globus pallidus) is localized. It is clear that the chances of benefit and the risks of complications are directly related to how close the electrode is to the correct target.

How can the target area be localized?

There are several ways in which the target is localized. One way is to rely only on computed tomography (CT) or magnetic resonance imaging (MRI) scans. Some teams also use micro-electrodes. Prior to placing the permanent stimulating electrode, micro-electrodes are used to record electrical activity generated by individual brain cells. Because these cells communicate by electrical impulses, micro-electrode recording is like eavesdropping on the conversation the brain cells are having. When just the right accent (just the right pattern of brain cell activity) is identified, the surgeon can be confident that the electrode is in the best location.

With modern CT and MRI techniques, the surgeon can get close, but the use of micro-electrode recordings will get the surgeon closer. While surgeons who use only the CT or MRI scans will have some success, the rate of success is greater and the risk of complications less when micro-electrode recordings are used. Micro-electrode recordings do take more time (and therefore, it is less popular with some surgeons).

There are two types of electrical recording that can be done. One type is with the micro-electrodes described. Another type is with macro-electrodes. These electrodes have a larger tip. Because of their size, they cannot record the electrical activity of individual brain cells but instead record the activity of many brain cells. Using macro-electrodes would be like hearing the roar of a crowd, whereas using the micro-electrodes is like listening to the individual conversations. The Cleveland Clinic believes that using the micro-electrodes and listening to the conversations of individual brain cells is more accurate.

Summary

One of the major problems in this area of medicine is that often patients and their physicians give up too early. Deep brain stimulation offers patients new hope. There is evidence that these surgeries are as effective as or more effective than the older thalamotomy and pallidotomy surgeries, which are well-established and accepted treatments. However, deep brain stimulation may be safer. Patients who fail to achieve satisfactory control with medications may consider deep brain stimulation, although it is also important for multiple sclerosis patients to have appropriate expectations regarding the potential benefits of deep brain stimulation.

Chapter 33

Rehabilitation for MS

Chapter Contents

Section 33.1

Physical Therapy

"Physiotherapy: Its Role in Rehabilitation," by Dawn Prasad, *MS in Focus, Issue 7*, 2006. © Multiple Sclerosis International Federation (www.msif.org). Reprinted with permission.

Physical therapy plays an important role in the management of multiple sclerosis (MS). In the early stages following diagnosis, there is a strong emphasis on education and self-management with advice on when it is beneficial to request a physical therapy assessment. The type of physical therapy approach and the intensity of the therapy will vary depending on the needs of the person with MS and the findings of the physical therapy assessment. People with MS do not require constant physical therapy input; however, there are benefits to bursts of rehabilitation following a relapse or a change in functional capacity. Physical therapy treatment may occur in a variety of settings such as hospital rehabilitation units as either an inpatient or outpatient, or in the community. In some countries, rehabilitation at home is available and may be organized by or through the national MS society.

Physical therapy for people with MS includes:

• comprehensive assessment of level of impairment due to MS;

• formation of functional and achievable goals;

• treatment;

• evaluation of response to treatment;

• education and promotion of healthy lifestyle; and

• plans for follow-up rehabilitation.

Physical therapy is beneficial in the treatment of many symptoms of MS and during rehabilitation the physical therapist will work with the person with MS to achieve functional goals. Some symptoms helped by physical therapy, often in conjunction with other disciplines, are listed here:

Weakness is a major symptom of MS and leads to a reduced ability in walking, standing, and transfers—as well as problems with daily living activities that involve the upper limbs. Physical therapy techniques to improve strength may involve the physical therapist handling the person with MS to provide manual resistance for movements; examples include, exercises using the weight of the body against gravity, or exercises using weights or elastic bands to provide progressive resistance. During the rehabilitation phase, strengthening exercises are often focused on regaining control of particularly weak muscles and correcting muscle imbalance to restore postural stability.

Weakness is thought to be a factor in fatigue because weak muscles work less efficiently and tire more quickly—therefore, strength training helps to reduce fatigue. Weakness also influences balance and coordination and recent research into the benefits of strength training have shown improvements with functional tasks.

Reduced motor control (or paralysis) of a leg or an arm may result from damage to the nerve pathway supplying the muscles that control the limb. Recovery of control will be dependent on where the damage occurs and the severity of the damage. Physical therapy may help restore lost movement when there is still the possibility of nerve impulses activating weak muscles. If restoration of movement is not possible, then the physical therapist may prescribe an external orthopaedic appliance that helps the movement of the limbs (an orthosis) such as a foot splint to improve walking.

Reduced balance occurs when there is a problem with the vestibular system of the brain, or sensory losses, or weakness. Physical therapists are skilled at assessing the contributing factors to the balance problem and prescribing remedial techniques. Education and promotion of some compensatory strategies are often part of the solution; for example, vision is very important for providing additional information to the brain—therefore, putting on a light when getting up to go to the toilet at night is very useful in reducing the risk of falling. People with MS who have impaired balance should be assessed by a physical therapist; without physical therapy input, people often adopt compensatory strategies to reduce the risk of falls. Over time these strategies can lead to greater secondary problems, such as joint strain, increased fatigue, and muscle imbalance.

Spasticity is a symptom experienced by many people with MS caused by changes in the nerve impulses to the muscles resulting in spasms and stiffness. Physical therapists are involved in teaching

327

people with MS and their caregivers stretching and positioning techniques which help to relieve spasms and prevent shortening in muscles that are prone to spasms. Often, medication such as baclofen or tizanidine is required to help control the spasticity, and physical therapists are important in monitoring the effectiveness of the prescribed medication over time.

Pain in MS may be related to the areas of the central nervous system that are affected, and is commonly termed neurogenic or neuropathic pain; this is treated by the use of medication such as gabapentin. Other types of pain in MS may be related to muscle spasms and joint strains and can be treated by physical therapy with success. For people with limited mobility, it is important for physical therapists to assess the level of seating and postural support required, and to provide advice on adequate pressure relief.

Tremor can be a difficult symptom that limits functional ability. A variety of treatments may be tried including, repetitive patterning movements which aim to improve coordination, adding weights to wrists to reduce the amplitude of the tremor, and education about positioning to increase stability of the arm or leg.

Liaison with Other Disciplines

Ideally physical therapists work closely with other health professionals on the rehabilitation team. Often, there is overlap with functional goals directed by one discipline helping the goals of another discipline become achievable. A good example of close collaboration is when physical therapists and occupational therapists perform joint wheelchair and seating assessments; the combined expertise of both disciplines ensures that postural needs, pressure care needs, and functional capacity are all met within the same assessment process.

Physical therapists are responsible for promoting a healthy and active lifestyle to people with MS to help reduce the impact of any relapses and to promote recovery. In the past, people with MS were not encouraged to exercise, particularly those with fatigue; however, more recent research into exercise has highlighted its positive effects and found that fatigue is actually reduced by a more active lifestyle. For people who are no longer able to exercise by themselves, physical therapists have an important role in teaching caregivers how to perform regular stretches and positioning techniques.

At the completion of an inpatient rehabilitation period, it is important for physical therapists to provide a suitable home program or advice on suitable exercise and activities to promote continued well-being. The physical therapist plays a primary role in a comprehensive rehabilitation program. Physical therapy is appropriate at different stages of the disease for people with various levels of impairment and can be effective for treating many problems due to or associated with MS.

Section 33.2

Occupational Therapy

"Occupational Therapy Helps to Manage Daily Life," by Marijke Duportail and Daphne Kos, *MS in Focus, Issue 7*, 2006. © Multiple Sclerosis International Federation (www.msif.org). Reprinted with permission

A compensatory rehabilitative approach can appropriately complement treatment with symptomatic and disease-modifying therapies for people with multiple sclerosis (MS). This process involves the modification of techniques and the development of new strategies to compensate for functional limitations. Occupational therapy is an important part of this approach and focuses on skills that are important for the occupations of daily life and on reducing participation restrictions and activity limitations.

Evidence from the Literature

The role of occupational therapy in multidisciplinary rehabilitation is well acknowledged. However, the multidisciplinary character of MS treatment means it is difficult to demonstrate the net effect of occupational therapy as people receiving multidisciplinary rehabilitation will be seen to benefit from interventions from a variety of fields. While currently there is no reliable scientific evidence available that occupational therapy helps people with MS in managing their disease, it is likely that most professionals and individuals with MS, based on experience, do see benefit from occupational therapy interventions. Small studies have found that fatigue can be relieved using energy conservation techniques.

Primary Objectives and Aims

The primary objective of occupational therapy is to enable individuals to participate in self-care, work, and leisure activities that they want or need to perform, thereby optimizing personal fulfillment, well-being, and quality of life. The occupational therapist evaluates whether people with MS are limited in the life domains that are important to them and determines strategies for overcoming these difficulties. Possible strategies include restoration, compensation, adaptation, and prevention.

Life domains include:

* personal care (washing, dressing);
* domestic activities (cooking meals, shopping, gardening);
* employment and education;
* recreation and leisure (sport, social activities, hobbies);
* communication (writing, computer use);
* mobility (walking, using public transportation).

Interventions

Evaluation is the first step in the occupational therapy program. The therapist assesses the performance skills in daily life activities, assesses general physical and cognitive abilities, discusses personal goals, and may assess the home and work environments to evaluate the potential need for modifications. A customized occupational therapy rehabilitation program improves the individual's ability to perform daily activities within his or her own unique situation, thus, often requiring a combination of different techniques.

Applicability at Different Stages of the Disease

For people in the early stage of MS who experience changes in their ability to function effectively at some tasks, the occupational therapist focuses on teaching new strategies for dealing with fatigue, information about home environment adjustments, modifications to the car or workplace, as well as job performance. Energy management courses may also be most appropriate at an early stage of the disease.

If functional loss increases, the occupational therapist assists the person with MS in maintaining and improving skills in different areas of the life domains. Depending on the functional abilities and needs of the individual, more attention may be focused on compensation techniques in combination with advice on obtaining an assistive device, as well as the opportunity to try out different devices and other options to meet short- and long-term needs.

Occupational Therapy in the Home

Meeting the individual and the family in their environment can provide the occupational therapist with valuable information that may not be readily available when assessing the person within a health care setting. The assessment includes an evaluation of the individual's current functional status in relation to the performance of activities of daily living. An assessment of the home situation includes the evaluation of the need for assistive equipment and training. Finally, the occupational therapist's visit to the home can serve to determine whether additional paid assistance may be useful.

Working with Other Disciplines

Collaboration with professionals promotes independence in all life domains. Occupational therapists work with social services for organizing home visits, with physical therapists regarding functional exercises, with speech and swallowing therapists on issues related to communication, with nurses in performing evaluations and improving performance in activities of daily living, and with neuropsychologists and speech therapists on cognitive training.

Conclusion

Occupational therapy focuses on learning strategies for managing daily life based on the person's physical, social, and psychological needs.

Section 33.3

Counseling Therapy

"The Role of Counseling in Rehabilitation," by C.N. Tromp and R. Petter, *MS in Focus, Issue 7*, 2006. © Multiple Sclerosis International Federation (www.msif.org). Reprinted with permission.

Counseling people with multiple sclerosis (MS) is more than just listening and giving advice. It is a form of helping an individual to deal with personal problems relating to the disease that is often absent from conversations with family, friends, and some health care professionals. It is about providing support and helping people change, and not primarily about promoting practical solutions.

A counselor is not committed to a certain medical treatment policy, and therefore, aspects of dealing with the disease can be discussed without direct consequences for treatment. Counselors can also be helpful in shaping the style of living with MS according to the person's wishes and needs. An optimal treatment program for a health care provider can be difficult and unsatisfactory for the individual treated. A person with MS can often exert more influence on his or her life and disease management than he or she may think. Helping people with MS realize their autonomy in decision-making is part of the counseling process.

Aims of Counseling

Counseling for people with MS focuses mainly on coping with the uncertainties and unpredictability of the illness. Each person with MS, regardless of the type and course of the illness, must adapt continuously to changing symptoms and find ways to live with relapses and remission. Learning to assess the effects of these changes (both physical and cognitive) on daily life, setting priorities for where energy should be concentrated and recognizing the need for new priorities for activities and tasks, making therapeutic decisions, redistributing responsibilities within the family, and making vocational choices, are some of the important topics that can be discussed during counseling with a professional counselor who has an understanding of MS.

After diagnosis, the need for information, advice, and reassurance—especially about the prognosis and therapy options—is foremost. Information about the illness, both from the medical side and regarding public resources—especially that taken from the internet—can be evaluated and interpreted with particular reference to the person's own opinion about it with the assistance of the counselor. When a person with MS is not followed and supported during this early period, dealing with the disease can be a lonely, isolating experience. A counselor can be an important resource during this time and at various times throughout life with MS.

Discussing Difficult Topics

No one can read the minds of others, so the need to be specific and clear when communicating about personal and perhaps difficult subjects such as the amount of help and support that is required, can put a strain on relationships, especially when support needs may fluctuate from one day to another. This constant effort to be both candid and tactful can be very challenging and discouraging both for the person with MS and those around him or her. The situation often creates a need for the person with MS to be outspoken and assertive in expressing needs and desires with family members. Assertiveness that is appropriate for the situation and contexts may require practice. The counselor can play a role in helping the person rehearse and prepare discussions on difficult topics with family members and can provide encouragement and feedback.

Topics of Counseling

Up to 50 percent of patients with MS in the relapsing-remitting condition develop serious, and sometimes permanent, psychological symptoms. Prevention or management of these symptoms is another aim of counseling efforts. Psychological problems include depression, stress reactions, and chronic fatigue. Cognitive problems can be a major concern, requiring an understanding of not only the individual, but also of those around the person with MS. Shifts in the competence and roles of parents or children within a family structure are sometimes difficult to accept. For parents, dealing with the requirements of younger family members, who often come home from school or work and expect attention and care exactly at a moment when their parent is most exhausted can be frustrating. Working out practical solutions can be part of the counseling process.

Counselors knowledgeable in MS can also have a role in working with children whose parent has MS. Meeting with the entire family, with the child or children individually, as well as participating in the development of programs and activities organized for children of people with MS, are all ways in which a counselor can help families to deal with the challenges of MS.

Counseling can be of value both for the person with MS as well as for those who are close to the individual who deals with MS in their personal lives—either directly or indirectly. Indications for counseling include a broad range of subjects which require close and timely cooperation with other professionals, including the nurse, neurologist, and social worker, in order to be a valuable supplement to regular care.

Chapter 34

Complementary and Alternative Medicine in MS

Separating the Help from the Hype

Once largely ignored, if not outright dismissed by most health care providers, complementary and alternative medicine (CAM) has become more popular now than ever. Patient use of herbal and other CAM remedies has risen significantly in recent years[1] and those with multiple sclerosis (MS) are no exception.

Popular among MS Patients

"Studies have routinely found that the majority of people with MS have tried some form of alternative therapy," noted Allen Bowling, MD, PhD, Medical Director of the Rocky Mountain Multiple Sclerosis Center in Englewood, Colorado, and Clinical Associate Professor of Neurology at the University of Colorado Health Sciences Center. Of the 3,140 respondents to a 2003 survey of MS patients, 57% reported using one or more CAM therapies.[2]

CAM use by MS patients was quite common during the 1970s, because clinicians had little to offer these individuals other than symptomatic management, noted June Halper, MSCN, ANP, FAAN, Executive

---

This chapter includes text from "Complementary and Alternative Medicine in MS," by Peter Doskoch, *MS Exchange*, February 2006. © 2006 Consortium of Multiple Sclerosis Centers. Reprinted with permission. Additional text from the Consortium of Multiple Sclerosis Centers is cited separately within the chapter.

Director of the Bernard W. Gimbel MS Comprehensive Care Center in Teaneck, New Jersey. "Some of our patients would spend fortunes on totally unproven therapies such as cobra venom or elemental calcium," she recalled. Today, the limitations of certain disease-modifying therapies—and the increased acceptance of CAM by health care professionals—have ensured that alternative therapies remain on the radar screen for most patients.

Helping Patients Make Informed Decisions

"There are very few alternative therapies for which definitive evidence of efficacy exists," Dr. Bowling admitted. Therefore, health care providers may feel that discussing alternative medicine is a waste of the patient's time. However, even MS clinicians who are skeptical about the efficacy of CAM may find a working knowledge of alternative therapies valuable. "We do know about many alternative therapies that could possibly be helpful—or harmful—and we can improve quality of care by sharing this information with our patients," said Dr. Bowling.

Discussing CAM with Patients

Some patients don't tell their clinicians that they're using CAM because they fear disapproval, Ms. Halper said. In turn, health care providers often don't raise the issue. "It's the job of the clinician to initiate a frank, open discussion of CAM," she stated.

Medical professionals need not provide or even endorse alternative therapies themselves. Indeed, given the liability and licensing issues associated with recommending therapies for which efficacy and safety data are lacking, the best approach for most clinicians may be to simply provide information and resources, according to Dr. Bowling.

Safety Concerns

Unfortunately, some patients assume that natural CAM therapies are completely safe. "Patients typically are not well-informed about the side effects and drug interactions that may occur with some vitamins and herbal supplements," said Pam Newland, RN, MSN, PhD, a Lecturer at Southern Illinois University School of Nursing in Edwardsville.

For example, some CAM therapies have immune-stimulating properties that could, in theory, provoke or worsen the symptoms of autoimmune diseases such as MS, added Dr. Bowling.

Other alternative therapies can have adverse effects not unlike those of conventional medications. For instance, ginkgo can increase the risk of bleeding and thus should be avoided by people who are using anticoagulants or have bleeding disorders. To cite a more extreme example, kava, used to treat mild anxiety, has been linked to fatal liver toxicity and has been banned in Canada and some European countries. "Thus, it is important that clinicians educate their patients on any side effects or interactions that may occur," stressed Dr. Newland.

CAM and the MS Treatment Plan

In formulating a treatment plan, Dr. Bowling advised focusing first on conventional pharmacologic therapies as well as accepted adjunctive approaches, such as physical therapy. "However, if patients ask whether there is anything else they can do, information about various interventions can be provided." Clinicians should be sure to stress that evidence-based data on CAM therapies are often limited, Dr. Bowling said.

While Dr. Bowling's center provides printed material and references for patients interested in a particular CAM modality, personal discussions with patients are invaluable. "If we're able to talk with patients about alternative therapies and make them aware of what might be helpful and what might be harmful, we can improve the quality of care that we provide," he said.

CAM Therapies of Note for the MS Practitioner

Following are some biologic and other CAM therapies that because of their effectiveness, potential for adverse effects, or popularity may be of interest to clinicians who treat MS patients.

Acupuncture: One large study of acupuncture in MS patients showed improvements in symptoms such as pain, fatigue, spasticity, and bowel problems; however, the study did not include a control group. More rigorous trials are underway.[4] Acupuncture is usually well-tolerated. When performed by a trained practitioner, serious side effects are rare.[5]

Cold remedies: It has been suggested that influenza and the common cold might worsen MS symptoms or trigger attacks. However, some CAM therapies for treating or preventing respiratory infections, such as echinacea, may pose similar risks because of their immunostimulatory effects.

Vitamins or calcium: In addition to helping maintain bone density, vitamin D may have mild immunosuppressive effects, which could be beneficial in MS (though no studies have confirmed such benefits).

Because research suggests that oxidative stress may play an important role in the etiology of MS,[6] it has been suggested that supplements containing antioxidants (such as vitamins A, C, and E) may also be beneficial to persons with MS. However, there is no evidence to support this theory. "Moreover, antioxidants increase the production and activity of immune cells and thus pose a theoretical risk to MS patients," said Dr. Bowling. "In addition, high intake of vitamins A (greater than 10,000 international units [IU] per day) can be toxic and doses of vitamin C above 1,000 milligrams (mg) per day can cause nausea and diarrhea."

Psyllium: Because many patients with MS experience constipation, psyllium (a form of dietary fiber) may be a useful symptomatic therapy.

St. John's Wort: Often used for mild depression, this herb should be taken under the guidance of a clinician because it is a cytochrome P450 inducer that alters the metabolism of many drugs. It may also be sedating.

Dietary fats: The omega-3 and omega-6 polyunsaturated fatty acids (PUFA) are the best-studied nonpharmacologic therapy for MS. One randomized trial involving 312 patients found a statistical trend ($P = .07$) for a lower progression rate in persons with MS treated with a combination of eicosapentaenoic acid and docosahexaenoic acid.[7] Epidemiologic evidence is consistent with these findings—countries with a high intake of polyunsaturated fatty acids have relatively low rates of MS.[8]

The best dietary source of omega-3 PUFA is fatty fish, said Dr. Bowling, though supplementation with fish oil is necessary to attain the intake levels used in most studies. Most Americans receive an adequate supply of omega-6 PUFA from dietary sources. "As regular use of PUFA supplements may cause deficiency in Vitamin E, modest supplementation (100 IU per day) is desirable," he added.

References

1. Kelly JP, Kaufman DW, Kelley K, et al. Recent trends in use of herbal and other natural products. *Arch Intern Med.* 2005;165:281–286.

2. Nayak S, Matheis RJ, Schoenberger NE, Shiflett SC. Use of unconventional therapies by individuals with multiple sclerosis. *Clin Rehabil.* 2003;17:181–191.

3. Rocky Mountain MS Center. Available at: www.mscam.org. Accessed December 28, 2005.

4. Wang H, Hashimoto S, Ramsum D. A pilot study of the use of alternative medicine in multiple sclerosis patients with special focus on acupuncture. *Neurology.* 1999;52:A550.

5. National Institutes of Health Consensus Conference. Acupuncture. *JAMA.* 1998;280:1518–1524.

6. Gilgun-Sherki Y, Barhum Y, Atlas D, et al. Analysis of gene expression in MOG-induced experimental autoimmune encephalomyelitis after treatment with a novel brain-penetrating antioxidant. *J Mol Neurosci.* 2005;27:125–135.

7. Bates D, Cartlidge NE, Franch JM, et al. A double-blind controlled trial of long chain n-3 polyunsaturated fatty acids in the treatment of multiple sclerosis. *J Neurol Neurosurg Psychiatry.* 1989;52:18–22.

8. Bates D. Lipids and multiple sclerosis. *Biochem Soc Trans.* 1989;17:289–291.

Alternative Medicines That "Could" Be Harmful in Patients with Multiple Sclerosis

Text in this section is from "Alternative Medicines that 'Could' Be Harmful in Patients with Multiple Sclerosis," by Ellen Guthrie, PharmD. © 2004 Consortium of Multiple Sclerosis Centers. Reprinted with permission.

Alternative medicine is widely used in the United States. In 1998, Dr. David Eisenberg estimated that 42% of Americans use some form of complimentary alternative medicine (CAM).[1] A similar study was conducted with multiple sclerosis (MS) patients at the Rocky Mountain MS Center in 1997. This study found that 67% of MS patients used some form of CAM.[2] One could conclude from this data that MS patients are more likely to use alternative or unconventional medicine than non-MS patients.

Concerning alternative medicine, patients with and without MS have one thing in common—they rarely admit to their doctors that they use it. This can be very dangerous because 90% of individuals who use alternative medicine also use conventional medicine.[2] Drug interactions can occur between conventional and unconventional medications just like they can occur between conventional medicines. The best way to avoid all drug interactions is to make your physicians aware of any and all medications (conventional and unconventional) that you use.

MS is a very complicated disease that affects both the immune and nervous systems. In order to understand which alternative medications are safe and unsafe in MS, it is necessary to examine the disease. Patients with MS have an up-regulated or excessively active immune system. CD4-TH1 cells in the immune system attack the myelin in the nervous system. Multiple sclerotic plaques then develop in the central nervous system (CNS) and axonal damage can result.

The immune system in the MS patient is the opposite from the immune system in a cancer or human immunodeficiency virus (HIV) patient. These patients have a suppressed immune system. Therefore, immune-stimulating therapies that would be helpful for cancer and HIV patients may actually be harmful in MS patients.

A general rule of thumb for alternative medicine and MS:

- If a particular product is recommended for a condition where the immune system is suppressed (for example, cancer, HIV, colds), avoid the product in MS.

Many alternative medications are known to stimulate the immune system. While these products are beneficial in treating conditions of a weaken immune system, they can possibly worsen MS since it is a disease of an up-regulated immune system. It is very important for MS patients to be aware of alternative medications that can up-regulate the immune system. The following alternative medications pose potential risks for the MS patient because of their immune stimulating properties.[3]

- alfalfa
- echinacea
- ginseng, Siberian

- green tea

- arnica

- garlic supplements

- golden seal

- licorice

- cat's claw

- ginseng, Asian

- grape seed extract

- saw palmetto

In high doses, certain vitamins may also stimulate the immune system. It is best to avoid high doses of vitamin A, vitamin C, beta-carotene, and zinc in MS patients. Taking the recommended daily allowance (RDA) of these products poses no risk to patients with MS. As mentioned, it is very important to talk with your doctor before you take alternative medications. This gives you and your physician the opportunity to weigh the pros and cons of the agents in question. This advice is especially true for MS patients since certain alternative medicines can theoretically worsen the course of the disease. Basically, when it comes to your body and your health, it is better to be safe than sorry.

Five Basic Truths Regarding CAM and MS

1. Tell your doctor about all medications that you take (conventional and unconventional).

2. Realize that information you read (in print or on the internet) may or may not be correct.

3. MS is a disease that involves an up-regulated immune system; therefore, products that stimulate the immune system may be contraindicated.

4. Anything that has a positive effect on the body can also have a negative effect on the body.

5. Just because an alternative medicine has scientific evidence to back up its claims does not mean that controlled clinical trials have proven its use.

341

References

1. Eisenberg D, Davis R, Ettner S, et al. Trends in alternative medicine use in the United States, 1990-1997. *JAMA* 1998; 280:1569–1575.

2. Bowling A. *Alternative Medicine and Multiple Sclerosis.* New York: Demos Medical Publishing, Inc., 2001:8.

3. Bowling A. *Alternative Medicine and Multiple Sclerosis.* New York: Demos Medical Publishing, Inc., 2001:118.

Additional Information

Consortium of MS Centers
718 Teaneck Road
Teaneck, NJ 07666
Phone: 201-837-0727
Fax: 201-837-9414
Website: http://www.mscare.org
E-mail: info@mscare.org

Chapter 35

Plasmapheresis: A Controversial Treatment for MS

Plasmapheresis is a process involving the following steps:

- Whole blood is withdrawn from the person.
- The liquid portion or plasma is removed from the blood and replaced.
- The blood, with all its red and white blood cells, is transfused back into the person.

This process is a successful method for treating autoimmune diseases such as myasthenia gravis and Guillain-Barré Syndrome, because it removes the circulating antibodies that are thought to be responsible for these diseases.

It is not clear whether plasmapheresis is of benefit in the short- or long-term treatment of MS, and its use in MS remains controversial.

Because MS may also involve an autoimmune process—where the body is attacked by its own immune system—and because demyelinating factors have been found in plasma from MS patients, plasmapheresis has been tried as a treatment for MS.

Mixed Results in Progressive Forms of MS

Studies using plasmapheresis in patients with primary and secondary progressive MS have yielded mixed results.

One carefully controlled study among MS patients who were also receiving medication that suppresses the immune system, suggests that patients who received both plasmapheresis and immunosuppressants did better than those receiving immunosuppressants alone. The apparent advantage of plasmapheresis was most pronounced within the first five months of treatment. The study was placebo-controlled to make sure that responses to treatment were based on therapeutic benefit, rather than a psychological effect of receiving treatment. The study was also double-blind-neither the researchers nor the patients knew who was receiving active treatment until the study was over.

Other studies by other investigators did not find plasmapheresis when combined with chemotherapy to be any more effective than chemotherapy alone.

Minimally Shortened Recovery Time from Exacerbations

A more recent clinical trial studied the effect of plasmapheresis in treating acute exacerbations. An exacerbation—also known as an attack, relapse, or flare—is a sudden worsening of an MS symptom or symptoms, or the appearance of new symptoms, which lasts at least 24 hours and is separated from a previous exacerbation by at least one month.

In this multicenter study, 116 patients having an exacerbation received adrenocorticotropic hormone (ACTH) and immunosuppressant medication, and either plasmapheresis or "sham" plasmapheresis (in which the plasma withdrawn from the patient was returned, instead of being replaced). The results indicated a minimally shortened time to recovery in the plasmapheresis treated group compared to the control group. No long-term benefits were observed, at a 12-month follow-up.

A Recent Study on Plasma Exchange

In a recent study on plasma exchange the investigators concluded that plasma exchange might contribute to recovery from an acute attack in people with MS or other inflammatory demyelinating diseases who have not responded to standard steroid treatment.

344

They recommend, therefore, that this treatment only be considered for individuals experiencing a severe, acute attack that is not responding to high-dose steroids. Since the vast majority (90%) of people experiencing acute attacks respond well to the standard steroid treatment, plasma exchange would be considered a treatment alternative only for the 10% or so who do not. For those 10%, however, plasma exchange may offer an important and beneficial treatment option.

Side Effects Include Infection and Blood Clotting Problems

Side effects of plasmapheresis therapy include occasional infection and blood clotting problems.

Chapter 36

Cooling Therapy for MS

A Randomized Controlled Study of the Acute and Chronic Effects of Cooling Therapy for MS

Background: Cooling demyelinated nerves can reduce conduction block, potentially improving symptoms of multiple sclerosis (MS). The therapeutic effects of cooling in patients with MS have not been convincingly demonstrated because prior studies were limited by uncontrolled designs, unblinded evaluations, reliance on subjective outcome measures, and small sample sizes.

Objective: To determine the effects of a single acute dose of cooling therapy using objective measures of neurologic function in a controlled, double-blinded setting, and to determine whether effects are sustained during daily cooling garment use.

Methods: Patients (n = 84) with definite MS, mild to moderate disability (Expanded Disability Status Scale [EDSS] score less than 6.0), and self-reported heat sensitivity were randomized into a multicenter, sham-treatment controlled, double-blind crossover study.

This chapter includes: Excerpts from Schwid, S., et al. "A randomized controlled study of the acute and chronic effects of cooling therapy for MS," *Neurology* 2003 June 24 60(12): 1955–60. © American Academy of Neurology. Reprinted by permission of WoltersKluwer. Text under the heading "Multiple Sclerosis and Cooling" is excerpted from *Multiple Sclerosis and Cooling, Third Edition*, © 2004 Multiple Sclerosis Association of America. All rights reserved. Reprinted with permission.

Patients had the MS Functional Composite (MSFC) and measures of visual acuity/contrast sensitivity assessed before and after high-dose or low-dose cooling for one hour with a liquid cooling garment. One week later, patients had identical assessments before and after the alternate treatment. Patients were then re-randomized to use the cooling garment one hour each day for a month or to have observation only. They completed self-rated assessments of fatigue, strength, and cognition during this time, and underwent another acute cooling session at the end of the period. After one week of rest, they had identical assessments during the alternate treatment.

Results: Body temperature declined during both high-dose and low-dose cooling, but high-dose produced a greater reduction ($p < 0.0001$). High-dose cooling produced a small improvement in the MSFC (0.076 ± 0.66, $p = 0.007$), whereas low-dose cooling produced only a trend toward improvement (0.053 ± 0.031, $p = 0.09$), but the difference between conditions was not significant. Timed gait testing and visual acuity/contrast sensitivity improved in both conditions as well. When patients underwent acute cooling following a month of daily cooling, treatment effects were similar. Patients reported less fatigue during the month of daily cooling, concurrently on the Rochester Fatigue Diary and retrospectively on the Modified Fatigue Impact Scale.

Conclusions: Cooling therapy was associated with objectively measurable but modest improvements in motor and visual function as well as persistent subjective benefits. Although other studies have demonstrated that continuous cooling can promote improvement in neurologic signs over several days, no other study has systematically assessed the long-term benefits of daily cooling, as patients would typically use it. We found no evidence that cooling effects changed over time. Given the lack of side effects observed in this study, modest improvements demonstrated using objective measures of motor and visual function, and persistent subjective benefits, cooling therapy could be considered as a potential adjunct to other symptomatic and disease-modifying treatments for patients with MS.

Multiple Sclerosis and Cooling

How to Use Active Cool Suits

The first step to safe cooling is to establish a baseline temperature. This is an average of temperatures over at least seven days. This is important because a maximum cooling of two-degrees Fahrenheit from a person's baseline is generally considered safe. A one-degree Fahrenheit drop in a person's temperature, however, has been found to be sufficient for effective active-cooling therapy.

The next step is to choose a room with a stable and moderate room temperature (70 to 75 degrees Fahrenheit). Room temperature plays a vital role in effective cooling. If the room is too cool, the body will react against the cooling. If the room is too warm, the cooling suit will be ineffective.

Active suits are always started at room temperature and then the temperature is slowly reduced during the first 15 minutes. Most in-home cooling sessions are conducted for one hour. They may be repeated with or without exercise (as recommended by one's physician) for up to three times per day, waiting at least two hours between each session. These units can also be used with a battery pack, enabling individuals who are heat intolerant to once again enjoy the outdoors.

Cooling therapy, when used correctly, may help reduce some symptoms of MS, including problems with fatigue, vision, spasticity, motor function, and cognition. As with any therapy, not all people receive the same benefit or any benefit at all. Cooling therapy should be viewed as an adjunct to disease modifying drugs, not as an alternative, and should only be done with the approval of a medical professional.

How Passive Cooling Can Help

Passive cooling refers to cooling with no active cooling mechanism, such as a separate pump. Passive cooling can be accomplished through a simple transfer of heat by wearing a garment containing a cooling source.

Evaporation garments include bandanas, skullcaps, and vests. These garments are usually soaked in water, rung out, and occasionally chilled in the refrigerator. As the water in the garments evaporates, they provide limited relief from heat, depending on climate conditions. These garments are less effective in areas with high humidity.

Most passive-cooling garments work by placing ice or gel packs into pockets of a vest. This type of system can provide immediate and simple relief from the heat. These vests allow many people with MS to enjoy outside activities that would otherwise be intolerable.

Studies have shown that the immediate loss of cognitive or physical function can occur due to an increase in either internal (through exercise) or external (room or outside) temperature. Passive cooling can significantly reduce the impact of these factors by providing a simple cooling mechanism. Passive cooling cannot be viewed as a symptomatic therapy, but can be seen as a valuable preventative tool to help reduce the impact of heat in people with MS.

349

Chapter 37

Clinical Studies of MS

What are clinical studies?

Clinical studies are research studies in which real people participate as volunteers. Clinical research studies (sometimes called trials
or protocols) are a means of developing new treatments and medications for diseases and conditions. There are strict rules for clinical
trials, which are monitored by the National Institutes of Health (NIH)
and the U.S. Food and Drug Administration (FDA).

Why should I participate?

The health of millions has been improved because of advances in
science and technology, and the willingness of thousands of individuals like you to take part in clinical research. The role of volunteer
subjects as partners in clinical research is crucial in the quest for
knowledge that will improve the health of future generations.

What are Phase I, Phase II, and Phase III studies?

The phase 1 study is used to learn the "maximum tolerated dose"
of a drug that does not produce unacceptable side effects. Patient volunteers are followed primarily for side effects, and not for how the
drug affects their disease. The first few volunteer subjects receive low

Excerpted from "FAQs about Clinical Studies," National Institutes of
Health (NIH) Clinical Center, 2006.

doses of the trial drug to see how the drug is tolerated and to learn how it acts in the body. The next group of volunteer subjects receives larger amounts. Phase 1 studies typically offer little or no benefit to the volunteer subjects.

The phase 2 study involves a drug whose dose and side effects are well-known. Many more volunteer subjects are tested, to define side effects, learn how it is used in the body, and learn how it helps the condition under study. Some volunteer subjects may benefit from a phase 2 study.

The phase 3 study compares the new drug against a commonly used drug. Some volunteer subjects will be given the new drug and some the commonly used drug. The trial is designed to find where the new drug fits in managing a particular condition. Determining the true benefit of a drug in a clinical trial is difficult.

What is a placebo?

Placebos are harmless, inactive substances made to look like the real medicine used in the clinical trial. Placebos allow the investigators to learn whether the medicine being given works better or no better than ordinary treatment. In many studies, there are successive time periods, with either the placebo or the real medicine. In order not to introduce bias, the patients, and sometimes the staff, are not told when or what the changes are. If a placebo is part of a study, you will always be informed in the consent form given to you before you agree to take part in the study. When you read the consent form, be sure that you understand what research approach is being used in the study you are entering.

What is the placebo effect?

Medical research is dogged by the placebo effect—the real or apparent improvement in a patient's condition due to wishful thinking by the investigator or the patient. Medical techniques use three ways to rid clinical trials of this problem. These methods have helped discredit some previously accepted treatments and validate new ones. Methods used are the following: randomization, single-blind or double-blind studies, and the use of a placebo.

What is randomization?

Randomization is when two or more alternative treatments are selected by chance, not by choice. The treatment chosen is given with the highest level of professional care and expertise, and the results of each treatment are compared. Analyses are done at intervals during a trial, which may last years. As soon as one treatment is found to be definitely superior, the trial is stopped. In this way, the fewest number of patients receive the less beneficial treatment.

What are single-blind and double-blind studies?

In single- or double-blind studies, the participants don't know which medicine is being used, and they can describe what happens without bias. Blind studies are designed to prevent anyone (doctors, nurses, or patients) from influencing the results. This allows scientifically accurate conclusions. In single-blind (single-masked) studies, only the patient is not told what is being given. In a double-blind study, only the pharmacist knows; the doctors, nurses, patients, and other health care staff are not informed. If medically necessary, however, it is always possible to find out what the patient is taking.

Are there risks involved in participating in clinical research?

Risks are involved in clinical research, as in routine medical care and activities of daily living. In thinking about the risks of research, it is helpful to focus on two things: the degree of harm that could result from taking part in the study, and the chance of any harm occurring. Most clinical studies pose risks of minor discomfort, lasting only a short time. Some volunteer subjects, however, experience complications that require medical attention. The specific risks associated with any research protocol are described in detail in the consent document, which you are asked to sign before taking part in research. In addition, the major risks of participating in a study will be explained to you by a member of the research team, who will answer your questions about the study. Before deciding to participate, you should carefully weigh these risks. Although you may not receive any direct benefit as a result of participating in research, the knowledge developed may help others.

What safeguards are there to protect participants in clinical research?

The following section describes safeguards that protect the safety and rights of volunteer subjects. These safeguards include:

Protocol review. As in any medical research facility, all new protocols produced at NIH must be approved by an institutional review board (IRB) before they can begin. The IRB, which consists of medical specialists, statisticians, nurses, social workers, and medical ethicists, is the advocate of the volunteer subject. The IRB will only approve protocols that address medically important questions in a scientific and responsible manner.

Informed consent. Your participation in any research protocol is voluntary. For every study in which you intend to participate, you will receive a document called "Consent to Participate in a Clinical Research Study" that explains the study in straightforward language. A member of the research team will discuss the protocol with you, explain its details, and answer your questions. Reading and understanding the protocol is your responsibility. You may discuss the protocol with family and friends. You will not be hurried into making a decision, and you will be asked to sign the document only after you understand the nature of the protocol and agree to the commitment. At any time after signing the protocol, you are free to change your mind and decide not to participate further. This means that you are free to withdraw from the study completely, or to refuse particular treatments or tests. Sometimes, however, this will make you ineligible to continue the study. If you are no longer eligible or no longer wish to continue the study, you will return to the care of the doctor who referred you to the trial.

Patient representative. The Patient Representative acts as a link between the patient and the hospital. The Patient Representative makes every effort to assure that patients are informed of their rights and responsibilities, and that they understand what the Clinical Center is, what it can offer, and how it operates. We realize that this setting is unique and may generate questions about the patient's role in the research process. As in any large and complex system, communication can be a problem and misunderstandings can occur. If any patient has an unanswered question or feels there is a problem they would like to discuss, they can call the Patient Representative.

Bill of Rights. Finally, whether you are a clinical research or a patient volunteer subject, you are protected by the Clinical Center Patients' Bill of Rights. This document is adapted from the one made by the American Hospital Association for use in all hospitals in the country. The bill of rights concerns the care you receive, privacy, confidentiality, and access to medical records.

Clinical Trials Recruiting Patients

For a complete listing of available clinical trials for MS patients, visit http://clinicaltrials.gov on the internet. Following is a small sample and brief summary of the types of MS clinical trials recruiting patients.

Combination Therapy in Patients with Relapsing-Remitting Multiple Sclerosis (MS) CombiRx

ClinicalTrials.gov Identifier: NCT00211887
Website: http://clinicaltrials.gov/ct/show/NCT00211887?order=1

This is a phase 3, randomized clinical trial to determine if the combined use of interferon beta-1a (IFN) and glatiramer acetate (GA) is a measurable better therapy than either agent used individually in patients with relapsing-remitting (RR) multiple sclerosis (MS).

Efficacy and Safety of MBP8298 in Subjects with Secondary Progressive Multiple Sclerosis (MAESTRO-03)

ClinicalTrials.gov Identifier: NCT00468611
Website: http://clinicaltrials.gov/ct/show/NCT0046811?order=7

This phase 3 study will assess the efficacy and safety of MBP8298 compared to placebo in subjects with secondary progressive multiple sclerosis (SPMS).

Trial of Memantine for Cognitive Impairment in Multiple Sclerosis

ClinicalTrials.gov Identifier: NCT00300716
Website: http://clinicaltrials.gov/ct/show/NCT00300716?order=13

This phase 2 and phase 3 study is designed to determine whether memantine is an effective treatment for memory and cognitive problems associated with multiple sclerosis when compared to placebo.

Additional Information about Clinical Trials

ClinicalTrials.gov
Toll-Free: 800-411-1222
Toll-Free TTY: 866-411-1010
Website: http://clinicaltrials.gov
E-mail: prpl@mail.cc.nih.gov

Part Four

Living with Multiple Sclerosis

Chapter 38

Telling Family, Friends, and Employers That You Have MS

Deciding whether or not to tell people that you have multiple sclerosis (MS) is a very personal decision. For many people with MS the disease is not clearly obvious, so there is a choice whether to disclose the diagnosis or not. If you need practical assistance, either daily or occasionally, this may dictate revealing to those close to you that you have MS. Your decision may depend on your relationships with others and how you think that they will react to the news.

Families

When you first learn that you have MS, you may feel able to discuss it with your family. For many people, it is a relief to be able to talk about it. Before you discuss your diagnosis with members of your family, you need to consider how you think that they will react. Family members generally are supportive. However, they may also be upset by the news, especially if they don't know anything about MS. It may be helpful to have informational pamphlets available to help talk about MS and how it affects you to ensure that people understand the disease. You may decide not to tell your family, or to tell only some of your relations, if you think that is could be detrimental to your relationships or lead to unwanted disclosure of your condition.

"Telling Family, Friends, and Employers," © 2007 Multiple Sclerosis International Federation (www.msif.org). Reprinted with permission.

Telling Young Children

It is probably not useful to make a formal announcement about MS to very young children, but it is important that their questions are answered as and when they occur. Instinctively children are aware that something is wrong and that you are worried. You need to be aware of this and understand that their behavior can sometimes be disturbed. The truth is hardly ever as frightening as their fears. A number of the national MS societies have booklets for children available that you may find helpful.

Telling Older Children

Older children and adolescents need to be informed but may require a more careful approach. Although they can appear outwardly calm and possibly even indifferent, they are most likely very concerned. Their anxiety can be helped by information. Their concerns need to be addressed as they arise and they need to know that you are willing to speak with them as issues come up. The opportunity to read selected literature from the national MS society may be helpful.

Adolescents feel that they should be treated as adults, and if they are not allowed to play a responsible part in a family problem, they can feel both hurt and resentful and as a result may start behaving in a destructive way. If, however, their cooperation is encouraged, they can become surprisingly mature and a source of strength. Trying to keep your problem to yourself will not spare them any anxiety.

Telling Parents

Telling parents of your diagnosis can also be difficult. It is very hard for parents to accept their child's diagnosis, and it is extremely important to be sensitive to their feelings and needs. Mothers, especially, will probably be extremely protective and many parents will feel that they are to blame.

When a Dependent Child or Adolescent Has MS

The parents of a child or adolescent with MS face enormous responsibility as to what to tell the young person about the disease and how much information and responsibility should be placed on their child. Many young people with MS are minimally affected initially and parents, both for their own sake and for the young person, resist public exposure when there may be many years before the effects are obvious. During this time, they hope the child or adolescent can mature into an adult, complete an education, set out on a career, and build relationships.

Usual counseling advice is based on the idea that all people diagnosed with MS are adults, and though not common, there are older children and adolescents who develop MS. The notion of immediate and full revelation of the nature of MS is a worthwhile generality that comes under some question in this particular cluster of persons with MS.

In the case of children under fifteen, particularly with minor symptoms and minimal disability, there is some argument for withholding the full nature and prospect of the disease. Obviously, the child is aware there is something wrong which comes and goes and often requires medical attention—but the parents can bear the responsibility of decisions and involvement with medical personnel while the child continues to lead a "normal" existence.

In the case of adolescents (fifteen years and older), they are old enough to be involved in the reality of the disease and the decisions which their parents make regarding treatment, education, etc. Nevertheless, it is important to remember that all adolescents are emotionally labile and have fragile self-images, MS being an additional burden for them to cope with.

Employers

The decision over whether to tell your employer could have an impact on your work. It may ensure more support or, in some cases, unfairly affect your career prospects. The legal requirements in relation to disclosure vary from country to country and you should check with your national MS society.

Advantages of Disclosure

1. Telling of your diagnosis can bring peace of mind. Many people with MS report that hiding is more stressful than telling. Disclosure also makes it easier, if the need arises, to discuss any workplace adaptations that might be necessary.

2. Having cleared the air, you will have an understanding of others' reaction to the fact that you have MS and of how you are likely to be perceived and treated by colleagues. You will be able to deal far more honestly with people.

3. You will be released from the worry that a past employer or reference might inadvertently reveal the fact that you have a disability.

4. Your apprehension about any proposed medical examination will be reduced because you will know that the employer, insurance company, and other relevant parties are aware of your MS before the examination.

5. Having told your employer that you have MS, you would find it much easier to educate him or her and colleagues regarding the true nature of the disease. As well, this allows you to discuss with your employer any future changes in your condition.

Disadvantages of Disclosure

1. Fear of being discriminated against because of having MS, for example, being denied promotion or training.

2. Fear of reaction of colleagues and others.

3. Fear of losing your job or not being offered a job (particularly if it has happened to you before).

4. Fear that, if something goes wrong in your job, it will be blamed on your disability.

What do I tell people about having MS?

Before you tell people that you have MS, you need to think about what they need to know. Many people will have no experience with MS or, on the other hand, know of someone with MS whose experience of the disease may be very different to yours. Your community includes people who are intimately connected to you and those whom you know casually. Your relatives, friends, and employer naturally will want to know what has happened to you, especially if you have visible symptoms. They may also want to know what they can do to help. If you are honest with those close to you and let them know you will accept help when you need it, you will allay their worries and probably find them very supportive.

You can start with a simple explanation of MS and how it is affecting you at this time, so that people are aware of any practical support which you may need without imagining that your MS is any worse than it is. If you have a standard description which you use, it can help to ensure that you feel confident giving the information and that the details you give are consistent. Certain general issues may need to be quickly refuted—for many people there are stereotypes which surround MS (for example, that everyone with MS ends up in a wheelchair) or misunderstandings (for example, that MS is contagious). MS societies have pamphlets and brochures that will make the task easier. Casual acquaintances can be told if it comes up in conversation or if you wish. In this case, there is probably no need for formal explanation.

Chapter 39

Can Disability, Chronic Conditions, Health, and Wellness Coexist?

Introduction

Can disability, chronic conditions, health, and wellness coexist? This question has broad and significant implications on the quality of life for people with chronic conditions and disabilities. Depending on personal beliefs, values, and current experience, people often emphasize one aspect over another in their own definitions of health. Traditional definitions describe health and disability at opposite ends of a single health continuum. Such definitions lead far too many people to view health and disability as mutually exclusive of each other, an either/or proposition. This view must be examined as it has damaging and lasting effects on people who live with disability and chronic conditions. As Bob Williams, Deputy Assistant Secretary for Disability, Aging, and Long-Term Care Policy in the U.S. Department of Health and Human Services puts it, "Learned helplessness truly is the greatest crippler anyone can experience. And, many people with disabilities have unfortunately learned to be passive, if not completely disengaged, where questions of their own health and well being are concerned." Many see health as just one more thing beyond their control, something they cannot change or influence. (Williams, p.5).

The ability to practice healthy behaviors, even in the presence of disability, has led to newer models of health. These newer definitions view health as multidimensional and see optimal health as defined within a given person's unique circumstances. Health is viewed as the maximizing of one's potential along various dimensions. Health includes a dynamic balance of physical, social, emotional, spiritual, and intellectual factors. When this definition is used, disability poses no obstacle to maximizing health and one's potential (Lanig, p.13). When health is viewed not as the absence of disability or chronic conditions, but as the ability to function effectively in given environments, to fulfill needs, and to adapt to major stresses, then, by definition, most people with disabilities are healthy.

Peg Nosek, Director, Center for Research on Women with Disabilities and Professor Department of Physical Medicine and Rehabilitation at Baylor College of Medicine, writes, that the stereotype of infirmity, sick people in wheelchairs covered with blankets, haunts people with disabilities. Curious new acquaintances or health providers will ask, "When did you first get sick?" Instead of, "How are you doing?" people with disabilities often get asked, "How are you feeling?" (Nosek, p. 2) Even in those situations where people are experiencing poor health, chronic fatigue, or pain, they don't want to be asked how they feel all the time.

Health care providers, like many others, are not free of the common disability stereotypes which cause discrimination and environmental and attitudinal barriers that people with disabilities encounter daily. Health providers, like society at large, have the same, if not stronger, misunderstandings about the health of people with disabilities. People working in medical settings constantly have these stereotypes reinforced, often because they are only exposed to people with disabilities and chronic conditions who are indeed sick. In addition, medical students report there is very little, if anything, taught about disability, living with disability, or health, wellness, and disability in medical school.

When the medical system does not understand the health needs of people with disabilities, this translates into practices and mistakes that affect people in the most important aspect of their lives, their health (Nosek, p. 6). A provider who equates disability and difference with dysfunction and illness, invalidates people with disabilities.

While disability and long-term conditions can involve pain or poor health, disability and health can and do coexist. Most people with disabilities are not sick. They are indeed healthy, when health is defined as the absence of illness and disease beyond disability. The assumption that health, wellness and disability cannot coexist is a myth. Providers who understand that people with disabilities can be healthy, active, and assertive participants and co-managers of their health and health care, can be of tremendous assistance in helping people select and practice tailored health promotion behaviors and activities directed at increasing a person's level of well-being.

Physical exercise, good nutrition, stress-management, and social support are important for every one, but they are actually more critical for people with disabilities who sometimes have been described as having "thinner margin of health" (Becker, p. 236). This does not imply that people with disabilities are sick. It means that people with disabilities are more vulnerable and more susceptible to certain health and secondary conditions depending on their disability. For example, some people with spinal cord injuries are more likely to have to deal with pressure sores, urinary tract infections, and kidney conditions. People with respiratory conditions can be more vulnerable to upper respiratory infections and pneumonia.

Health promotion activities are critical for people with disabilities who are prone to have a more sedentary lifestyle and have a tendency for under, over, or misuse of various muscle groups. Although we cannot yet replace the cells we lose as we age, "research is showing us that we can improve the efficiency of the remaining cells by staying as flexible as possible and by challenging our heart, lungs, and muscles to maximize in strength and endurance through exercise (Ontario Federation for Cerebral Palsy, p. 9)"

Questions That Need to Be Addressed

People with disabilities have many questions about strategies pertaining to weight control, diet, fitness, and exercise. Some of these key questions include:

- Where do people with disabilities go for fitness information that has a disability filter? How should we exercise? How much?

- What is the effect of exercise on preventing increasing disability for specific types of disability groups?

- How important is conditioning, flexibility, and endurance for people with disabilities? Is it more important that conditioning and flexibility be maintained because many people with disabilities work harder to physically function?

- Does active and consistent participation in various physical activities (i.e., sports, fitness) for people with disabilities accelerate musculoskeletal injury or pain or does it slow or prevent pain or injury?"

- How do people with disabilities maintain cardiopulmonary conditioning, physical strength, bone density, coordination, and joint mobility?

- Should aerobic conditioning come before specific muscle strengthening or the reverse?

- What type of strengthening program is best for people with significant spasticity?

- Where do people with disabilities find affordable personal trainers with disability expertise?

- What exercise books should people with disabilities read?

- What exercise videos should people with disabilities use?

- Which strengthening and aerobic equipment should people with disabilities use?

- Is a weight-lifting program going to strengthen muscles or will it cause or exacerbate pain and stiffness and lead to arthritis?

- Will osteoporosis become a major problem for people with mobility disabilities? Should screening be conducted earlier for people with disabilities than for people without disabilities? What interventions are effective? When should they be started?

- Since living with disability often means continual body strain and stress, should specialized diets be tailored to people with specific types of disabilities? For example, do wheelchair users need a greater intake of calcium than the recommended daily allowance to prevent bone loss? Are peak performance diets more relevant for people with disabilities?

- What are the implications for people with disabilities, of the fact that people without disabilities who have been athletic all their lives, and who have continued to eat and exercise properly, seem to age less rapidly and are healthier than their non-athletic counterparts?

When health care providers take the time to explore and understand negative misconceptions and stereotypes surrounding disability, many will be discarded. Providers who invest time in understanding issues related the health, wellness, and health care needs of people with disabilities can be strong supporters and advocates. Providers need to encourage people with disabilities to be healthy and active, as well as assertive participants and co-managers of their health and health care.

Unfortunately health promotion and preventative health care has received little attention, in part due to the strong perception that health and disability are mutually exclusive. As a friend, Kathleen Lankasky put it, "The lack of knowledge and understanding on the part of health care professionals concerning my disability and how it is affecting me as I age is extremely frightening to me....We are tired of reacting to pain and stiffness rather than preventing them."

The inability of people with disabilities to get helpful information regarding what types of exercises are best suited to their specific limitations is exasperating. This information gap is extremely troubling given the vast amount of existing evidence that indicates that many physical difficulties which accompany aging in people without disabilities can be prevented or lessened by exercise. Although good health habits, including exercise, do not guarantee a long life, they do greatly increase chances for a good quality of life.

What People with Disabilities Need

People with disabilities need:

• Exercise guidelines that are age and functional limitation-sensitive, to help assess how "fit" we are using appropriate standards and measures, fitness facilities we can get to, enter and use, integrated and convenient, not special or separate;

• Exercise facilities (YMCAs and other community-based fitness centers and programs) that are aware of and comply with their legal obligations under the Americans Disability Act;

• Exercise equipment that incorporates universally designed features so the equipment can then be used by people with a broad spectrum of strength and abilities without reducing the equipment's usability or attractiveness for all exercisers.

Everyone agrees that exercise and good nutrition is important, but helpful and specific information for people with disabilities is difficult to find. Although scarce, scientific and practical information does exist, it is poorly organized and spread over a wide range of disciplines. Answers that will help people with disabilities deal with these issues are needed. It's up to you to help fill these research, service, and information gaps.

~June Isaacson Kailes

June Isaacson Kailes, MSW, LCSW, is a Disability Policy Consultant in Playa del Rey, who works with the Center for Disability Issues and the Health Professions.

Note: The information provided here is offered as a service only. The National Center on Physical Activity and Disability, University of Illinois at Chicago, the National Center on Accessibility, and the Rehabilitation Institute of Chicago do not formally recommend or endorse the equipment listed. As with any products or services, consumers should investigate and determine on their own which equipment best fits their needs and budget.

National Center on Physical Activity and Disability
1640 W. Roosevelt Rd., Suite 711
Chicago, IL 60608-6904
Toll-Free Voice/TTY: 800-900-8086; Fax: 312-355-4058
Website: http://www.ncpad.org
E-mail: ncpad@uic.edu

Additional Information

Books

1. Indira S. Lanig (Eds.). (1996). *A Practical Guide to Health Promotion After Spinal Cord Injury*. Aspen Publishers.

2. Becker, E.F. and Mauro, R. (1994). *How to Live Longer with a Disability*. Bloomington, IL: Accent Press.

Journal

Nosek, P. (1992). Point of View: Primary Care Issues for Women with Severe Disabilities. *Journal of Women's Health*, 1(4).

Newsletter

NCPAD. *NCPAD Monthly Newsletter*.

Pamphlet

(1992). *Aging with a Lifelong Physical Disability: A Self-Help Guide*. Ontario Federation for Cerebral Palsy.

Chapter 40

MS and Nutrition

Introduction

Multiple sclerosis (MS) is a chronic degenerative inflammatory neurological disease that affects the brain and spinal cord. Dietary recommendations for people with MS are similar to those for the general population. Recommendations are based on the Food Guide Pyramid.

Growth, Nutrient, and Energy Needs

Detailed attention has been paid to the role of dietary fat and their possible therapeutic effects on people with MS. High consumption of saturated fat, such as animal fat, butterfat, shortening, and hydrogenated oils, may be involved in the cause and course of MS. Most of the findings still remain controversial and further research is needed in order to establish more precise recommendations. Individuals with MS should follow the American Heart Association guidelines:

- 30% of total calories should come from fat
- 7%–10% saturated fat sources

"Multiple Sclerosis and Nutrition," December 2005. This article is reproduced from the National Center on Physical Activity and Disability at www.ncpad.org. It may be freely distributed in its entirety as long as it includes this notice but cannot be edited, modified, otherwise altered without the express written permission of NCPAD. Contact NCPAD at 1-800-900-8086 for additional details. Copyright 2006 The Board of Trustees of the University of Illinois.

- 10% polyunsaturated fat sources
- 10% monounsaturated fat sources

Fat Types and Common Sources

Saturated fat—limit intake: Butter, cheese, whole milk, ice cream, cream, fatty meats, or coconut and palm oils

Polyunsaturated fat: Seeds, nuts, avocado, lean meat, eggs, legumes, fish such as salmon, mackerel, or sardines, seafood, or safflower, sunflower, corn, and soybean oils

Monounsaturated fat: Olive and canola oils

Common Health Concerns Related to Multiple Sclerosis

1. Fatigue

2. Pressure Sores

3. Constipation: People with MS frequently experience bowel dysfunction. Even though both diarrhea and constipation may occur, constipation is a more common problem. This is the result of demyelination of the central nervous system pathways responsible for bowel movement, weakened abdominal muscles, medications, insufficient fiber and fluid intake, and decreased mobility.

- Suggestions:
  - Adequate fluid intake, preferably water—six to eight 8-ounce glasses per day.
  - Raw fruits and vegetables: Leave skin on—it is a great source of fiber.
  - Dried fruits such as raisins, prunes, or figs.
  - High fiber grains/cereal products: bran, whole wheat flour, whole cornmeal, wheat bran cereals (All Bran, Bran Buds, Bran Chex), bran flakes (Raisin Bran), Grape-Nuts, or Shredded Wheat.
  - Regular meals during the day.
  - If these do not work, consult with a registered dietitian or physician about taking high fiber supplements such as Metamucil.

4. Dysphagia: As the disease progresses, swallowing problems may occur. Swallowing problems may result in weight loss, malnutrition, dehydration, constipation, loose dentures, reduced strength, tiredness, and loss of general well-being.

- Foods to avoid:
    - mixed textured foods and liquids (i.e., vegetable soup);
    - food that needs lots of chewing (i.e., caramel candy or taffy);
    - stringy food (i.e., bacon or celery);
    - hard, coarse food (i.e., nuts, toast, crackers, or chips);
    - foods that can become sticky in the mouth (i.e., bread or lettuce);
    - thicker drinks may not be appropriate, depending on the dysphasia.

- Meal ideas:
    - Have 4–6 smaller meals throughout the day—it may be less tiring than three large meals.
    - Allow ample time for each meal.
    - Don't rush—rest between courses.
    - Concentrate on eating.
    - See and smell the food.
    - Garnishes make food more tempting.
    - If the food needs to be pureed, process each item separately to retain individual flavors and colors.
    - Cold, iced drinks stimulate greater swallowing reflex—sip on a cold drink before and during each meal.

5. Vitamin and Mineral Supplements

An increasing number of people use vitamin and mineral supplements. Supplements should be taken with caution. Careless supplementation can cause toxicity and deficiency of micronutrients. The best source of vitamins and minerals is food. Following are some vitamins and minerals that you may want to keep in mind:

Micronutrient Food Sources

Zinc: Whole grains, wheat, oysters, or dark meat of turkeys and chickens

Calcium: Dairy products (choose low-fat kind), salmon, almonds, fish (small fish such as sardines can be eaten with bones), beans, or green vegetables

Vitamin B_6: Bananas, navy beans, or walnuts (heating, freezing, and canning may alter the availability of this vitamin)

Vitamin C: Brightly colored fruits and vegetables such as oranges, broccoli, strawberries, or kiwi

Vitamin E: Vegetable oils, nuts, or green, leafy vegetables

Vitamin B_{12}: Poultry, fish, shellfish, eggs, or fortified breakfast cereals

Approaches for Healthy Lifestyles

Social Aspects of Eating

- Allow ample time for each meal.
- Do not feel pressure to hurry and finish.
- Focus on eating—try to relax and enjoy the meal.

Ideas for Increasing Physical Activity

Exercise to increase strength, sharpen reflexes, and maintain balance. Below are some creative ways of doing exercise. Remember to start slowly.

- Play swing ball.
- Knit.
- Make pastries.
- Wax a car.
- Play miniature golf.
- Pull weeds in the garden.
- Go dancing.
- Take a walk.
- Play computer games—it sharpens reflexes.

Journals

1. Zhang, S. M., Willett, W. C., Hernan, M. A., Olek, M. J., and Ascherio, A. (2000). Dietary fat in relation to risk of multiple sclerosis among two large cohorts of women. *American Journal of Epidemiology*, 152(11), 1056–1064.

2. Riise, T., and Wolfson, C. (1997). Diet and multiple sclerosis. *Neurology*, 49(2), Supplement (2), S55–S61.

3. Ghadirian, P., Jain, M., Ducic, S., Shatenstein, B., and Morisset, R. (1998). Nutritional factors in the aetiology of multiple sclerosis: A case-control study in Montreal, Canada. *International Journal of Epidemiology*, 27, 845–852.

4. Caldis-Coutris, N., Namaka, M., and Melanson, M. (2002). Nutritional management of multiple sclerosis. *CPJ/RPC*, 135(5), 31–40.

Chapter 41

Exercise Guidelines for People with MS

Multiple Sclerosis

Multiple sclerosis is a chronic, inflammatory disease that affects the central nervous system and causes gradual destruction of myelin (demyelination) and transection of neuron axons patches throughout the brain and spinal cord. Myelin, the fatty material surrounding the nerves, is destroyed, leading to symptoms such as muscle weakness/paresis/paralysis, spasticity/tremor, and impaired balance, lack of coordination, heat sensitivity, and fatigue.

Importance of Exercise

In addition to improving overall health, cardiovascular fitness, range of motion, and flexibility, exercise can help one increase energy, improve balance, manage spasticity, decrease muscle atrophy, and better perform activities of daily living.

Types of Training

- cardiovascular to increase stamina

- strength to improve function, and to help prevent contractures, muscle imbalance, and atrophy

- flexibility to increase range of motion and maintain joint flexibility

- coordination and balance

Important Considerations when Exercising

- **Cardiovascular dysautonomia:** Irregular function of the autonomic nervous system (ANS) leads to a blunted heart rate and decreased blood pressure in response to exercise. If this condition is present, heart rate and blood pressure must be monitored throughout the exercise program, and intensity might need to be decreased.

- **Heat sensitivity:** This can include fatigue, loss of balance, and visual changes. Create a cool environment with fans, air temperature between 72° and 76° F, pool temperature between 80° and 85° F, and if exercising outdoors, exercise during early morning or evening hours. Wear clothing that breathes (i.e., cotton), and use cooling aids as needed (i.e., cool vests, ice packs, cool baths at 84° F or less, etc.). To counter dehydration, experiment with using sports drinks instead of water, depending on problems with incontinence.

- **Incontinence:** Loss of control of bowel/bladder. Void bladder before exercise and monitor urinary cycle. Try drinking sports drinks instead of water.

- **Spasticity/tremors:** Choose supportive exercise modalities such as upright or recumbent bicycle instead of the treadmill, and use equipment such as toe clips and heel straps for foot stability. Avoid water temperatures below 80° F and placing toes in a pointed position. When strength training, focus on areas of muscle imbalance, engage in gentle rhythmical/active flexibility exercises before exercise and in static flexibility movements after exercise that focus on increasing mobility and lengthening of tight areas (pelvis, chest, calf, and hip flexors).

- **Balance and coordination:** As problems with balance and coordination can lead to dangerous falls, choose exercises providing maximum support (i.e., swimming, recumbent bicycle) and check with a physical health professional (i.e., clinical exercise specialist, kinesiologist, exercise physiologist, or other fitness/

health professional trained in exercise program design for individuals living with neurological conditions) to design a physical activity program that incorporates balance and coordination training.

- **Medication:** Be aware of side effects of medication you are taking and how this will affect your exercise program. Medication can affect energy level, muscle coordination, and muscle strength.

General Cardiovascular Training Guidelines

- Set an exercise pace that is feels good to you. Rate your level of exertion by the Rate of Perceived Exertion scale (range of 6 to 20 where 6 = very, very light, and 20 = very, very hard); 12 to 14 is a good target zone.

- Vary cardiovascular training to prevent boredom and avoid muscle imbalance by using a variety of machines (appropriate to level of ability).

- General cardiovascular exercise can be done daily and is recommended at least three to four days per week for 20 to 60 minutes per session.

Examples of Beneficial Cardiovascular Training

- swimming/aquatic fitness classes
- stationary recumbent or upright bicycle
- walking

Strength Training Guidelines

- Begin strength training at 70% of a 10-repetition maximum. This is 70% of the weight that one can perform an exercise ten times. When this weight can be performed for 25 repetitions for two consecutive sessions, increase the weight 10%.

- Training should be performed two to three times per week, for three sets, eight to 12 repetitions per exercise, 10 to 15 minutes per session.

- Do not strength-train the same muscle groups on consecutive days.

A variety of equipment can be used, depending on the levels of balance/coordination, plasticity/tremor, strength, and/or fatigue:

- free weights
- isokinetic machines
- stretch band exercises
- sandbag weights
- water resistance exercises

General Flexibility Training Guidelines

- Stretching should be performed daily for at least 10 to 15 minutes.
- Stretching should be performed before and after every cardio-vascular and strength workout (rhythmical/active flexibility training before exercise and static flexibility training after exercise).
- Every muscle group used in a workout should be thoroughly stretched before and after.
- Spend more time on tight muscle groups.
- Stretches should be held for a minimum of 15 to 30 seconds for maximum benefit.
- Static stretches should be held for a minimum of 5 to 15 seconds for maximum benefit.
- Stretching should not be painful.

Recommended Activities that Address Flexibility

- yoga
- tai chi

Note: The information provided here is offered as a service only. The National Center on Physical Activity and Disability, University of Illinois at Chicago, the National Center on Accessibility, and the Rehabilitation Institute of Chicago do not formally recommend or endorse the equipment listed. As with any products or services, consumers should investigate and determine on their own which equipment best fits their needs and budget.

Additional Information

National Center on Physical Activity and Disability
1640 W. Roosevelt Rd. Suite 711
Chicago, IL 60608-6904
Toll-Free Voice/TTY: 800-900-8086
Fax: 312-355-4058
Website: http://www.ncpad.org
E-mail: ncpad@uic.edu

Organizations

Multiple Sclerosis Foundation
6350 North Andrews Avenue
Ft. Lauderdale, FL 33309-2130
Toll-Free: 888-MSFOCUS (673-6287)
Phone: 954-776-6805
Fax: 954-351-0630
Website: http://www.msfocus.org
E-mail: support@msfocus.org

National Multiple Sclerosis Society
733 Third Ave., 6th Fl.
New York, NY 10017-3288
Toll-Free: 800-344-4867 (FIGHTMS)
Phone: 212-986-3240
Fax: 212-986-7981
Website: http://www.nationalmssociety.org
E-mail: nat@nmss.org

Book

American College of Sports Medicine. (1997). *ACSM's exercise management for persons with chronic diseases and disabilities.* Champaign, Illinois: Human Kinetics Publishers.

Pamphlets

1. National Multiple Sclerosis Society. *Staying Well Series: Exercise as Part of Everyday Life.* Harmon, M.

2. National Multiple Sclerosis Society. *"Moving With Multiple Sclerosis".* Kimberg, I.

Videos

1. (2003). *Yogability and You with Shelley Sidelman.*
2. Mobility Limited. Yoga for MS and Related Conditions.

Chapter 42

Managing Fatigue

You Can Manage Fatigue

Many factors are involved in causing fatigue including medications you may take, sleep disturbances, and depression. In addition, abnormal nerve conduction can cause fatigue. And so can lack of exercise which causes deconditioning. (Your muscles become weak when they are not used.) Finally, MS can cause a unique "MS fatigue" or lassitude. This type of fatigue occurs daily, worsens as the day goes on, and is often aggravated by heat.

Yes, fatigue is a difficult symptom to treat, but you can manage your fatigue.

How to Make the Most of a Nap

A nap is any quiet rest period—not necessarily sleep—during daylight hours when you'd normally be awake. An occupational therapist can help you determine whether your nap schedule is helpful for your situation. Naps are helpful only if they don't interfere with your nighttime sleep. (Excerpted from "Fatigue: What You Should Know").

Suggestions under the heading "You CAN Manage Fatigue!" are tips from The Heuga Center that promotes health and creates hope for people with MS and from the National MS Society. © 2005 National Multiple Sclerosis Society. Contributing editors are Brian Hutchinson, PT, President, The Heuga Center, and *Inside MS* Magazine. Additional text from the Consortium of Multiple Sclerosis Centers is cited separately within the chapter.

You Can

- Learn energy management techniques. Consult a physical or occupational therapist.

- Prioritize. You can be realistic and responsible.

- Pace yourself. Remember the tortoise and hare.

- Delegate. Asking for help can be difficult but it will help conserve your energy.

- Exercise. Sounds contradictory when you want rest, but it can increase your energy level and decrease deconditioning. Talk to your physician or rehabilitation professional about your options.

- Use technology. Consider assistive devices. Wheels on a laundry cart. Wheels on a chair. They can help with both efficiency and mobility.

- Take medication. Speak with your physician about what is available for MS fatigue. Medications can be helpful, but may not be enough.

Use your health care team to differentiate MS fatigue from secondary causes, such as depression, pain, or an overactive bladder that is robbing you of sleep. Many secondary causes can be treated. A guided program of regular physical activity will help you manage MS fatigue.

Evidence that Energy Conservation Education is an Effective Strategy for Managing Fatigue of Persons with Multiple Sclerosis

"Evidence that Energy Conservation Education is an Effective Strategy for Managing Fatigue of Persons with Multiple Sclerosis," by Cindy Jacobs, MS, OTR/L and Virgil Mathiowetz, Ph.D., OTR/L. © 2006 Consortium of Multiple Sclerosis Centers. Reprinted with permission.

The Multiple Sclerosis (MS) Council for Clinical Practice Guidelines. (1998) reported fatigue as the most common symptom experienced by people with MS. One approach used by occupational therapists for clients with fatigue is energy conservation education; however, in 1998, the MS Council in reviewing the literature for their Clinical Practice Guidelines "did not find any scientifically-based evidence to establish the efficacy" of such education.

Since that time, several studies have evaluated the effects of a specific energy conservation course, *Managing Fatigue: A Six-Week Course for Energy Conservation* (Packer, Brink, and Sauriol, 1995). This course, which was evaluated in three studies, consisted of six weeks of highly structured, two-hour classes taught in community settings with 7–10 participants per group. This energy conservation course was based on the theory of psychoeducational group development and used a variety of teaching methods including lectures, discussions, long-term and short-term goal setting, practice activities, and homework activities to assist participants' integration of energy conservation principles into their performance of everyday tasks. The six sessions addressed the importance of rest throughout the day, positive and effective communication, proper body mechanics, ergonomic principles, modification of the environment, changing standards, setting priorities, activity analysis and modification, and living a balanced lifestyle.

Mathiowetz, Matuska, and Murphy (2001) reported evidence that this energy conservation course (Packer et al., 1995) was effective in reducing the impact of fatigue and some aspects of quality of life in persons with mild to moderate symptoms of MS (number in sample [N]=54). Likewise, Vanage, Gilbertson, and Mathiowetz (2003) reported a significant decrease in fatigue impact for persons with moderate to severe MS (N=37). Participants in both of these studies were taught by occupational therapy practitioners, certified assistants, and students using the course or a modified version of the course. In both studies, participants' scores on the Fatigue Impact Scale (Fisk et al., 1994) decreased significantly from pre- to post-course assessments and beneficial effects were maintained six to eight weeks after completion of the course. These relatively small studies provided beginning evidence to support energy conservation education as a strategy for managing fatigue for persons with MS.

Recently, Mathiowetz, Finlayson, Matuska, Chen, and Luo (2005) conducted a much larger study funded by the National Multiple Sclerosis Society (NMSS). This randomized clinical trial was conducted at two sites: Minnesota (Twin cities area) and Illinois (Chicago area). One-hundred sixty-nine persons with MS were randomly assigned to either immediate or delayed treatment groups. One-hundred thirty-one of these participants completed the course and the follow-up assessments. Results of this study support the efficacy and effectiveness of the energy conservation course to decrease the impact of fatigue, increase self-efficacy, and improve some aspects of quality of life. In addition, greater than 70% of participants implemented eight out of fourteen energy conservation strategies taught in the course and effectiveness of the strategies were rated highly (7–8.2 on a 10-point scale)(Matuska, Mathiowetz, and Finlayson, 2007). On written evaluations given at the final class session, participants' comments included the following:

- "Felt course was good eye opener on ways to conserve/organize life to get advantage over fatigue."

- "Would recommend course to others with MS. I feel I have a little more control over fatigue than it has on me (on most days)."

- "Good for spelling out things I'd been thinking about."

- "Had unrealistic expectations—was wanting magic cure, so at first was disappointed, but by third week realized there were benefits to course."

- "Helped me be even better at watching/monitoring my fatigue."

The research team working on the grant developed many additional tools for use with the course including Self-Efficacy for Performing Energy Conservation Strategies Assessment (Leopold and Mathiowetz, 2005), Energy Conservation Strategies Survey (Mallik, Finlayson, Mathiowetz, and Fogg, 2005), which measures behavioral change due to the course, biweekly quizzes on course content, and treatment fidelity measures designed to ensure similar administration of the course across instructors. In addition, self-study modules of each session (Lamb, Finlayson, Mathiowetz, and Chen, 2005) were developed for persons who missed a session and a teleconference version of the course (Finlayson, Holberg, Van Denend, and Frakes, 2004; Finlayson, 2005) was also developed. Professionals serving persons with MS are encouraged to read the referenced articles for further details regarding the studies as well as to watch for future related publications and resources to serve as support in educating consumers on matters of energy conservation.

Unfortunately, the Packer et al. (1995) manual is currently out of print. The author is exploring the possibility of reprinting with another publisher. Until it is republished, contact the author, Tanya Packer, (e-mail: T.Packer@exchange.curtin.edu.au) for the latest information on how to obtain a copy of the manual.

References

Finlayson, M. (2005). Pilot study of an energy conservation education program delivered by telephone conference call to people with multiple sclerosis. *NeuroRehabilitation*, 20, 267–277.

Finlayson, M., Holberg, C., Van Denend, T., and Frakes, J. (2004). *Telephone Energy Management Program for People with Multiple Sclerosis* (Newsletter). Chicago: University of Illinois at Chicago.

Fisk JD, Ritvo PG, Ross L, Haase DA, Marrie TJ, and Schlech WF. (1994). Measuring the functional impact of fatigue: Initial validation of the fatigue impact scale. *Clinical Infectious Diseases*, 18 (Suppl 1), S79–83.

Lamb, A. L., Finlayson, M., Mathiowetz, V., and Chen, H. Y. (2005).The outcomes of using self-study modules in energy conservation education for people with multiple sclerosis. *Clinical Rehabilitation,* 19, 475–481.

Leopold A. and Mathiowetz V. (2005). Reliability and validity of the Self-Efficacy for Performing Energy Conservation Strategies Assessment for persons with multiple sclerosis. *Occupational Therapy International*, 12, 234–249.

Mallik, P. S., Finlayson, M., Mathiowetz, V., and Fogg, L. (2005). Psychometric evaluation of the Energy Conservation Strategies Survey. *Clinical Rehabilitation*, 19, 583–543.

Mathiowetz, V. G., Finlayson, M. L., Matuska, K. M., Chen, H. Y., and Luo, P. (2005). Randomized controlled trial of an energy conservation course for persons with multiple sclerosis. *Multiple Sclerosis*, 11, 592–601.

Mathiowetz V, Matuska KM, and Murphy ME. (2001). Efficacy of an energy conservation course for persons with multiple sclerosis. *Archives of Physical Medicine and Rehabilitation*, 82, 449–456.

Matuska, K., Mathiowetz, V., and Finlayson, M. (2007). Use and perceived effectiveness of energy conservation strategies for managing multiple sclerosis fatigue. *American Journal of Occupational Therapy*, 61, 62–69.

Multiple Sclerosis Council for Clinical Practice Guidelines. (1998). *Fatigue and multiple sclerosis: Evidence-based management strategies for fatigue in multiple sclerosis.* Washington, DC: Paralyzed Veterans of America.

Packer, T. L., Brink, N., and Sauriol, A. (1995). *Managing fatigue: A six-week course for energy conservation.* Tucson, Arizona: Therapy Skill Builders.

Vanage SM, Gilbertson KK, Mathiowetz V. (2003). Effects of an energy conservation course on fatigue impact for persons with progressive multiple sclerosis. *American Journal of Occupational Therapy*, 57, 315–323.

Chapter 43

Stress and MS

You've heard that stress is bad for people with multiple sclerosis (MS). Even the most conservative doctors and researchers would agree to that. The real question is: Do stressful life events trigger exacerbations? Doctors and researchers can't give a definite yes or no to that question yet, but here is what they can tell you.

There have been numerous studies and papers over the last 20 years about the effects of stress on MS symptoms, and while the methodology and focus of the studies varies greatly, the vast majority agree that the risk of exacerbation after a stressful life event is significantly increased.

It has been a struggle to achieve even this much consensus, because of the vague nature of the term stress and the difficulty in singling out its effects. Most studies decided to focus on particular events that are viewed as stressful, such as illness in the family, job stress, death of a relative or friend, problems in a relationship or marriage, etc. When we are in stressful situations such as these, our body produces stress hormones—adrenalin and glucocorticoids. Adrenalin raises blood pressure and heart rate, making more energy available. Glucocorticoids enhance memory and immune function. While these responses can be helpful in the short term, continuing high levels of

This chapter includes: "Stress and MS" by Laurie Long, © 2004 Multiple Sclerosis Association of King County. Reprinted with permission. And, excerpts from "Stress and Your Health," National Women's Health Information Center, August 2004.

these hormones may have adverse affects on health. According to a panel of experts speaking at Experimental Biology 2004, the body's hormonal response to stress alters immune system function and influences susceptibility, onset, and exacerbation of mental and physical diseases, including autoimmune diseases such as multiple sclerosis.[1]

Dr. William Malarkey, while speaking to the panel, described how the perception of stress activates the interaction between the endocrine system and the immune system, initiating a cascade of physiological events. If the stress is short-term, these hormonal changes fade away. But if the stress persists, the resulting dysregulation of the immune system initiates an inflammatory state that, if not stabilized, leads to symptoms and then established disease processes.[2]

A new study by David C. Mohr et al., which combines the findings of 14 studies on stress and exacerbations in MS from 1965 to 2003, concluded: "There is a consistent association between stressful life events and subsequent exacerbation in multiple sclerosis."[3] Another study completed in 2003 by D. Buljevac et al., and reported in the *British Medical Journal* showed that, "occurrence of stress was associated with a doubling of the exacerbation rate during the subsequent four weeks."[4]

How to Deal with Stress

The signs and symptoms of stress cover a broad spectrum including irritability, headaches, anxiety, fatigue, worrying, distractibility, feeling overwhelmed, stomach aches or nausea, clenched muscles, feeling demoralized, constant worrying, and more. Doctors and researchers say that stress can be helped by preventative strategies such as regular exercise, good social support, and stress coping behaviors. Some of these include deep breathing exercises, visualization exercises, meditation, yoga, tai chi, chi gung, stretching exercises or physical therapy, regular exercise of any kind such as walking, swimming, or gardening, and by eating a healthy diet. Recent studies have also found that certain drugs used to treat depression can also help protect the brain against the effects of stress.[5]

If you think that you are suffering from the effects of ongoing stress, consult with your doctor on ways of relieving and coping with it. Remember that there are many different coping strategies. Find the approach that works for you to evaluate and manage your stress.

Endnotes and Bibliography

[1, 2] Rabin, Dr. Bruce S. et al., PsychoNeuroImmunology Research Society, Alteration of Health by the Hormonal Response to Stress. *Experimental Biology* 2004.

[3] Mohr, David C, et al., Association Between Stressful Life Events and Exacerbation in Multiple Sclerosis: a Meta-Analysis. *British Medical Journal*, Vol. 328, March 27, 2004.

[4] Buljevac, D. et al., Self Reported Stressful Life Events and Exacerbations in Multiple Sclerosis: Prospective Study. *British Medical Journal*, Vol. 327, Sept. 20, 2003, 646–9.

[5] Ackerman, Sandra J., New Research Stresses the Response to Stress. *BrainWork—The Neuroscience Newsletter*, Vol. 14, No.2, March–April 2004.

Goodwin, Sarah, *Hormonal Response to Stress Alters Immune System Function and Alters Mental and Physical Disease.* Federation of American Societies for Experimental Biology, April 18, 2004.

Ackerman Dr. Kurt, et al, Stressful Life Events Precede Exacerbations of Multiple Sclerosis. *Psychosomatic Medicine*, 64:916–920 (2002).

Mohr, David C., et al, Psychological Stress and the Subsequent Appearance of New Brain Lesions in MS. *Journal of Neurology*, 2000;55:55–61.

Nisipeanu P, Korczyn, AD, Psychological Stress as Risk Factor for Exacerbations in Multiple Sclerosis. *Neurology* 1993;43:1311–2.

Foley, Dr. Frederick and Sarnoff, Jane, *Taming Stress in Multiple Sclerosis.* National Multiple Sclerosis Society, 1996.

Stress and Your Health

What are some early signs of stress?

Stress can take on many different forms, and can contribute to symptoms of illness. Common symptoms include: headache, sleep disorders, difficulty concentrating, short temper, upset stomach, job dissatisfaction, low morale, depression, and anxiety.

How do men and women tend to react to stress?

During stress, women tend to care for their children and find support from their female friends. Women's bodies make chemicals that are believed to promote these responses. One of these chemicals is oxytocin, which has a calming effect during stress. This is the same chemical released during childbirth and found at higher levels in breast feeding mothers, who are believed to be calmer and more social than women who do not breast feed. Women also have the hormone estrogen, which boosts the effects of oxytocin. Men, however, have high levels of testosterone during stress, which blocks the calming effects of oxytocin and causes hostility, withdrawal, and anger.

How does stress affect my body and my health?

Everyone has stress. We have short-term stress, like getting lost while driving or missing the bus. Even everyday events, such as planning a meal or making time for errands, can be stressful. This kind of stress can make us feel worried or anxious.

Other times, we face long-term stress, such as racial discrimination, a life-threatening illness, or divorce. These stressful events also affect your health on many levels. Long-term stress is real and can increase your risk for some health problems, like depression.

Both short and long-term stress can have effects on your body. Research is starting to show the serious effects of stress on our bodies. Stress triggers changes in our bodies and makes us more likely to get sick. It can also make problems we already have worse. It can play a part in these problems:

- trouble sleeping
- headaches
- constipation
- diarrhea
- irritability
- lack of energy
- lack of concentration
- eating too much or not at all
- anger
- sadness
- stomach cramping
- stomach bloating
- skin problems, like hives
- depression
- anxiety
- weight gain or loss
- heart problems
- high blood pressure
- irritable bowel syndrome
- diabetes

- higher risk of asthma and arthritis flare-ups
- tension
- neck or back pain
- less sexual desire
- harder to get pregnant

What are some of the most stressful life events?

Any change in our lives can be stressful—even some of the happiest ones like having a baby or taking a new job. Following are some of life's most stressful events.

- death of a spouse
- divorce
- marital separation
- spending time in jail
- death of a close family member
- personal illness or injury
- marriage
- pregnancy
- retirement

Source: From the *Holmes and Rahe Scale of Life Events* (1967)

How can I help handle my stress?

Do not let stress make you sick. Often we are not even aware of our stress levels. Listen to your body, so that you know when stress is affecting your health. Following are ways to help you handle your stress.

- **Relax:** It's important to unwind. Each person has her own way to relax. Some ways include deep breathing, yoga, meditation, and massage therapy. If you cannot do these things, take a few minutes to sit, listen to soothing music, or read a book.

- **Make time for yourself:** It is important to care for yourself. Think of this as an order from your doctor, so you do not feel guilty. No matter how busy you are, you can try to set aside at least 15 minutes each day in your schedule to do something for yourself, like taking a bubble bath, going for a walk, or calling a friend.

- **Sleep:** Sleeping is a great way to help both your body and mind. Your stress could get worse if you do not get enough sleep. You also cannot fight off sickness as well when you sleep poorly. With enough sleep, you can tackle your problems better and lower your risk for illness. Try to get seven to nine hours of sleep every night.

- **Eat right:** Try to fuel up with fruits, vegetables, and proteins. Good sources of protein can be peanut butter, chicken, or tuna salad. Eat whole-grains, such as wheat breads and wheat crackers. Don't be fooled by the jolt you get from caffeine or sugar. Your energy will wear off.

- **Get moving:** Believe it or not, getting physical activity not only helps relieve your tense muscles, but helps your mood too. Your body makes certain chemicals, called endorphins, before and after you work out. They relieve stress and improve your mood.

- **Talk to friends:** Talk to your friends to help you work through your stress. Friends are good listeners. Finding someone who will let you talk freely about your problems and feelings without judging you does a world of good. It also helps to hear a different point of view. Friends will remind you that you're not alone.

- **Get help from a professional if you need it:** Talk to a therapist. A therapist can help you work through stress and find better ways to deal with problems. For more serious stress-related disorders, like post traumatic stress disorder (PTSD), therapy can be helpful. There also are medications that can help ease symptoms of depression and anxiety and help promote sleep.

- **Compromise:** Sometimes, it is not always worth the stress to argue. Give in once in awhile.

- **Write down your thoughts:** Have you ever typed an e-mail to a friend about your lousy day and felt better afterward? Why not grab a pen and paper and write down what is going on in your life. Keeping a journal can be a great way to get things off your chest and work through issues. Later, you can go back and read through your journal and see how you have made progress.

- **Help others:** Helping someone else can help you. Help your neighbor, or volunteer in your community.

- **Get a hobby:** Find something you enjoy. Make sure to give yourself time to explore your interests.

- **Set limits:** When it comes to things like work and family, figure out what expectations are realistic. There are only so many hours in the day. Set limits with yourself and others. Do not be afraid to say no to requests for your time and energy.

- **Plan your time:** Think ahead about how you are going to spend your time. Write a to-do list. Figure out what is most important to do.

- **Do not deal with stress in unhealthy ways:** This includes drinking too much alcohol, using drugs, smoking, or overeating.

Deep Breathing

Deep breathing is a good way to relax. Try it a couple of times every day. Here is how to do it.

1. Lie down or sit in a chair.

2. Rest your hands on your stomach.

3. Slowly count to four and inhale through your nose. Feel your stomach rise. Hold it for a second.

4. Slowly count to four while you exhale through your mouth. To control how fast you exhale, purse your lips like you're going to whistle. Your stomach will slowly fall.

5. Repeat five to ten times.

For More Information

American Institute of Stress
124 Park Ave.
Yonkers, NY 10703
Phone: 914-963-1200
Fax: 914-965-6267
Website: http://www.stress.org
E-mail: stress125@optonline.net

Anxiety Disorders Association of America
8730 Georgia Ave., Suite 600
Silver Spring, MD 20910
Phone: 240-485-1001
Fax: 240-485-1035
Website: http://www.adaa.org

Mental Health America (formerly known as National Mental Health Association)
2000 N. Beauregard St., 6th Floor
Alexandria, VA 22311
Toll-Free: 800-969-6642
Toll-Free TTY: 800-433-5959
Phone: 703-684-7722
Fax: 703-684-5968
Website: http://www.mentalhealthamerica.net

National Mental Health Consumers' Self-Help Clearinghouse
1211 Chestnut St., Suite 1207
Philadelphia, PA 19107
Toll-Free: 800-553-4539
Phone: 215-751-1810
Fax: 215-636-6312
Website: http://www.mhselfhelp.org
E-mail: info@mhselfhelp.org

National Mental Health Information Center
P.O. Box 42557
Washington, DC 20015
Toll-Free: 800-789-2647
Toll-Free TDD: 866-889-2647
International Calls: 240-221-4021
Fax: 240-747-5470
Website: http://www.mentalhealth.org
E-mail: info@mentalhealth.org

Chapter 44

Maintaining Intimacy and Sexuality If You Have MS

"Although more than 56 million people with disabilities are currently living in the United States, and Congress passed sweeping disability rights legislation in 1990, the right to sexual expression and satisfaction for disabled people remains the last taboo, the last frontier on the long road to equality." (Source: Ken Kroll and Erica Levy Klein, *Enabling Romance.*)

Everyone is a sexual being. From the moment of birth until the moment of death, our capacity for communication, relatedness, and intimacy unfolds in a natural developmental sequence. As such, it is natural for everyone to desire affection and intimacy. Whether you are newly diagnosed, young, mature, single, or in a committed relationship, chronic illnesses and disability do not diminish these needs and desires.

With multiple sclerosis (MS), symptoms can occur that may present obstacles in your capacity for emotional relatedness and sexual intimacy. By approaching these obstacles as challenges rather than burdens, you can empower yourself to explore the variety of possible solutions in relating intimately. Educate yourself. Overcome your embarrassment and ask questions of yourself, your health care team, and your partner. Experiment and even challenge yourself to change

"Intimacy and Sexuality with Multiple Sclerosis," by Frederick W. Foley, Ph.D., reviewed 2005. © Multiple Sclerosis Foundation (www.msfacts.org). Reprinted with permission.

some of your ideas about what intimacy and sexuality really means to you. Think about yourself as a sexual being, acknowledging that part of yourself, is the first step.

Prevalence of Sexual Changes in MS

Although normal sexual function changes throughout the lifespan, MS can affect an individual's sexual experience in a variety of ways. Studies on the prevalence of perceived sexual concerns or problems in MS range from approximately 40 to 80 percent in women and 50 to 90 percent in men. Reports of sexual problems in the general U.S. population range from 30 to 50 percent, depending on the study reflecting the widespread prevalence of sexual complaints in general.

How Does MS Affect Sexuality?

The ways in which MS can affect sexuality and expressions of intimacy can be divided into primary, secondary, and tertiary sexual dysfunction.

Primary sexual dysfunction stems directly from MS-related changes in the brain and spinal cord that affect the sexual response or the ability to feel sexual pleasure. In both men and women, this can include a decrease or loss of sex drive, decreased or unpleasant genital sensations, and diminished capacity for orgasm. Men may experience difficulty achieving or maintaining an erection and a decrease in or loss of ejaculatory force or frequency. Women may experience decreased vaginal lubrication, loss of vaginal muscle tone, and/ or diminished clitoral engorgement.

Secondary sexual dysfunction stems from MS-related symptoms that do not directly involve nerve pathways to the genital system, but nevertheless impair sexual pleasure or the sexual response. Secondary symptoms may include bladder and bowel problems, fatigue, spasticity, muscle weakness, body or hand tremors, impairments in attention and concentration, and non-genital sensory changes.

Tertiary sexual dysfunction results from disability-related psychosocial and cultural issues that can interfere with one's sexual feelings and experiences. For example, some people find it difficult to reconcile the idea of being disabled with being fully sexually expressive. Changes in self-esteem—including the way one feels about one's body—depression, demoralization, or mood swings can all interfere with intimacy and sexuality. The sexual partnership can be severely challenged by changes within a relationship, such as one person becoming the other person's caregiver. Similarly, changes in employment status or role performance within the household are often associated with emotional adjustments that can temporarily interfere with sexual expression. The strain of coping with MS challenges a couple's efforts to communicate openly about their respective experiences and their changing needs for sexual expression and fulfillment.

Assessing Sexual Problems

Diagnosis of sexual dysfunction is usually based upon the self-reports of the person with MS or the sexual partner. Determining the etiology, or cause, of the dysfunction, and whether it stems from primary, secondary, and/or tertiary sources, requires medical assessment by a health care professional knowledgeable about MS and sexual function. The diagnostic process may include a physical and neurological exam, sexual history interview, and review of all prescribed medications. Screening for depression and other contributing tertiary factors may be done. Occasionally, additional medical tests may be given. Proper assessment of the contributing factors to the problem sets the stage for effective clinical management. Valid self-reports of sexual function, such as the Multiple Sclerosis Intimacy and Sexuality Questionnaire-19 (MSISQ-19) (Sanders et al., 2000), can be very helpful to both the person with MS and their health care team.

Treatment

Published treatment studies on MS and sexual dysfunction with rigorous research controls are limited, although better information is available for men than women. Most treatment reports constitute clinical guidelines that describe diagnosis and treatment of the various MS symptoms as they impact sexual function.

For Men

Treatment for Erectile Problems

For men, complaints of erectile dysfunction are the most common sexual problem in MS, and the most frequent reason men seek sexual help. Oral medicines, such as Viagra® (sildenafil citrate), Levitra® (vardenafil), and the recently approved Cialis ™ (tadalafil), work by blocking a chemical in the erectile tissues that causes erections to become flaccid. They do not improve sex drive, but are helpful in maintaining erections when they occur. Although these three drugs are similar in action, their dosage, onset of action time, and duration of action differ.

There are a number of other oral medications in clinical trials for erectile dysfunction, including Vasomax® and IC351®. These medications work by chemically inducing the relaxation of the smooth muscle in the penis, which enhances the ability to develop and maintain erections. Further testing is required on these medications, and it is not yet known whether they will be helpful in MS. Other medications, currently in the testing process, work directly in the brain to increase neurotransmitters that facilitate erectile capacity.

Other medical approaches for erectile dysfunction in MS involve the injection of medications into the penis, such as alprostadil (Prostin VR®) or papaverine, which increase blood flow and help maintain blood volume within the spongy erectile tissues. The injection usually causes only mild discomfort. Side effects are minimal for most users.

Alprostadil can also be used via urethral suppository (MUSE®), in addition to the penile injection. With this approach, a small plastic applicator is used to insert the drug into the urethra. The direct application of alprostadil to the surface of the penis in the form of a cream or gel is undergoing testing. Alprox-TD® and Topiglan® are both applied directly to the penis, and are rapidly absorbed. Preliminary data indicates that these are helpful in non-MS populations, although further testing is needed.

A device that aids in erections is the vacuum tube and constriction band. With this method, a plastic tube is fitted over the flaccid penis, and a suction pump is operated to create a vacuum that produces an erection. A latex band is slipped from the base of the tube onto the base of the penis. The band maintains engorgement of the penis for sexual activities.

More invasive forms of treatment for erectile problems include the surgical implantation of a penile prosthesis. A penile prosthesis is a mechanical device designed to give a man with erectile dysfunction the option of having an erection. However, there can be significant side effects and complications with implant surgery. Because many other alternatives for erectile dysfunction have become widely available, this option is utilized only as a last resort for men in whom less invasive procedures have failed.

For Women

Treatment of Orgasmic Loss and Sexual Response

From a research perspective, treatment of orgasmic loss in women with MS has been poorly studied. From a clinical perspective, treatment recommendations depend on developing an understanding of what primary, secondary, and/or tertiary factors are contributing to the loss. For example, if sensation is disturbed in the genitals or lower body areas (a primary symptom), it is essential to develop a sensory body map with one's partner to explore the exact locations of pleasant, decreased, or altered sensations. Developing a body map requires one to systematically touch the body from head to toe (or all those places one can comfortably reach). By varying the rate, rhythm, and pressure of touch, areas of sensual pleasure, discomfort, or sensory change can be noted. Altering patterns of touch in subsequent exercises is then conducted to maximize pleasure. Instructing one's sexual partner to touch in a similar manner sets the stage for rediscovering sensual and erotic pleasure. As with the treatment of all sexual symptoms in MS, experimentation and communication are the keys to maximizing sexual response and pleasure.

If diminished genital sensation occurs, stimulation can be increased through oral stimulation or via mechanical vibrators, which are widely available by mail order. Increasing stimulation to other erogenous zones, such as breasts, ears, and lips may enhance the orgasmic response. Increasing cerebral stimulation by watching sexually oriented videos, exploring fantasies, and introducing new kinds of sexual play into sexual activities can sometimes promote an orgasmic response.

Painful or irritating genital or body sensations can sometimes be treated with medication. Amitriptyline (Elavil®), carbamazepine (Tegretol®) and phenytoin (Dilantin®) are sometimes prescribed to help manage this difficult symptom.

It is not yet known whether oral medicines, such as Viagra, Levitra, or Cialis, are helpful for women with MS. A woman's sexual identity tends to be more complex than a man's, so it is not yet clear how helpful medicines that increase blood flow to the genitals will be for women with MS. However, since increased blood flow to the clitoris and labia occurs during the sexual response, it is possible that enhancing blood flow via oral or topical medicines, or via a vacuum device, will enhance sexual pleasure.

Coping with Lowered Libido

Loss of libido, or sex drive, is the most frequently reported sexual symptom among women with MS. Currently, there are no medicines that are effective for this symptom. There have been case reports that have addressed this topic in MS. In one, sex therapy in combination with MS symptom management and communication skills training, reported anecdotal success in women with MS. Behavioral retraining that targets redevelopment of sexual pleasure in the absence of libido has been reported. The rationale for behavioral retraining is that partially differing neural pathways mediate sexual drive and sexual pleasure or response. In the absence of libido, a different set of behaviors and attitudes are required to stimulate sexual pleasure. In other words, the nervous system is often sufficiently intact to respond to sexual stimulation even when libido is absent. The issue thus becomes one of sexually getting started without libido, which is taught via behavior therapy.

Coping with Vaginal Dryness and Tightness

Similar to the erectile response in men, vaginal lubrication is controlled by multiple pathways in the brain and spinal cord, some of which may be compromised in MS. The simplest method to cope with vaginal dryness is to apply generous amounts of water-soluble lubricants (for example, K-Y® Jelly, Astroglide®, Replens®). However, most women who use lubricants do not use sufficient amounts. If dryness persists with lubricant use, more generous dosing is needed.

Communication with Your MS Health Care Team

Fatigue, spasticity, weakness, bladder or bowel disturbance, depression, and cognitive changes are MS-related symptoms that have been widely reported as impairing sexual response. There are numerous protocols and medications available to manage these symptoms. Communication with an MS health care provider on aggressive symptom management with sexual health in mind can be helpful in restoring sexual function. Although treatment of these symptoms frequently eases associated sexual complaints, it is necessary for the MS health care provider to know that sexual function is an ongoing concern. For example, some antidepressant medications have excellent efficacy in treating symptoms of depression, but can also cause impairments in libido and capacity for orgasm. If the person with MS and the health care provider have had an open dialogue about sexual function, appropriate medications and dosing strategies can be implemented to minimize or eliminate the sexual side effects.

In coping with sexual dysfunction, it is very important to include the sex partner in the discussion when a long-term relationship is present. This enhances intimacy by allowing both partners to learn and explore together. If partners feel inhibited about talking through these issues, counseling with a mental health professional that is knowledgeable about MS can prove helpful.

Reference

Sanders A, Foley FW, LaRocca NG, and Zemon V (2000). The Multiple Sclerosis Intimacy and Sexuality Questionnaire-19(MSISQ-19). *Sexuality and Disability*, Vol. 18 (1):3–26.

For More Information

American Association of Sexuality Educators, Counselors, and Therapists (AASECT)
P.O. Box 1960
Ashland, VA 23005-1960
Phone: 804-752-0026
Fax: 804-752-0056
Website: http://www.aasect.org
E-mail: aasect@aasect.org

AASECT certifies professional sex therapists who have met their criteria for minimum educational and clinical experience standards. AASECT-certified therapists also must agree to adhere to a code of ethics. Although many highly qualified sex therapists do not choose to join AASECT, you can obtain a list of AASECT-certified sex therapists by contacting AASECT.

Chapter 45

Developing a Support Group If You Have MS

What Is a Mutual Support Group and What Can It Do for You?

A mutual support group is a gathering of people with multiple sclerosis (MS). The purpose of the group is to provide support to the members and thus allow them to cope better by:

- sharing their feelings and experiences;

- learning more about MS;

- obtaining accurate information;

- giving people with MS an opportunity to talk through problems they are facing or choices they have to make;

- listening to others who share similar feelings and experiences;

- helping others through the sharing of ideas and information and providing support;

- knowing they are not alone.

The roles of an MS group are mutual support and information, but it can also serve to identify professional help.

Excerpted from "How to Develop a Mutual Support Group," February 2002. © Multiple Sclerosis International Federation (www.msif.org). Reprinted with permission. The information offered is deemed pertinent despite the date of this document.

What a Mutual Support Group Cannot Do

An MS group cannot solve all problems, nor can it replace the services of a doctor or other health care professionals. It is important to remember that an MS group is not helpful to everyone. Some people are not comfortable sharing personal feelings with others.

"My group can't replace the support I get from my family, but it is so great to talk about things I'm going through that my family just can't understand."

Types of MS Groups

Some MS groups develop with characteristics in common. The most important factor is that any decision to develop MS groups with particular members should be a decision made by the group. Examples include:

- newly diagnosed
- women
- men
- different ages
- couples

In addition, MS groups may also be developed for spouses, caregivers, and family members of people with MS, following the same basic steps outlined in this chapter.

How to Get Started

If it appears that there is no suitable group in your area to meet your particular needs, you might consider the following questions before starting.

First ask yourself:

- Do I have the necessary time and energy?
- Do I have the needed support from family and friends?
- Can I cope with the additional demands of organizing a support group?
- Do I wish to hear about other people's experiences and to share my own?

Getting Help

Don't try to do it all yourself. Are there other people with MS you can talk to? Will they help you share responsibilities?

Are there local or national organizations that might help, for example, a national MS Society or local branch? If there is an MS Society in your country, they should be contacted about forming the MS group as they could also help identify professionals, advertise the MS group, and provide support.

Are there any professionals, doctors, social workers, health workers, or nurses who might help by:

- spreading the word about the group;

- serving as invited speakers on various topics; or

- providing information about MS?

Planning the First Meeting

Getting started can take some planning and effort. The following are some of the issues to consider when preparing for the first meeting:

Aims of the Group

It is a good idea to work out what the aims of your group might be. This will help you in explaining your ideas to others and enlisting their help. Group members should review these aims once the group is formed.

Aims can be very simple such as:

- to provide people with MS with an opportunity to learn more about the disease;

- to enable people with MS to meet on a regular basis to provide mutual support;

- to enable people with MS to meet others in a similar situation and share their feelings and experiences.

Who Might Be in the Group?

An MS group is not for everyone, but many people with MS find them helpful. Publicizing the meeting is important in order to recruit those who might be interested in taking part.

The following are a few of the many ways to advertise a meeting:

* the national MS society magazine or newsletter;

* radio and television stations that often provide free advertising for community events;

* local newspapers that publish notices of meetings—check first to see if there is a charge for this;

* places of worship are also a good source of new members, mention might be made of the meeting in their regular bulletin or notice board;

* posters can be placed in doctors' offices, community centers, nursing homes, libraries, pharmacies, and food stores; and,

* by word of mouth.

There may also be others that are specific to your community. Any publicity should include:

* date, place, and time of meeting; and

* name, telephone number, or place where a contact person can be found.

Numbers

It is probably best not to worry about the numbers at first. It will be impossible for all members to attend every meeting, but some level of commitment is necessary. Attendance may also drop after the initial meetings. If the numbers become too large and it becomes difficult for everyone to participate, then dividing into two groups might be considered. Do not be upset about too few people attending the first meeting.

Open or Closed

During the first meeting, it should be decided by the MS group whether it will be an open or closed group. An open group will allow new members at every meeting, while a closed group will consist of those people who attended the first few meetings only. Once the decision has been made, it has to be kept. If after three months this method develops problems, then it can be revised.

Place

In selecting a place to hold the meetings you might want to consider:

- accessibility—is the location and its facilities fully accessible?

- convenience—can people get there easily?

- size—is it large enough? Is there enough space for wheelchairs and are there enough chairs?

- comfort—is it quiet and private enough to allow for a comfortable exchange between group members?

- cost—is there a charge for its use?

Schools, places of worship, community centers, libraries, or someone's home can be considered. It is essential for someone to visit the place where a meeting is to be held beforehand, to inspect it, and be sure that the listed considerations have been met.

Time

How often should the group meet? Monthly? Every two months? Usually members of the group will make this decision at the first meeting. Most groups meet on a regular basis. It is easier for everyone to remember if the day of the week and the time are the same for each meeting. The frequency of the meetings should be reviewed on a regular basis.

What time? Morning? Afternoon? Evening? It all depends on what is convenient to members of the group. A note about choosing a convenient time—it is impossible to find a time that is always convenient for everyone. However, if members exchange telephone numbers, a member who is unable to attend a meeting still has a way of being in touch with others.

Cost

MS groups should be free of charge. Finding a free room and having members take turns bringing refreshments is a good idea. If you do end up with expenses, it is usually preferable that these are paid for by the group, not by one or two individuals. If you have a national MS society, it or its local branch should be approached for financial assistance.

Recommendations

- The group should decide how often to meet, how long the meeting will last, and for how many months (for example, the group could meet once a week for a period of three months and each meeting could be 90 minutes in duration). This decision should be reviewed by the group on a regular basis.

- A member of the group should keep track of the time to make sure that the meeting starts promptly and does not go on too long. The length of the meeting should be agreed beforehand.

- After three months the group should evaluate whether or not it is possible and useful to continue. At this time new members can be invited to participate.

- Remember that all groups must eventually come to an end. The participants themselves need to decide when the group no longer offers clear benefits to the members. This is not a sign of failure, rather it is an accomplishment.

Chapter 46

Tips and Tools
for MS Caregivers

Caring Skills and Tools

Caregivers of people with multiple sclerosis (MS) are involved in a range of assistance and support activities throughout the course of the disease. The result is that often caregivers evolve and learn skills in their caring role. For many, this means a gradual change to adapt to MS care needs rather than the sudden and urgent care needs that are more common in other situations, for example following a head or spinal cord injury.

When a person with MS experiences difficulty such as weakness, spasticity, or other functional loss in the upper or lower limbs, he or she may require assistance with the activities of daily living (often referred to as ADL). These include any daily activity a person performs for self-care (feeding, grooming, bathing, dressing), work, homemaking, and leisure. Depending on the specific needs of the individual, a caregiver may provide assistance with activities of daily living at different times during the day and night.

The personal and sometimes intimate nature of assistance with activities of daily living requires mutual trust and respect between the

This chapter includes: "Caring Skills and Tools," by Margit Böehmker, *MS in Focus, Issue 9*, 2007. © Multiple Sclerosis International Federation (www.msif.org). Reprinted with permission. And, "National Family Caregiver Support Program: Because We Care: Living Day to Day," Administration on Aging, September 2004.

person providing care and assistance and the person with MS. In order for caregivers to be as effective as possible, it is helpful for them to be knowledgeable about safe transferring techniques, personal hygiene techniques, basic motion exercises that can be performed at home, and some of the professionals who may be involved in the support and care of people with MS.

Transferring

Transferring refers to an action that moves a person from one place to another, for example, from a wheelchair to a bed, toilet, or car. Many people with MS are completely independent in performing safe transfers within their own homes and in other environments. Others require assistance in transferring. Unsafe transferring techniques can be harmful for both for the person with MS and for their caregiver, resulting in falls and stress on the back and other parts of the body. The caregiver and person with MS can learn safe transfer techniques from a physical therapist.

For people who experience spasticity (particularly upon waking in the morning) and require assistance moving from a bed to a standing position, wheelchair, or other type of chair, the transfer can be made less uncomfortable with the help of the caregiver. Moving the legs, hips, and knees, using light stretching exercises, done in a slow and rhythmical manner, can help to ease spasticity and can also help to conserve energy for when the transfer is carried out.

Important issues regarding transfers:

• The caregiver should be sure to prepare everything necessary prior to beginning the transfer technique, for example, positioning the wheelchair correctly.

• It is important that the caregiver communicates with the person with MS throughout the transfer the actions or movements he or she is planning on performing, so the person with MS knows exactly what to expect as the transfer is occurring.

• When transferring from a sitting to standing position, the feet of the person with MS should always be in firm contact with the ground.

• The caregiver assisting the transfer should keep his or her feet apart, providing a wide and stable base.

Personal Hygiene and Motion Exercises

It is important to discuss personal hygiene techniques with a MS nurse or other health care professional. It is also important to get professional advice from a physical therapist with regard to motion exercises, as these vary for different individuals.

Working with the Physical Therapist and Occupational Therapist

Involvement of the caregiver in assessments and visits with the physical therapist and occupational therapist is essential. While the person with MS is ultimately responsible for accepting or rejecting suggestions for therapy, adaptations, and assistive technology, the caregiver's involvement in this process will increase adherence to suggestions made by professionals, particularly within the home environment. This is especially true when suggestions require the assistance of, or input from, the caregiver. Examples include a home exercise program or installation of equipment, such as a lift.

Further, an occupational therapist or other professional may evaluate the home environment and give suggestions for eliminating architectural barriers, adding accommodations, and may make recommendations for improving caregiving techniques. These all require active participation from the person with MS and their caregiver, who may both be able to enrich the evaluation of the professional by providing important information regarding the home setting, use of home appliances, and the caregiving routine.

Home Accommodations

Making accommodations to the home can help ensure that care and assistance are efficient and safe. These accommodations can include, among many others, strategically placed hand or grab rails in the bathroom, kitchen, and hallways; shower and bathtub chairs; electric lifts and ramps; widened doorways; and adjustable beds.

Assistive Technology

Assistive technology includes any item, piece of equipment, or product system, whether acquired commercially from a retailer or customized, that is used to maintain or improve functional capabilities of disabled people. There are many different types of assistive technology that can make providing care to the person with MS safer and more efficient.

There are many factors that can influence whether or not devices are used, such as taking the user's opinion into account when selecting assistive technology, changes in the needs of the person with MS, training, and an opportunity to test equipment. Involvement of the person with MS and his or her caregiver throughout the process of evaluating and choosing assistive technology also helps to assure proper, safe use.

Further, due to the changing nature of MS, assistive devices may not be long-term solutions, and invariably some types of devices become obsolete. The preferences and lifestyle of the person with MS may also change. For these reasons, regular assessment for assistive technology needs is important.

When Particular Attention Is Needed

For people with MS who experience a loss of sensation, attention to certain caregiving activities is very important. Loss of sensation can result in an inaccurate or lack of perception to temperature, pressure, and pain. If not adequately identified and considered, loss of feeling can result in skin breakdown, scalding from hot bath water, and other complications.

Regarding insensitivity to pressure, the buttocks, heels, and elbows are particularly at risk. For people with MS who require assistance in positioning while lying down or sitting, continual turning and repositioning by the caregiver is often necessary so that skin breakdown does not occur. This task can be particularly trying for both people, especially during the night. The physical therapist can provide advice on pressure mattresses, the positioning of pillows, and a repositioning schedule.

Conclusion

Effective caregiving can be achieved with the use of skills and tools that are acquired through collaboration with the physical therapist and occupational therapist. These professionals have an important role in evaluating the caregiving situation and in making recommendations for optimizing caregiving activities, as well as in supporting caregivers through information, training, and encouragement.

Because We Care: Living Day to Day

As caregivers, we sometimes become so involved in the day-to-day efforts to keep things going that we tend to forget that each day can be an opportunity to try new approaches and activities that will make a positive difference in our life and the life of those we care for. Some things that can bring about positive changes for the better include:

- standing back and taking a look at your situation—what is working well and what isn't—and finding ways to make changes for the better;

- establishing routines that effectively meet your care receiver's needs;

- improving your physical surroundings;

- physical, speech and occupational therapy, and exercise;

- assistive devices, which range from special eating utensils to specially equipped telephones, that increase independence and safety;

- improved nutrition;

- carefully monitoring medications and their interactions;

- intellectual stimulation;

- social interaction;

- spiritual renewal;

- employing home or health care personnel who demonstrate that they really do care and who will work to foster independence;

- finding ways to economize on your work load;

- filling each day with activities to which you can both look forward.

Hands-On Caregiving

If your older relative or friend needs considerable help, a well-planned routine can make the more demanding parts of your caregiving day go more smoothly, take less time, and help to ensure that your care receiver does not develop problems which could be prevented.

- Make a list of all the things you need for morning and bedtime routines, buy several of these items and have them close at hand, such as bathing items, medications, and clothing. This saves time and keeps you from having to search or leave the room for them when you are helping your older family member.

413

If you use items in several different places, have duplicate items stored in these rooms, such as the bathroom and bedroom.

- If possible, have someone help you with the morning and bedtime routines if your older relative needs a lot of assistance since getting up and going to bed often are the most challenging times of the day.

- Practice good oral hygiene that includes tooth brushing, denture cleaning, and cleaning around the gums, preferably after every meal. Good oral hygiene helps to prevent tooth decay, tooth loss, and gum diseases, as well as secondary infections that can result from poor dental care. Persons with disabilities or medical problems may need special care in addition to daily hygiene routines.

- If your older family member is disabled, has poor eyesight, or cognitive impairments, you may need to remind them about personal hygiene or assist them. If your care receiver is incontinent, it is especially important to ensure that he or she is clean at all times, to use protective (barrier) creams, and to change incontinence aids and clothing as often as needed. Poor hygiene can result in diaper rash and blistering of the skin. Poor hygiene also can contribute to the development of decubitus ulcers (pressure sores) and other problems that cause pain, discomfort, and serious, even life-threatening infections. In older women, tight fitting clothing and diapers can lead to yeast infections. There are commercial products that make incontinence much less of a problem than it once was because they keep clothes and bed linens clean and dry. You also can discuss ways in which your care receiver's incontinence may be corrected with your health care provider, including exercises and surgical procedures.

- Older persons with limited movement should be turned in bed on a regular basis to prevent pressure sores. Correct bedding, such as sheepskin or egg carton bed coverings, or an air mattress, helps to prevent pressure sores. It is important to move older persons with disabilities at least once an hour, even if it just to reposition them, to do range of motion exercises, and to have them sit in various chairs that offer sufficient support.

- Make lists of:
    - morning and bed time routines;

- medical personnel with their area of expertise, addresses, and telephone numbers;

- home health agencies;

- other people who can help or fill in, if you need additional help;

- lawyers and financial advisors;

- where needed items are kept, such as thermometers and blood pressure monitors;

- medications—when they are to be taken, and where they are stored;

- exercise schedules and directions;

- emergency contacts in addition to 911.

These lists and other needed information can be put into a clearly marked notebook and kept where others can easily find them in your older relative's room. This book should be complete enough so that someone filling in for you will know exactly what is needed and what to do.

Tips on Safety

Quick, easy, and readily available ways to communicate with others that can help in an emergency are a must for you and your older family member or friend. Helpful items might include:

- a cordless speaker phone with memory so that you can simply hit one button in an emergency and get help without compromising the safety of your care receiver;

- a cellular phone, if you and your care receiver travel;

- a signal system which will summon help with the push of a button to use if you leave your care receiver alone at times;

- a specially equipped telephone with speed dialing, a large digital display for easy reading, and ring and voice enhancer, if your care receiver has hearing problems;

- an intercom, that will alert you if your care receiver is having problems when you are in another room;

- smoke detectors on each floor which should be periodically checked to ensure that they are operating properly.

If your family member is disabled, you will want to ensure that he or she:

- Has a clear path through each room, that there are no rugs or raised room dividers to trip over, and no slippery floors. You can carpet the bathroom with all weather carpeting to help prevent falls. This can be pulled up in sections if it is wet.

- Uses a cane or walker if needed.

- Is secure in his or her wheelchair. If your older relative is weak, a tray that attaches to the wheelchair can prevent falls and gives your care receiver a place for drinks, magazines, and mail. It is important to ensure that the wheels are securely locked when doing transfers, or if the older person's chair is on an incline.

- Cannot fall out of bed. If the bed does not have guardrails, you can place the wheel chair or other guards next to the bed, and position your older relative in the middle of the bed so that she or he can turn over without fear of falling.

Meals

As people age, they sometimes experience problems with chewing and swallowing, but there are ways to minimize these problems. The need for certain nutrients in older person's diets may also change. Avoid foods that are high in:

- saturated fats;

- salts, chemical preservatives, and additives;

- sugar and calories that do not enhance nutrition, but may add to excessive weight gain.

There are numerous ways to obtain prepared and easy to prepare meals that are nutritious time savers.

For older people who are homebound, meal times can be pleasant social events, when you can be together and talk. If your relative or friend is confined to bed, you can sit and talk while he or she eats—

416

bring a tray in for yourself. There are a host of eating utensils and accessories that make eating easier for persons with disabilities.

Caring for Your Home

- Use an attractive plastic tablecloth or place mats that are easy to clean and an attractive towel, apron, or other covering for your care receiver's clothes, if there is a tendency to spill food. Be sure that it is large and long enough to cover their laps and fold it inward before taking it off to avoid spillage on the floor. Consider having a vase of flowers (even if they are artificial) on the table or next to the bed, if your older relative is confined to bed, and open the curtains and let the sun shine in.

- Use light-weight, plastic, easy-grip glasses, or cups with handles. If there is a lot of spillage, try a drink holder with a lid and plastic straw insert.

- If clothes are wrinkled, you can put them in the dryer with a wet towel or sponge on a warm setting. This often saves a lot of time ironing.

- If your care receiver is incontinent, you can use:

  - washable or disposable pads on the bed above the sheet;

  - rubberized sheets underneath the bed sheet;

  - a stain and water resistant mattress pad.

- If the mattress does become soiled, it will need to be thoroughly cleaned and aired after being sprayed with a safe (always read the label) antibacterial cleaning agent. You can ask your doctor or pharmacist for recommendations.

- You can use water-resistant pads or heavy towels on the wheelchair or furniture that your care receiver uses. If you travel, keep pads in the car for use on the car seat and when visiting other places.

- When buying towel sets, you may want to purchase extra wash cloths since these are used more frequently and wear out faster. Thermal blankets also are useful because they are warm, lightweight, and easy to wash.

Exercise

In consultation with your care receiver's physician and physical therapist, you can plan a routine of exercises. Exercises even for bed and wheelchair-bound older persons help to improve:

• circulation,

• lung and heart function,

• posture,

• mental alertness.

Exercises help to prevent:

• diabetes,

• pressure sores,

• osteoporosis,

• heart disease,

• stroke.

If appropriate, encourage your relative to do a little more physical activity each week. Vary the exercises and challenge them to do better. Exercise with them. If they are confined to a bed or wheelchair, try to get them to exercise at least five minutes every hour, and again, regularly change their position to prevent pressure sores.

Clothing

Regardless of age or physical condition, people want to look and feel their best. Today's clothing options make that a much easier goal to reach. When buying clothing, consider the following:

• Clothing that is washable and wrinkle-free saves on dry cleaning bills and ironing time.

• Slacks and skirts that have elasticized waistbands or tie waistbands are easier to get on and off and are more comfortable.

• Clothing with snaps or zippers and some that button down the front are easier to manipulate.

• Shoes that will not slip off easily, and have a non-skid tread.

• Interchangeable and color coordinated clothing for example, slacks and tops that can go with several others.

Entertainment, Entertaining, and Travel

Boredom can sap our intellect and spirit, but you can change this by creating activities that you and your care receiver look forward to and by sharing these with others. There are many activities that frail and disabled older people can enjoy. You can:

- Check the television listings and choose your favorite programs to watch each day rather than having the television going nonstop.

- Get large print and talking books from the library and read together.

- Check for special events that are low-cost or free. Invite a friend or family member to join you, preferably one who can drive or help you if your care receiver has a disability.

- Go out to lunch or the early-bird specials at restaurants.

- Visit an art and hobby store and see what is available in the way of arts or crafts projects that you and your care receiver can enjoy.

- Invite family or friends over for dinner or lunch. If you have limited funds to entertain or do not have time to prepare food have them over for dessert or snacks, ask each of them to bring something, or to chip in on a carryout meal.

- Plan day trips to local places of interest. Again invite a friend or family member to join you.

- If you can afford to do so, go on a vacation. You can share the adventure and expense with other family members or friends. Many places offer senior discounts. Make sure that they can accommodate your needs, especially if your care receiver is disabled. Large hotel and motel chains now go out of their way to help, if you make your needs known to them. In addition, there are companies and organizations that plan trips for persons with limitations in their mobility. Many travel books have special sections on accommodations, travel, and activities for those with limited mobility.

- If you have the room, invite friends or family members to come and stay with you for awhile in your home.

- Check colleges, religious organizations, and community centers for free courses and other activities.

419

- Visit museums, galleries, botanical and zoological parks, or a petting zoo.

- If appropriate, get a pet. Your local shelter or humane society has many nice pets available for adoption.

- Get a computer with internet access so that you can e-mail friends, join in chat rooms, learn about things that are of interest to you, and enjoy computer games.

- Ask your local Area Agency on Aging about friendly visitor, volunteer, and telephone reassurance programs.

- Many fraternal, religious, and social organizations have activities specifically for older people. This can be a great way to extend your circle of friends and supportive network.

Additional Resources

Administration on Aging
Washington, DC 20201
Phone: 202-619-0724
Fax: 202-357-3556
Website: http://www.aoa.gov
E-mail: aoainfo@aoa.gov

Family Caregiver Alliance
180 Montgomery St., Suite 1100
San Francisco, CA 94104
Toll-Free: 800-445-8106
Phone: 415-434-3388
Fax: 415-434-3508
Website: http://www.caregiver.org
E-mail: info@caregiver.org

Well Spouse Association
63 W. Main St., Suite H
Freehold, NJ 07728
Toll-Free: 800-838-0879
Phone: 732-577-8899
Website: http://www.wellspouse.org
E-mail: info@wellspouse.org

Chapter 47

Features of Home Accessibility

Summary of Universal Design Home Features

"Universal design" considers a broad range of people and abilities throughout one's lifespan and incorporates those needs into an accessible design to limit obstacles and maximize independence. These design features increase the usability of the home by people of all ages and abilities. It also enhances the ability of all who reside there to live independently in their own home for as long as possible.

Summary of General Features to Incorporate in a Universal/Accessible Design Home

* Level entrance to the home, including the route to parking.

* Thirty-six-inch doors at the entrance to the home, as well as within the home. If unable to widen, evaluate use of "swing-clear" hinges to add an extra two inches or installation of pocket doors within the home.

* Sidelights at entrance door, or peepholes at heights for adults, children, and people using a wheelchair.

* Door locks that are easy to operate.

Excerpted from "Home Accessibility = Greater Independence," by Cindy Gackle, OTR/L MSCS, University of Minnesota Medical Center, Fairview © 2003 Consortium of Multiple Sclerosis Centers. Reprinted with permission.

- Eighteen–twenty-four inches of clear space on the opening side of entrance doors for wheelchair approach.

- Windows that can be accessed from a wheelchair. Windowsills that are about 24–30 inches above the floor allow people to see outdoors while seated, or standing.

- One-quarter to one-half inch maximum vertical rise at thresholds.

- At least 36-inch width hallways. Forty-two-inch wide hallways are recommended.

- Elimination of throw rugs.

- Use of hardwood floors, tile, linoleum, or carpeting that is sturdy, low pile, and tightly woven for easy maneuverability with or without mobility devices. Floors should be level with a non-slip surface, not sunken or raised.

- Clear, level route through the home, with enough room to turn all the way around in a wheelchair.

- Five-foot diameter turning spaces in bathrooms, kitchens, and at entrances.

- Counters placed at a lower height.

- Clear knee space at sinks and countertops. If plumbing is present, insulate pipes to avoid burns.

- Toilet seat heights at 17–19 inches from the floor.

- Lever handles on doors and water faucets instead of knob style.

- Water faucet and controls set off to the side of sink and shower.

- Anti-scald device for water faucets. Temperature can be turned down to 115 degrees Fahrenheit or less on the hot water heater.

- Grab bars securely fastened in bathroom walls.

- Railings as needed throughout the house.

- Front located controls on appliances (for example, stove, washer, and dryer), for easy reading and easy reach.

- Use of adjustable hanging closet rod and shelf systems for several heights.

- Placement of light switches, thermostat controls, and power outlets 32–36 inches above the floor.

- Electrical outlets placed 18–24 inches above the floor. Extra electrical outlets throughout the house can also accommodate possible future needs with use of assistive technology devices.

- Use of light switches that can be operated by a single touch using little force (for example, toggle, rocker, or touch sensitive electronic switches).

- Telephone jacks accessible and located in necessary rooms. Use of portable phones is desired.

- Good, overall lighting with extra, focused lighting as needed for task areas. Also, include lighting in closets.

- Use of bold and contrasting colors to make things easier to see. Rather than remodel or build a new home, it may be more desirable to move to an existing house that is more accessible. Use of a realtor who has experience with wheelchair-accessible housing can be invaluable with the purchase process. Identification of necessary features will be of assistance to the realtor.

Conclusion

Use of occupational and physical therapy services can influence positive accessibility decisions. Completing an in-home evaluation can often be the first step to identify accessibility barriers, solutions, modifications, and appropriate equipment recommendations. Referral to the services of an accessibility specialist, or other qualified professional who understands accessibility issues, can be especially helpful to determine design options that are desirable, functional, and create an atmosphere of wellness rather than disability.

It is essential that patients and their family or caregivers be educated about accessibility options. Researching and reading information and talking with others who have already made changes in their living situation is an excellent means of learning.

Home modifications are often completed to meet a change of one's immediate specific physical ability and are frequently planned quickly and without adequate research. Consequently, work can be done in haste and may not fully meet one's needs. Planning ahead to include universal design features can make the changes affordable, as well as make one's home more functional and accessible now, and in the future.

Developing an accessible plan that provides for future flexibility and also creates a home that is safe, desirable, and comfortable is worth the effort. Greater independence through improved home accessibility is a goal that is worth pursuing.

References

Burgess, L. (1999). Home Modifications: Bridging the Gap Between Inpatient and Community Practice. *OT Practice, July/August 1999*, 38–42.

Christenson, M.A. (1999). Embracing Universal Design. *OT Practice, November 8, 1999*, 12–15, 25.

East Metro SAIL (Seniors Agenda for Independent Living) (2002). Practical Guide to Universal Home Design: Convenience, Ease and Livability; Remodeling, Building, Buying a Home. June 2002

Eberhardt, K. (1998). Home Modifications for Persons with Spinal Cord Injury. *OT Practice, November 1998*, 24–27.

Ficocelli, M. (1994). Blueprints for Success Part 2: A Look at the specific home modification issues surrounding the bathroom and kitchen. *TeamRehab Report, November 1994*, 51–54.

Minnesota Housing Finance Agency/Home Accessibility Information Series.

National Multiple Sclerosis Society. *At Home with MS: Adapting Your Environment.* 2/01.

Residential Remodeling and Universal Design: Making Homes More Comfortable and Accessible (1996). U.S. Dept. of Housing and Urban Development. HUD User #HUD 7338, May 1996.

Rothenburg, Ronald S. Keys to Finding an Accessible Apartment. *Paraplegia News, August 1991.*

Shamberg, S., and Shamberg, A. (1996). Blueprints for Independence: Carefully Planned Environmental Modifications Can Improve Functional Performance. *OT Practice, June 1996.*

Sundstrom, I (1997). No Restrictions Apply, Home and Garden Editor, *Minneapolis Star Tribune, Thursday, October 16, 1997.*

The Ramp Project, Metropolitan Center for Independent Living. *How To Build Ramps–Reasonable–Economical–Safe.*

Whirlpool Corporation. *The Less Challenging Home: Kitchen and Laundry Guide for Builders and Remodelers.*

For Additional Information

Note: These are general resources, not endorsements of products or services.

Accessible Space, Inc. (ASI)
2550 University Ave., Suite 330N
St. Paul, MN 55114
Toll-Free: 800-466-7722.
Phone: 651-645-7271
Website: http://www.accessiblespace.org
E-mail: info@accessiblespace.org

The mission of Accessible Space, Inc. (ASI) is to provide accessible, affordable, independent and supportive living opportunities for persons with physical disabilities and brain injuries, as well as seniors. ASI services are available across the country.

AARP (formerly known as American Association of Retired Persons)
601 E Street, N.W.
Washington, DC 20049
Toll-Free: 888-687-2277
Website: http://www.aarp.org

The national seniors' advocacy organization offers printed materials and web resources on home accessibility and universal design (search "home accessibility").

Center for Universal Design
College of Design
North Carolina State University
Campus Box 8613
Raleigh, NC 27695-8613
Toll-Free: 800-647-6777
Phone: 919-515-3082
Fax: 919-515-8951
Website: http://www.centerforuniversaldesign.org

The Center for Universal Design (CUD) is a national information, technical assistance, and research center that evaluates, develops, and promotes accessible and universal design in housing, commercial and public facilities, outdoor environments, and products.

HUD (U.S. Dept. of Housing and Urban Development)
451 7th Street S.W.
Washington, DC 20410
Phone: 202-708-1112
TTY: 202-708-1455
Website: http://www.hud.gov/groups/disabilities.cfm

HUD works to strengthen communities in America in a variety of ways. This website was created for people with disabilities. Resources listed include (but are not limited to): independent living centers, modification funds, HUD's accessibility guidelines, supportive housing for persons with disabilities, accessible housing designs, and The Fair Housing Act.

Chapter 48

Equipment That Promotes Self-Care, Mobility, and Independence

Chapter Contents

427

Section 48.1

Assistive Technology

U.S. Department of Health and Human Resources (HHS), July 2005.

Assistive technology is any service or tool that helps the elderly or disabled do the activities they have always done but must now do differently. These tools are also sometimes called adaptive devices.

Such technology may be something as simple as a walker to make moving around easier or an amplification device to make sounds easier to hear (for talking on the telephone or watching television, for instance). It could also include a magnifying glass that helps someone who has poor vision read the newspaper or a small motor scooter that makes it possible to travel over distances that are too far to walk. In short, anything that helps the elderly continue to participate in daily activities is considered assistive technology.

Just as older people may have many different types of disabilities, many different categories of assistive devices and services are available to help overcome those disabilities. These include the following:

- **Adaptive switches:** Modified switches used to adjust air conditioners, computers, telephone answering machines, power wheelchairs, and other types of equipment. These switches might be activated by the tongue or the voice.

- **Communication equipment:** Anything that enables a person to send and receive messages, such as a telephone amplifier.

- **Computer access:** Special software that helps to access the internet, for example, or basic hardware, such as a modified keyboard or mouse that makes the computer more user-friendly.

- **Education:** Audio books or Braille writing tools for the blind come under this category, along with resources that allow people to get additional vocational training.

- **Home modifications:** Construction or remodeling work, such as building a ramp for wheelchair access that allows a person to overcome physical barriers and live more comfortably with a disability or recover from an accident or injury.

- **Tools for independent living:** Anything that empowers people to enjoy the normal activities of daily living without assistance from others, such as a handicapped-accessible bathroom with grab bars in the bathtub.

- **Job-related items:** Any device or process that a person needs to do his or her job better or easier. Examples might include a special type of chair or pillow for someone who works at a desk or a back brace for someone who does physical labor.

- **Mobility aids:** Any piece of equipment that helps a person get around more easily, such as a power wheelchair, wheelchair lift, or stair elevator.

- **Orthotic or prosthetic equipment:** A device that compensates for a missing or disabled body part. This could range from orthopedic shoe inserts for someone who has fallen arches to an artificial arm for someone whose limb has been amputated.

- **Recreational assistance:** New methods and tools to enable people who have disabilities to enjoy a wide range of fun activities. Examples include swimming lessons provided by recreational therapists or specially equipped skis for individuals who have lost a limb as a result of accident or illness.

- **Seating aids:** Any modifications to regular chairs, wheelchairs, or motor scooters that help a person stay upright or get up and down unaided or that help to reduce pressure on the skin. This could be something as simple as an extra pillow or as complex as a motorized seat.

- **Sensory enhancements:** Anything that makes it easier for those who are partially or fully blind or deaf to better appreciate the world around them. For instance, a Telecaption decoder for a television set would be an assistive device for a senior who is hard of hearing.

- **Therapy:** Equipment or processes that help someone recover as much as possible from an illness or injury. Therapy might involve a combination of services and technology, such as having a physical therapist use a special massage unit to restore a wider range of motion to stiff muscles.

- **Transportation assistance:** Devices for individuals that make it easier for them to get into and out of their cars or trucks and drive more safely, such as adjustable mirrors, seats, and steering wheels. Services that help people maintain and register their vehicles, such as a drive-up window at the department of motor vehicles, would also fall into this category.

What are the benefits of assistive technology?

For many individuals, assistive technology makes the difference between being able to live independently and having to get long-term nursing or home-health care. For others, assistive technology is critical to the ability to perform simple activities of daily living, such as bathing and going to the bathroom.

How can I tell if assistive technology is right for me?

People must carefully evaluate their needs before deciding to purchase assistive technology. Using assistive technology may change the mix of services that a person requires or may affect the way that those services are provided. For this reason, the process of needs assessment and planning is important.

Usually, needs assessment has the most value when it is done by a team working with the individual in the place where the assistive technology will be used. For example, a person who has trouble communicating or is hard of hearing should consult with his or her doctor, an audiology specialist, a speech-language therapist, and family and friends. Together, these people can identify the problem precisely and determine a course of action to solve the problem.

By performing the needs assessment, defining goals, and determining what would help the individual communicate more easily in the home, the team can decide what assistive technology tools are appropriate. After that, the team can help select the most effective devices available at the lowest cost. A professional member of the team, such as the audiology specialist, can also arrange for any training that the individual and his or her family may require to use the equipment needed.

When considering all the options of assistive technology, it is often useful to look at the issue in terms of high-tech and low-tech solutions. Each person must also remember to plan ahead and think about how their needs might change over time. High-tech devices tend to be more expensive but may be able to assist with many different needs. Low-tech equipment is usually cheaper but less adaptable for multiple purposes. Before buying any expensive piece of assistive technology, such as a computer, be sure to find out if it can be upgraded as improvements are introduced.

Whether you are conducting a needs assessment or trying to make a decision after such an assessment, it is always a good idea to ask the following questions about assistive technology:

- Does a more advanced device meet more than one of my needs?

- Does the manufacturer of the assistive technology have a preview policy that will let me try out a device and return it for credit if it does not work as expected?

- How are my needs likely to change over the next six months? How about over the next six years or longer?

- How up-to-date is this piece of assistive equipment? Is it likely to become obsolete in the immediate future?

- What are the tasks that I need help with, and how often do I need help with these tasks?

- What types of assistive technology are available to meet my needs?

- What, if any, types of assistive technology have I used before, and how did that equipment work?

- What type of assistive technology will give me the greatest personal independence?

- Will I always need help with this task? If so, can I adjust this device and continue to use it as my condition changes?

How can I pay for assistive technology?

Right now, no single private insurance plan or public program will pay for all types of assistive technology under any circumstances. However, Medicare Part B will cover up to 80 percent of the cost of assistive technology if the items being purchased meet the definition of durable medical equipment. This is defined as devices that are primarily and customarily used to serve a medical purpose, and generally are not useful to a person in the absence of illness or injury. To find out if Medicare will cover the cost of a particular piece of assistive technology, call 1-800-633-4227, TTY/TDD: 1-877-486-2048). You can also find answers to your questions by visiting the website at http://www.medicare.gov on the internet.

Depending on where you live, the state-run Medicaid program may pay for some assistive technology. Keep in mind, though, that even when Medicaid does cover part of the cost, the benefits usually do not provide the amount of financial aid needed to buy an expensive piece of equipment, such as a power wheelchair. To find out more about Medicaid visit http://www.cms.hhs.gov/home/medicaid.asp.

Seniors who are eligible for veterans' benefits should definitely look into whether they can receive assistance from the Department of Veterans Affairs (DVA). Many people consider the DVA to have a model payment system for assistive technology because the agency has a structure in place to pay for the large volume of equipment that it buys. The DVA also invests in training people in how to use assistive devices. For more information about DVA benefits for assistive technology, call the VA Health Benefits Service Center toll-free at 1-877-222-8387 or visit the department's website at http://www.va.gov/health.

Private health insurance and out-of-pocket payment are two other options for purchasing assistive technology. Out-of-pocket payment is just that; you buy the assistive technology yourself. This is affordable for small, simple items, such as modified eating utensils, but most people find that they need financial aid for more costly equipment. The problem is that private health insurance often does not cover the full price of expensive devices, such as power wheelchairs and motor scooters.

Subsidy programs provide some types of assistive technology at a reduced cost or for free. Many businesses and not-for-profit groups have set up subsidy programs that include discounts, grants, or rebates to get consumers to try a specific product. The idea is that by offering this benefit, the program sponsors can encourage people with disabilities to use an item that they otherwise might not consider. Obviously, people should be careful about participating in subsidy programs that are run by businesses with commercial interests in the product or service because of the potential for fraud.

Where can I learn more about assistive technology?

Most states have at least one agency that deals specifically with assistive technology issues. The Assistive Technology Act (Tech Act) provides funds to states for the development of statewide consumer information and training programs. A listing of state tech act programs is available at http://www.abledata.com.

Some area agencies on aging (AAA) have programs or link to services that assist older people obtain low-cost assistive technology.

You can call the Eldercare Locator at 1-800-677-1116 or visit the website at http://www.eldercare.gov to locate your local AAA. In addition local civic groups, religious and veterans' organizations, and senior centers may be able to refer you to assistive technology resources.

Additional Information

The following resources provide information on assistive technology products and services.

DisabilityInfo.gov
Toll-Free: 800-FED-INFO (333-4636)
 (Mon.–Fri., 8:00 a.m.–8:00 p.m. EST)
Website: http://www.disabilityinfo.gov
E-mail: disabilityinfo@dol.gov

This site is designed to serve as a "one-stop" electronic link to an enormous range of useful information to people with disabilities and their families.

ABLEDATA
8630 Fenton St., Suite 930
Silver Spring, MD 20910
Toll-Free: 800-227-0216
TTY: 301-608-8912
Fax: 301-608-8958
Website: http://www.abledata.com
E-mail: abledata@verizon.net

ABLEDATA is a federally funded project whose primary mission is to provide information on assistive technology and rehabilitation equipment available from domestic and international sources to consumers, organizations, professionals, and caregivers within the United States.

Eldercare Locator
Toll-Free: 800-677-1116
(Mon.–Fri., 9:00 a.m.–8:00 p.m. EST)
Toll-Free TTY: 800-677-1116
Phone: 301-419-3900
Website: http://www.eldercare.gov

Section 48.2

Tips for Dressing When Mobility Is Limited

"Dressing with Ease, Style, and Comfort." © 2007 Pamela A. Cazzolli, R.N. All rights reserved. Reprinted with permission. For additional information, visit www.alscareproject.org, or e-mail PCazzolliRN@aol.com.

Dressing and undressing are often challenging tasks for people with limited mobility. While buttoning buttons and zipping zippers are frustrating for some, others may have difficulty reaching arms through armholes or inserting legs through leg holes. Selecting attire to meet individual needs can make dressing easier and may eliminate unnecessary aggravation and fatigue. Getting dressed everyday will boost one's self-esteem, even if one is homebound.

In general, clothing should not restrict joint motion. Lightweight or stretch knit fabrics permit greater freedom of movement. Roomy armholes and garments that open in the front prevent the need to raise arms over the head and are easier to put on and take off. Large buttons, hooks and snaps are fasteners that are easy to use. Velcro closures require little finger or hand coordination, can replace standard fasteners, and are concealed under the openings of shirts, blouses, dresses, and pants. Zippered fronts on tops and dresses also offer accessibility. Buttons sewn on with elastic thread make buttoning less tedious.

Fabric loops, sewn inside pants and underwear, make it simpler to pull pants up and down. Trousers with elastic waistbands or drawstrings and underpants with wide leg openings or boxer shorts make dressing easier. Leg-brace wearers should choose knit pants loose enough to pull over braces.

Wraparound skirts go on better than skirts that fasten in the back and the style can accommodate weight changes. Wearing a wraparound skirt (with the opening in the back), as well as drop-easy pants, are ideal when using the toilet. By wearing culottes, ladies can enjoy the look of a skirt and the convenience of pants. Pulling a slip over the head can be avoided by wearing a half-slip. Front-fastening bras or all-stretch bras permit more independence in dressing.

Some people find dressing safer and easier while lying down, especially when pulling up pants; while others prefer to sit on the edge of the bed or chair. Those with one side weaker than the other should dress the weaker side first. Dressing aids are also available to help persons dress and undress. Some devices include:

- a dressing stick with a hook on the end to assist in pulling up pants without bending over;

- buttoners to pull buttons through button holes;[1]

- zipper pulls to open and close zippers;

- stocking aids to pull on socks or stockings;

- long wooden scissors for reaching clothing;

- long-handled shoehorn to help slide the foot into the shoe.

What to wear on the feet depends on one's ability to walk. Persons with weak ankles and feet may benefit from an evaluation by a physical therapist. Lightweight, supportive shoes may be recommended for walking, and possibly for brace support. Some persons prefer smooth-soled shoes or moccasins because rubber-soled shoes may cause tripping. However, wheelchair users may prefer shoes with rubber soles to help keep the feet from slipping off wheelchair footplates.

To put laced shoes on and off with ease and without having to retie them, use elastic laces. Other types of easy-access shoes are loafers or shoes with Velcro fasteners across the top. For added convenience, women can wear thigh-high hosiery or knee socks with skirts instead of pantyhose. Wearing knee-high fashion boots or calf-high leg warmers are ideas for hiding leg braces when wearing a skirt.

Persons who are sedentary should choose accessible clothing that not only feels comfortable, but also looks attractive. A flexible fabric, such as a soft cotton and polyester blend, moves with the body and provides the most comfort. Loose tops, which are worn on the outside of pants and skirts, look and feel the best. Wheelchair users find short jackets, ponchos, or capes more convenient than long coats. Men who wear suits may need to alter their suits by adding extra room in the shoulders and the seat. Many men find it helpful to use clip-on ties or ready-tied ties with a Velcro fastener. Dresses and skirts that are cut fuller in the hips prevent riding up when sitting.

Although outfits with fullness are comfortable, excess fullness in the sleeves, pant legs, and skirts can get caught in wheelchair spokes and cause tripping. Sitters should avoid wearing pants with heavy seams that may cause pressure areas when sitting.

The comfortableness of a fabric depends on the way it feels, the amount of heat it retains, and the manner in which it absorbs moisture. Because immobility and loss of subcutaneous fat can cause some persons to feel cold, wearing several layers of lightweight clothing retains heat and is more effective in keeping warm than wearing heavy clothing. Lightweight clothing made of terry cloth or cotton flannelette may feel comfortable both in the summer and winter.

Color and texture are important factors for dressing with ease, style, and comfort. Colorful tops add brilliance to basic slacks and skirts. Fleece wear is both functional and fashionable, and is easy to wear anytime, anywhere. The young-at-heart who like denims will find stone-washed cotton the softest.

Slippery fabrics, such as nylon, allow the body to glide easier from one surface to another, which includes transferring from bed to the chair. Wearing nylon or satin pajamas helps a person with limited mobility to move, turn, and slide more easily in bed. Persons with breathing problems should wear loose-fitting tops or have wide-open necklines. They should also avoid hairy fabrics, like mohair, as floating filaments could be inhaled.

Dressing for success means wearing clothes that are easy to wear, attractive, and comfortable all the time. Finding solutions to dressing problems will take the stress out of dressing. And feeling your best begins by looking your best.

Reference

[1] ButtonAngel. Solutions for Living LTD.

Section 48.3

Medicare Coverage of Durable Medical Equipment

Excerpted from "Medicare Coverage of Durable Medical Equipment," Centers for Medicare and Medicaid Services (CMS), Publication No. CMS–11045, February 2004.

Do you need durable medical equipment? Medicare can help. This section explains Medicare coverage for durable medical equipment in the Original Medicare Plan (sometimes called fee-for-service) and what you might need to pay.

Durable medical equipment includes things like:

* home oxygen equipment,
* hospital beds,
* walkers, and
* wheelchairs.

It's important for you to know that Medicare covers durable medical equipment and what you may need to pay. Talk to your doctor if you think you need some type of durable medical equipment to improve your health.

What is durable medical equipment?

Durable medical equipment is medical equipment that is prescribed by a doctor (or, if Medicare allows, a nurse practitioner, physician's assistant, or clinical nurse specialist can order the equipment) for use in the home. These items must be durable and primarily for medical purposes, such as walkers, wheelchairs, or hospital beds. This type of equipment is for someone who is sick or injured.

Who can get durable medical equipment?

Anyone who has Medicare Part B under the Original Medicare Plan can get durable medical equipment as long as the equipment is medically necessary.

Does the Original Medicare Plan cover durable medical equipment?

Under Medicare Part B, the Original Medicare Plan covers durable medical equipment that your doctor prescribes for use in your home. Medicare may require your doctor (or a nurse practitioner, physician's assistant, or clinical nurse specialist) to examine you in-person before you can get durable medical equipment. A hospital or nursing home that mostly provides skilled care can't qualify as your home in this situation.

Note: If you are in a skilled nursing facility and the facility provides you with durable medical equipment, the facility is responsible for this equipment.

What if I need durable medical equipment and I am in a Medicare + Choice Plan?

If you are in a Medicare + Choice Plan (pronounced Medicare plus Choice) and you need durable medical equipment, call your plan to find out if the equipment is covered and how much you will have to pay. If your plan leaves the Medicare program and you are using medical equipment such as oxygen or a wheelchair, call the telephone number on your Medicare + Choice Plan card. Ask for Utilization Management. They will tell you how you can get care under the Original Medicare Plan or under a new Medicare + Choice Plan.

If you are getting home care or using medical equipment and you choose to join a new Medicare + Choice Plan, you should call the new plan as soon as possible and ask for Utilization Management. They can tell if your equipment is covered and how much it will cost. If you return to the Original Medicare Plan, you should tell your supplier to bill Medicare directly after the date your coverage in the Medicare + Choice Plan ends.

How do I get the durable medical equipment I need?

To get the durable medical equipment you need to:

- see your doctor, and
- go to a supplier enrolled in Medicare.

If you need durable medical equipment, your doctor (or, if Medicare allows, a nurse practitioner, physician's assistant, or clinical nurse specialist) must prescribe the type of equipment you need for use in

438

your home. For some equipment, Medicare also requires your doctor or one of the doctor's office staff to fill out a special form and send it to Medicare to get approval for the equipment. This is called a Certificate of Medical Necessity. Your supplier will work with your doctor to see that all required information is submitted to Medicare. If your prescription or condition changes, your doctor must complete and submit a new, updated certificate.

The following durable medical equipment items require a Certificate of Medical Necessity.

- air-fluidized beds
- bone growth (or osteogenesis) stimulators
- external infusion pumps
- hospital beds
- lymphedema pumps/pneumatic compression devices
- oxygen
- power operated vehicles (POV) or scooters
- seat lift mechanisms
- transcutaneous electronic nerve stimulators (TENS)
- wheelchairs

You should go to a participating supplier or an enrolled supplier to get your durable medical equipment. You must go to a supplier enrolled in the Medicare program for Medicare to cover the equipment.

A supplier enrolled in the Medicare program will have a Medicare supplier number. Suppliers have to meet strict standards to qualify for a Medicare supplier number. If your supplier doesn't have a supplier number, Medicare won't pay your claim, even if your supplier is a large chain or department store that sells more than just durable medical equipment.

Special note about power wheelchairs and scooters: For Medicare to cover a power wheelchair or scooter, your doctor must state that you need it because of your medical condition. Medicare won't cover a power wheelchair or scooter only for your convenience or for leisure activities. Most suppliers who work with Medicare are honest. There are a few who aren't honest. Medicare is working very hard with other government agencies to protect you and the Medicare program from dishonest suppliers of power wheelchairs and scooters.

What is assignment in the Original Medicare Plan and why is it important?

Assignment is an agreement between Medicare and doctors, other health care providers, and suppliers of health care equipment and supplies (like wheelchairs, oxygen, braces, and ostomy supplies). Doctors, providers, and suppliers who agree to accept assignment accept the Medicare-approved amount as full payment. You pay the coinsurance (usually 20 percent of the approved amount) and deductible amounts.

If the supplier accepts assignment, you pay 20 percent of the Medicare-approved amount after you pay your $100 Medicare Part B deductible for the year. Medicare pays the other 80 percent. Suppliers who agree to accept assignment on all durable medical equipment claims are called participating suppliers.

If a durable medical equipment supplier doesn't accept assignment, there is no limit to what they can charge. You may have to pay the entire bill (your share and Medicare's share) at the time you get the durable medical equipment. The supplier will send the bill to Medicare. Then, Medicare will reimburse you for its share of the charge later.

Note: Ask if the supplier is a participating supplier in the Medicare program before you get durable medical equipment. If the supplier is a participating supplier, they must accept assignment. If the supplier is enrolled in Medicare, but isn't participating they have the option to accept assignment. If the supplier isn't enrolled in Medicare, Medicare won't pay your claim.

How will I know if I can buy or rent durable medical equipment?

If your supplier is a Medicare-enrolled supplier, they will know whether Medicare allows you to buy or rent durable medical equipment. Medicare pays for most durable medical equipment on a rental basis. Payment on a purchase basis is only allowed for inexpensive or routinely purchased items, such as canes, power wheelchairs, and in rare cases, items that must be made specifically for you.

Buying equipment: If you buy Medicare-covered durable medical equipment, Medicare may also cover repairs and replacement parts. Medicare will pay 80 percent of the Medicare-approved amount for purchase of the item. Medicare will also pay 80 percent of the

Medicare-approved amount (up to the cost of replacing the item) for repairs. You pay the other 20 percent. Your costs may be higher if the supplier doesn't accept assignment.

Note: The equipment you buy may be replaced if it's lost, stolen, damaged beyond repair, or used for more than the reasonable useful lifetime of the equipment.

Renting equipment: If you rent durable medical equipment, Medicare makes monthly payments for use of the equipment, but the rules for how long monthly payments continue varies based on the type of equipment. Total rental payments for inexpensive or routinely purchased items are limited to the fee Medicare sets to purchase the item. If you will need these items for more than a few months, you may decide to purchase these items rather than rent them. Monthly payments for oxygen and oxygen equipment, and frequently serviced items, such as ventilators, are made as long as the equipment is medically necessary. The payment rules for rented equipment called capped rental items follow. Medicare will pay 80 percent of the Medicare-approved amount each month for use of the item. You pay the other 20 percent after you pay the $100 Medicare Part B deductible.

The supplier will pick up the equipment when you no longer need it. Any costs for repairs or replacement parts for the rented equipment are the supplier's responsibility. The supplier will also pick up the rented equipment if it needs repairs. You don't have to bring the rented equipment back to the supplier.

Capped Rental Items

For certain kinds of durable medical equipment, like wheelchairs or hospital beds, Medicare requires the supplier to send you a purchase option letter in the tenth rental month (after you have rented an item for nine continuous months). You should respond to the purchase option letter within 30 days and indicate whether you would like to buy or continue renting the equipment.

If you choose the purchase option for your capped rental item, 13 monthly rental payments must be made as follows:

1. You pay your $100 Medicare Part B deductible for the year.

2. Medicare pays 80 percent of each of the 13 monthly rental payments.

3. You pay 20 percent of each of the 13 monthly rental payments.

After these 13 rental payments are made, you own the equipment. The amount you pay may be higher if the supplier doesn't accept assignment.

Note: Any rental payments you made before getting the purchase option letter counts towards the 13 rental payments.

If you choose to continue to rent the equipment or don't respond to the purchase option letter, Medicare will pay 80 percent of 15 rental payments. You pay the other 20 percent after you pay the $100 Medicare Part B deductible.

After 15 monthly rental payments, you can use the equipment without being charged a rental fee. However, beginning six months after the 15th rental payment, your supplier may charge a maintenance and servicing fee which you may have to pay to the supplier twice a year (whether or not service is provided). Medicare pays 80 percent of this fee (up to the amount of the rental payment for the first month of the equipment's use). You pay the other 20 percent. If the supplier doesn't accept assignment, your costs may be higher. Even though the supplier still owns the equipment, you can keep it as long as it's medically necessary.

Note: If your doctor prescribes a capped rental item (like a nebulizer or manual wheelchair) and you decide to buy it without first renting for 13 months, Medicare won't pay for any portion of it. The only exception to this rule is power or motorized wheelchairs, which you can buy as soon as you start using the equipment. Medicare will pay 80 percent of the costs.

Additional Information

Centers for Medicare and Medicaid Services (CMS)
7500 Security Blvd.
Baltimore, MD 21244-1850
Toll-Free: 877-267-2323
Toll-Free TTY: 866-226-1819
Phone: 410-786-3000
TTY: 410-786-0727
Website: http://cms.hhs.gov

Part Five

Multiple Sclerosis and Work, Financial, and Legal Issues

Chapter 49

Navigating the Workplace with MS

Chapter Contents

Section 49.1

Identifying and Managing the Challenges

Your ability to live and work successfully with multiple sclerosis (MS) depends on whether you can minimize your limitations and maximize your strengths. You face the fact that your life is different from what you prepared for or could have expected. This section is intended to challenge your thinking and to give you the information, resources, and tools you need to meet this challenge. But it doesn't supply answers. That's your job. Today is the moment to take charge of this life.

Unpredictable and Invisible Symptoms Affect How You Work and How Others Perceive You

Unpredictable Symptoms

The challenges you face living with MS symptoms are multiplied in the workplace, where your presence and delivery often are required on an ongoing, predictable basis. MS is unpredictable by nature, and there are several ways this can affect you. MS symptoms can flare at seemingly random times and you have no idea if and when they'll get better. Also, no two people present with the same disease course and for that reason, there isn't a roadmap to follow. Symptoms change in nature (like numbness in your hand one time and difficulty moving your foot the next), where they affect you (first your finger is numb and then your belly) and duration (symptoms can last for one week or six months).

Invisible Symptoms

MS symptoms are often not visible. This can mean that you look healthy, regardless of how you feel. You might think a limp or uneven gait is obvious, but the truth is, many people won't notice it. This can work in your favor when there's no need for others to know. But it can also make it more difficult for others to recognize what you're going through. Just because you might have told people about the disease, doesn't mean they will necessarily remember. It's easy for others to forget what they don't see.

Here are some tips to get the support you need from others:

- Keep any discussion about your health matter-of-fact. This is not the time to share your own feelings about having MS. Instead, focus the conversation on how the symptoms affect your work.

- Let others know you're doing the best you can not to be a burden. When you can't do something, be prepared with alternatives rather than expecting others to solve the problem.

- You can help others understand the variability of your symptoms by explaining that there will be times when you can't do something today that you could do yesterday, even though you look the same.

- Try to keep your expectations low regarding the emotional support you get from others, particularly if your situation makes their work harder. If everyone shares the same goals for the organization and you've demonstrated your willingness to do your part, you're more likely to get what you need to do your job, which is most important.

- Many people know someone with MS and this often shapes their ideas about what you can and cannot do. When you hear a comment that you find offensive, you have two choices: you can ignore it and go about your business. Or you can take the opportunity to educate others about this illness. Either way, when someone notices that you've developed some good tactics to manage your health, make sure you pat yourself on the back for the good work.

Cultivate Allies and Advocates for Support

It's difficult to devote time to personal relationships at work when you're exhausted from just doing your job. Socializing, which can be a satisfying part of the workday and is often a critical part of an organization's culture (think: lunchroom, voluntary meetings, group events), can become a low priority. Don't let this happen.

Allies Are Your Friends and Supporters

Surveys show that having friends at work plays a key factor in employee satisfaction. It's easy to fall into the trap of worrying that living with MS makes you less desirable as a friend, but that doesn't have to be the case if you don't let it interfere with your social interactions. Allies can be a valuable source of information when you're in doubt about your performance or how MS might be affecting your work. It's easy to feel isolated when you're sick in a healthy world; it's even more isolating when your illness is not visible. Allies can help you feel less isolated and alone.

Advocates Are People with Whom You Have a Professional Relationship

They know your work and will "go to bat" for you. Perhaps they've been your supervisor, a colleague, or someone with whom you collaborated on a project. Advocates have influence with others and are willing to use it in your support. With variable and unpredictable health, the time is likely to come when you will need an advocate's support and help.

Failing to Meet Expectations, Your Own and Those of Others, Is Something That No One Can Completely Avoid

Unpredictable health makes this more likely, but there are things you can do to keep it to a minimum.

Look at deadlines as something you can control, no matter how much others pressure you. Be rigorous in creating reasonable deadlines that you can meet, because you know the unexpected can and does happen.

Avoid the trap of thinking you're able to push yourself the way you used to. If you work in a highly pressured environment where everyone lives with high-performance expectations, you have to be very careful to know your limits. This is especially difficult because your health limits can be a moving target. But remember: just because others can afford to push themselves to meet tight deadlines on too little sleep, that doesn't mean you can. It can be tough to accept this idea of yourself, but it's a small price to pay to stay well and in the workforce.

It's no longer okay to be a procrastinator; you can't afford to pull an "all-nighter." If you know this about yourself, then it's something you can change. Here's a simple tool: With each project, large or small, create a plan for how and when the work is going to get done and build in extra time for the unexpected. Stick to your plan, because that's the only way you can be sure the work will get done on time. Create back-up plans.

Accept that there are things you just can't plan for. This is especially difficult because you've already lost so much that you used to be able to control. The most you can do is create a plan and stick to it the best you can. And then remind yourself that, as with your health, work-related things happen that are out of your control. Accepting this is all you can do—and that's a lot.

An Advocate Can Help You Get What You Need

Sharon found that her MS symptoms made it increasingly difficult for her to do the multi-tasking that was essential to her job as an internet technology (IT) project manager. She knew about a different job in another department in her company, one that she could manage much more easily, but she knew her boss would oppose the move. So she asked Alan, a former colleague (now a director), if he would help her. Alan advised her about what to say to her boss. When Sharon's boss refused her request, Alan wrote a letter of support to senior leadership. She was transferred and is doing much better in her current position.

Working on a Team Versus Working Solo

Many people don't have the option to make this choice, but if you can, you owe it to yourself to work on a team because it can increase the possibility of your success tremendously.

Working as Part of a Team

A supportive and flexible team in which members are trained and equipped to step in and do each other's jobs can be an ideal situation. That's true for anyone, and particularly so for a person living with unpredictable health. It can give you the camaraderie that is so helpful, especially in tough times. It can also provide the emotional and physical support you need to continue to work when you're unable to do the job on your own.

Unfortunately, teamwork situations don't always fit this description. If team members have clearly defined roles and expectations with little, if any, cross-training, it poses a problem when one member is unable to deliver. A "weak link" makes everyone look bad, creating tension and conflict.

Steps you can take to prepare your team in the event that your health becomes a problem:

- Be realistic about deadlines and try to build in a "fudge" factor to allow for the unexpected.

- Encourage cross-training on your team wherever possible.

- Develop an ally who is willing to help when you need it, with the understanding that you will do the same for them.

Self-Employment

Many people who live with MS, or any chronic illness, dream of self-employment. Self-employment means working solo. It can sound like the answer to your dreams, because it eliminates having to answer to a boss who doesn't understand your physical challenges, and offers the possibility of flexible scheduling. Self-employment allows you to follow your dreams, with no one there to argue with your ideas.

But self-employment also has some demanding requirements. You need financial backing while you're building a business, particularly to pay for health benefits. You need the discipline to stick to a schedule when you aren't accountable to anyone but yourself. You have to allow for the times that you aren't well, which might mean hiring a layer of support or creating a job that allows you to intermittently slow down or stop. You must consider a short-term (and maybe long-term) decrease in salary. And you most likely will pay for benefits out of your own salary.

If you can manage all of the mentioned steps and have a solid business idea, self-employment offers a strong opportunity for success.

- You can create your own schedule (if you allow yourself, that is, and don't give in to other people's demands).

- You can ramp up or pull back when you need to, as health or other needs require.

- You have the opportunity to do only what you can do (with your health in mind) without being forced to participate in activities that are draining.

Getting Help from Teammates

Consider these five tips when discussing what you need from your teammates in order to accomplish your job more effectively:

1. Decide who needs to know, and who doesn't need to know, about your illness. Make it clear that, although this isn't a secret, it's not public information, either.

2. Massage your message. Think of the concerns others have regarding your illness and give them a positive, upbeat message so they don't feel you're dumping your problem on them. Keep the details minimal but get your facts straight to maintain your credibility.

3. Be prepared with scenario planning. When health-related problems crop up, rather than force teammates to adjust to new information and face an unplanned situation, offer Plan B. If you keep it matter-of-fact, that's how most people will receive it.

4. There's a big difference between frequent complaints about your illness, and telling teammates when and how you need their help. If everyone shares the same goals for getting the work done, then they'll respect that you're working to accomplish the goal. You can't do anything about those who don't feel the same way.

5. Keep your guilty feelings to yourself. Your guilt or shame regarding something which you can do little to control only makes others uncomfortable. Don't be an emotional burden in the workplace.

Section 49.2

Asking for Accommodations or Different Job Duties

Excerpted from "Working with Multiple Sclerosis: Your Guide to Navigating the Workplace in a Healthy Way," by Rosalind Joffe. © 2006 Accelerated Cure Project for Multiple Sclerosis (www.acceleratedcure.org). All rights reserved. Reprinted with permission.

Improving Your Chances for Success

When you first get a diagnosis of multiple sclerosis (MS) it's easy to imagine yourself in a wheelchair someday, because that's a picture many of us associate with the disease. In fact, only 25% of those who live with MS ever need to use a wheelchair, and with improvements in treatment, that number is decreasing.

That doesn't mean you will never have debilitating (that which impairs your physical or intellectual strength) or disabling (that which deprives you of strength) symptoms. The fact is, at some point, you could experience MS symptoms that interfere with performing tasks that are necessary for your job.

Steps You Can Take to Try to Continue in Your Job

Even when symptoms disable you from doing part or all of your job, asking for accommodations is a factor both when interviewing for a job and when you already have a job.

The first step in getting accommodations is to accept that you have limitations that could be temporary or permanent. If they affect how you work or whether you can accomplish a task, you have three options:

1. Figure out how to get the job done in a different way without discussing the issue with anyone at work.

2. Figure out what you need, whether it is an accommodation to do this job differently or to do a different job, and ask for it.

3. Quit your job, or choose not to apply for a job that will not accommodate to your needs.

Clearly, option #1 is the easiest route, if it doesn't jeopardize your employment or your health.

In most cases, an accommodation or a job change requires the involvement and support of others. That's when you should employ option #2. Before you ask for an accommodation that would allow you to do your job (because a disability currently prevents you from doing it), take a good, hard look at yourself, your history at this job, and the culture of the workplace. Think about these issues:

-   If you have a good track record, you have a better chance of getting what you need because people regard you positively.

-   If your work has been sliding recently and you've received a warning or negative feedback, it could be more difficult to get the support you need.

-   If the environment has always been a difficult one for you to succeed within, ask yourself: Do I want this job enough to make a request? Do I believe it's worth it to negotiate or even face conflict to get what I need to stay?

-   If you get these accommodations, will you be able to be successful here? If you can say yes, you'll know it's worth the effort.

There may come a time when you employ option #3 because you know it's the best choice you've got. It's rarely easy to quit a job (especially if you don't have another one lined up). But when you just can't get the accommodations you need to be effective in your job, it's time to move on. Similarly, it's just as important to recognize job situations that don't offer the flexibility or environment that you need to thrive in before you take or start the job.

Increase Your Chances of Getting the Accommodations You Need

Do your research and be prepared. Here are some steps to take:

1. Do a functional analysis of your job.

    -   Make a list of job responsibilities.

- Break each responsibility down into tasks.
- List what is functionally required to do each task.

2. List activities that you can't do because of disabling symptoms.

  - Include all tasks or activities that you can't do, regardless of your job. This will be helpful if your supervisor wants to place you in a different position.

  - Get any documentation from a specialist that will support your claim of disabling symptoms.

3. Determine what you need to continue to be effective in your current job. Some examples:

  - You need more time for tasks.

  - You need a workstation that fits your ergonomic requirements.

  - You need a half-time person to fill in when there is additional work.

4. Develop one or several solutions. This helps you decide what's possible, while demonstrating that you aren't trying to dump your problem on others.

  - Identify who would be involved in different solutions.

  - Identify what tasks or functions would be affected.

  - Research any costs involved.

5. Gather supporting documentation.

  - Ask your doctor to write a letter that supports your claim by describing your current health challenges and how they affect your ability to function.

  - Gather annual reviews and other documentation supporting your positive work history (this is not mandatory, but it is helpful).

  - Determine if there are other jobs in your workgroup (or elsewhere) that you could try, ones that would eliminate the need for an accommodation that could create "undue hardship" according to the Americans with Disabilities Act (ADA). Doing this demonstrates your willingness to be flexible. (For more, see the ADA online: http://www.usdoj .gov/crt/ada/adahom1.htm)

6. Meet with your boss (or other decision-maker) to discuss the situation.

   • Identify the problem and present your ideas for a solution. Have as much information as possible regarding costs and who the changes could affect.

   • Frame your case to demonstrate how the positive outcomes outweigh the negative logistics and costs.

   • Stick to the facts and don't let the discussion become personal or emotional. It's not about you. It's about the job you do.

It is usually easier to get reasonable accommodations from your current employer than to find a new job that offers the accommodations you need. Option #3 should only be exercised when you have fully explored options #1 and #2.

Sample Job Functional Analysis

Job Responsibility: Handle customer complaints

Responsibilities

• Listen to customer complaints.

• Write reports of complaints and get customers to sign off on them.

• Deliver reports to the proper departments.

• Follow up on responses from those departments.

• Follow up with responses, in writing, to customers.

Functional Tasks

• Hearing and listening; excellent comprehension skills.

- Ability to empathize with people.

- Ability to have patience with angry people.

- Ability to take a complex story, simplify it, and write a report that another person will find usable.

- Ability to work with other people in the organization to get complaints resolved.

- Self-starter personality.

- Ability to organize and track complaints and follow-ups.

Sample of a "Non-Functional List"

Functions I cannot currently perform:

- writing legibly

- walking long distances (such as between departments in different buildings)

- climbing stairs (in buildings that don't have elevators)

Some Thoughts about Claiming an Accommodation as Your "Right" Under the Americans with Disabilities Act (ADA)

There are numerous resources available that explain the ADA and its obligations and benefits. In particular, the handbook "Know Your Rights: A Handbook for Patients with Chronic Illness," offers excellent guidance. It offers comprehensive information on such topics as health and disability insurance, types of discrimination, and equity issues, to name a few. One piece of good news about the ADA is that in addition to protecting the rights of the disabled, the Act has raised corporate awareness about disabilities.

On the other hand, most people don't think of chronic illness as a disability, especially one that falls under ADA guidelines. (In fact, such cases have not always been successful in litigation.) If you believe your rights are being violated, it's important to check with a lawyer. In the long run, if you can get the accommodations you need to perform your job without turning the process into a legal dispute; it will be less expensive, less adversarial, and less unpleasant for you.

For More Information

Accelerated Cure Project for Multiple Sclerosis
300 Fifth Avenue
Waltham, MA 02451
Phone: 781-487-0008
Fax: 781-487-0009
Website: http://www.acceleratedcure.org
E-mail: info-wwms@acceleratedcure.org

U.S. Department of Justice
950 Pennsylvania Ave., N.W.
Civil Rights Division
Disability Rights Section–NYA
Washington, DC 20530
Toll-Free: 800-514-0301
Toll-Free TTY: 800-514-0383
Fax: 202-307-1198
Website: http://www.usdoj.gov/crt/ada/adahom1.htm

Section 49.3

Regaining Power in the Workplace with Chronic Illness

7 Habits for Regaining Power in the Workplace with Chronic Illness

1. Focus on What You Can Control

You may not be able to control the course of your illness. You can, however, control the direction you take and the choices you make regarding that illness in the workplace. View your chronic illness as a challenge to be met, not an obstacle in the way.

2. Ignore the Nay Sayers

Many people will tell you that work is stressful and that rest is best for people with chronic illness. Ignore them. Unpleasant work or too much work can be bad for anyone's health but stress or lack of rest does not cause chronic illness. Yes, you have more challenges now than you did before, but throwing in the towel is not the only option. Shape your work environment to meet your needs and you can't harm yourself.

3. Come Out of the Closet

Chronic illness is nothing to be ashamed of. Keeping it a secret depletes your precious energy and gets in your way. Maintain your right to privacy and be judicious with your information, but don't take on the added burden of pretending that you don't have a chronic illness. Be as public as you need to be and as private as you want to be.

4. Don't Just Survive; Thrive

It's easy to feel that survival is enough with chronic illness, and most of the people who love you won't expect any more than that. But chronic illness or not, you weren't born for mediocrity. Raising the bar doesn't have to mean doing more than you can, it simply means aim high and seek out the resources you need to thrive. Reach beyond relief; go for the satisfaction.

5. Control the Message

Other people on the job will be looking to you to set the tone, and you can influence the way they respond to your illness. Design and control your message: What and how much do you want to say? Who do you want or need to say it to? When and where do you want to talk? Get out in front of the conversation.

6. Don't Let Your Illness Define Who You Are

Some people might try to paint you as a martyr; others may consider you less worthy of recognition or promotion. Neither extreme works to your advantage; each gets in your way. The message you want to convey is that your chronic illness is simply one of several cards in your deck; just like everybody else. Having a chronic illness is neither a source of shame nor a source of pride.

7. Look for the Silver Lining

Although you may not believe it now, workplace success in the face of illness is transforming. Many of us have found new strength and confidence—qualities we never knew we had—as a result of our illnesses. We have used this new found power to face other life challenges. It need not all be about the bad news.

Section 49.4

Employment Support and Opportunities for People with Disabilities

This section includes text excerpted from: Kaye, H. Stephen, (2003). "Improved Employment Opportunities for People with Disabilities," *Disability Statistics Report (17)*. Washington, DC: U.S. Department of Education, National Institute on Disability and Rehabilitation Research. Also included is "How does the federal government define disability?" U.S. Department of Labor (DOL), 2007; and, excerpts from "Ticket to Work Program Questions and Answers," Social Security Administration (SSA), 2007.

Employment Opportunities for People with Disabilities

More than a decade has passed since American businesses were put on notice that people with disabilities were to be afforded equal employment opportunity, and it has been ten years since the Americans with Disabilities Act's first employment provisions went into effect. By now, we would have expected definite indications of progress to have emerged from the data: Once opportunities improved, people with disabilities would take advantage of them in great numbers, and the result would be a steady, upward trend in the employment rate, perhaps even a reduction in the Social Security disability benefit rolls. Alas, our society is more complicated than that. Major social, economic, demographic, and perhaps epidemiologic shifts have occurred during the past decade, changes that affect not only those working and seeking work but also the base population classified as having activity limitations. These changes force us to dig far deeper if we want to find evidence of real improvements in the employment picture for people with disabilities.

The population with disabilities grew dramatically during the early 1990s, and the most pronounced and persistent increase occurred among those declaring themselves unable to work. This change is reflected consistently across survey measures, which suggest that the underlying cause was a real decline in health and functional ability among working-age adults.

Only when we account for the growth in the proportion of working-age adults with disabilities who see themselves as unable to work—most straightforwardly by calculating employment statistics exclusive of those who cannot work—do we find indications that progress has been made. Indeed, when we look at the population with disabilities who actively participate in the labor force or desire to do so, we find clear evidence that opportunities for employment have improved substantially for this group. By some measures, people with disabilities finally appear to be gaining ground in comparison with their non-disabled peers.

Employers appear to be doing better—perhaps only modestly in terms of giving breaks to job applicants who present themselves with disabilities, but significantly better at retaining workers with disabilities, probably (one suspects) in particular for those who acquire disabilities while already employed. Even if this is only a partial victory, it is surely a positive development.

Workers with disabilities employed in thriving industries, or those who have been able to switch over to such industries, have especially benefited from these improvements. Opportunities for people with disabilities in growth industries have risen to almost equal those of non-disabled workers. But economic expansion doesn't explain all of the gains we have seen: Of particular note is the fact that larger businesses, despite their relative decline in importance to our economy, appear to have increased opportunities for workers and applicants with disabilities, relative to those for non-disabled people, more significantly than smaller businesses.

Do these data offer evidence that the ADA is working? Or could they simply be a consequence of the booming economy during the latter part of the decade? This is a crucial distinction, not only because we still await statistical proof that the ADA has truly benefited our society, but also because we want to be reassured that these gains will not vanish in the current sluggish economy. Although no analysis of population statistics can answer questions of employer motivations, we can make a reasonable argument that economic and legal factors both played a role in improving the employment prospects of working-age Americans with disabilities.

Although we find cause for some measure of optimism, it manifests itself only when we restrict our focus to measuring opportunities for employment rather than overall employment rates—in other words, when we limit the scope of the analysis to people who regard themselves as able to work. We must keep in mind that, when we look at the larger picture, we find only stagnation, with no hint of the mass transition into the labor force we had hoped for among the population with disabilities as a whole. All in all, the gains in employment opportunities would seem to be only a glimmer of a silver lining within a very dark cloud.

Gloomier still is the prospect that these improvements may well prove transitory. The economic boom of the late 1990s has ended, and our economy has slowed down. To the extent that the progress we have seen was the result of economic expansion, it is in danger of leveling off or even of being reversed. Furthermore, various court decisions have narrowed the scope of the ADA, so that many people who are limited in activity (and therefore, by our definition, have disabilities) no longer appear to be covered under the law. Some employers, who provided opportunities and accommodations for a broad spectrum of people they considered to have disabilities, may now feel free to abandon those practices for those workers not deemed eligible by the courts. Just as we are finally beginning to produce evidence that this legislation has truly benefited people with disabilities in the employment arena, the protections under the ADA are being restricted and weakened.

Federal Government Definition of Disability

The definition of disability varies depending on the purpose for which it is being used. Federal and state agencies generally use a definition that is specific to a particular program or service. For example:

• For purposes of nondiscrimination laws (for example, the Americans with Disabilities Act, Section 503 of the Rehabilitation Act of 1973 and Section 188 of the Workforce Investment Act), a person with a disability is generally defined as someone who (1) has a physical or mental impairment that substantially limits one or more "major life activities," (2) has a record of such an impairment, or (3) is regarded as having such an impairment.

• To be found disabled for purposes of Social Security disability benefits, individuals must have a severe disability (or combination of disabilities) that has lasted, or is expected to last, at least 12 months or result in death, and which prevents working at a "substantial gainful activity" level.

- State vocational rehabilitation (VR) offices will find a person with a disability to be eligible for VR services if he or she has a physical or mental impairment that constitutes or results in a "substantial impediment" to employment for the applicant.

Some of these definitions include words or phrases that have been the subject of lawsuits, as individuals, agencies, and courts try to clarify the terms used in some of these definitions of disability. If you want to find out if a particular disability or condition gives you certain rights, contact the federal or state agency that enforces the law in question. If you want to find out if you qualify for a particular program or service, contact the federal or state agency that administers the program to find out the specifics of the disability definition they use.

Ticket to Work Program

The Ticket to Work and Work Incentive Improvement Act was enacted on December 17, 1999. This law included several important new incentives and opportunities for successful work experiences for people who receive Social Security disability benefits who want to go to work.

What is the Ticket to Work Program?

Ticket to Work is a voluntary program that offers Social Security Administration (SSA) disability beneficiaries greater choice in obtaining the support and services they need to help them go to work and achieve their employment goals. If you receive Social Security Disability Insurance (SSDI) or Supplemental Security Income (SSI) benefits based on disability or blindness and would like to work or increase your current earnings, this program can help you get vocational rehabilitation, training, job referrals, and other ongoing support and services to do so.

When did the Ticket to Work Program begin?

The regulations implementing this new program were published in the Federal Register on December 28, 2001, and they were effective 30 days after that date. The program was phased in beginning in February 2002. As of September 2004, the Ticket to Work program is available in all 50 States, the District of Columbia, as well as all the U.S. territories.

Are there age limits for participating in the Ticket to Work Program?

Yes. You must be age 18 or older and have not reached age 65 to be eligible for a Ticket.

What will a Ticket look like?

The Ticket is a paper document that has some personal information about the person receiving it and some general information about the Ticket Program. You can find an example of the Ticket at www.socialsecurity.gov/work/Ticket/newTicketImage.html

How will I get my Ticket?

If you are eligible to receive a Ticket, we will automatically send the Ticket to you in the mail, along with a notice and a booklet explaining the Ticket Program.

If I get a Ticket, do I have to use it?

No. The Ticket to Work Program is voluntary. If you would like to work or increase your current earnings, this program can help you get vocational rehabilitation, training, job referrals, and other ongoing support and services to do so.

Can a replacement Ticket be issued if the original Ticket has been lost or destroyed?

Absolutely, the Social Security Administration recognizes that a Ticket-holder may misplace or destroy his or her Ticket before having an opportunity to assign it to an Employment Network. Even without the Ticket in hand, you can still go to an Employment Network or State VR Agency and arrange to use your ticket with them. However if you would like a replacement ticket, contact Ticket to Work toll-free at 866-968-7842 or 866-833-2967 (TDD) to request a Ticket on Demand (TOD). The Ticket-holder should receive the TOD by mail within 7–10 business days of the request.

Where would I take my Ticket to get services?

You would take your Ticket to an Employment Network or to the State Vocational Rehabilitation Agency that offers the services you believe will best help you to meet your rehabilitation and employment goals. The Employment Networks are private organizations or public agencies, that have agreed to work with Social Security to provide services under this program.

You may contact MAXIMUS, Inc. for information about Employment Networks. If you are a ticket holder, upon request MAXIMUS will send a list of the Employment Networks that serve the area where you live. You can find this information on the internet at: http://www.socialsecurity.gov/work, or, http://www.yourtickettowork.com. Also, some Employment Networks may contact you to offer their services.

How will I find out about the Employment Networks?

You may contact MAXIMUS, Inc. for information about Employment Networks that serve the area where you live. You can contact any Employment Network in your area to see if it is the right one for you. Both you and the Employment Network have to agree to work together to attain your employment goals. You are free to talk with as many Employment Networks as you choose without having to give one your Ticket. And you can stop working with one Employment Network and begin working with another one, or with the State Vocational Rehabilitation Agency.

If you need help in choosing an Employment Network, you may contact the Protection and Advocacy System in your State. There are also Work Incentive Planning and Assistance projects in your area. These projects have specially trained staff that can help you with your ticket questions.

How can I find out about expanded availability of health care services?

The Ticket law included changes in Medicaid and Medicare. Effective October 1, 2000, the law extended Medicare Part A (Hospital) premium-free coverage for four and one-half years beyond the current limit for disability beneficiaries who work.

The law also included several important changes to Medicaid. For example, it gives States the option of providing Medicaid coverage to more people ages 16–64 with disabilities who work. To find out if this coverage is available in your State, call the State Medicaid office in your area.

Does the Ticket remove work disincentives?

SSA will not conduct a medical review of a person receiving disability benefits if that person is using a Ticket. Benefits can still be terminated if earnings are above the limits.

Effective January 1, 2002, Social Security disability beneficiaries who have received benefits for at least 24 months will not be medically reviewed solely because of work activity. However, regularly scheduled medical reviews can still be performed and, again, benefits terminated if earnings are above the limits.

Work Incentives Rules: The new law has not changed SSA work incentives rules. While participating in the Ticket Program, you may be able to use a combination of work incentives to help protect you from loss of income until you begin to earn enough to support yourself.

To find out specifically how your participation in the Ticket Program could affect your disability benefits, you may contact a Work Incentives Planning and Assistance (WIPA) agency in your state. If you use the internet, you can find a list of the WIPA agencies by state at WIPA directory. Or you can contact your local Social Security Office.

If my disability benefits stop because I go back to work, will I have to file a new application if I can't work anymore?

Effective January 1, 2001, if your benefits have ended because of work, you can request that we start your benefits again without having to file a new application. There are some important conditions:

- You have to be unable to work because of your medical condition. The medical condition must be the same as or related to the condition you had when we first decided that you should receive disability benefits.

- You have to file your request to start your benefits again within 60 months of the date you were last entitled to benefits.

- While we determine whether you can receive benefits again, you can receive up to six months of temporary benefits as well as Medicare or Medicaid. If your request is denied, you will not have to repay the temporary benefits.

Additional Information

Social Security Administration
Office of Public Inquiries
Windsor Park Building
6401 Security Blvd.
Baltimore, MD 21235
Toll-Free: 800-772-1213
Toll-Free TTY: 800-325-0778
Website: http://www.socialsecurity.gov
SSA Work Site: http://www.socialsecurity.gov/work

Ticket to Work Program
Toll-Free: 866-968-7842
Toll-Free TDD: 866-833-2967
Website: http://www.yourtickettowork.com

Chapter 50

Social Security Disability Benefits

Qualify and Apply Overview

The Social Security Administration (SSA) pays disability benefits under two programs:

* The Social Security disability insurance (SSDI) program pays benefits to you and certain family members if you worked long enough and paid Social Security taxes. Your adult child also may qualify for benefits on your earnings record if he or she has a disability that started before age 22.

* The Supplemental Security Income (SSI) program pays benefits to disabled adults and children who have limited income and resources. SSI benefits also are payable to people 65 and older without disabilities who meet the financial limits.

For most people, the medical requirements for disability payments are the same under both programs and disability is determined by the same process. Whether you apply for Social Security or SSI disability, you will be asked for information about your medical condition, work and education history to help SSA decide if you are disabled under their rules.

This chapter includes: "Qualify and Apply for Disability and SSI," Social Security Administration (SSA), April 2007; excerpts from "Part I: General Information, Disability Evaluation under Social Security," SSA Pub. No. 64–039, June 2006; and excerpts from "Listing of Impairments (Overview)," SSA, June 2006.

Applying for Benefits

Apply as soon as you become disabled. Most of the application forms can be completed online, depending on the type of benefit for which you apply:

- **Social Security Disability Benefits:** You can complete both the application and Adult Disability and Work History Report online.

- **Supplemental Security Income (SSI):** You can complete the online Adult Disability and Work History Report. Call 1-800-772-1213 (TTY 1-800-325-0778) or contact your local Social Security Office to set up an appointment to complete the SSI application form in person or over the phone.

- **Disability benefits for children:** You can complete the Child Disability Report online. Call 1-800-772-1213 (TTY 1-800-325-0778) or contact your local Social Security Office to set up an appointment to complete the rest of the application in person or over the phone.

NOTE: If your disability application was recently denied, the notice you received from SSA will explain how to request a review of the decision. The Appeal Disability Report is a starting point to request a review of the decision about your eligibility for disability benefits claim.

If you are an advocate, attorney, or third party representative and you are helping someone prepare an Internet Social Security Benefit Application and/or an Internet Disability Report, SSA will need additional information from you on the application.

General Information about Disability Evaluation under Social Security

The Social Security Administration (SSA) administers two programs that provide benefits based on disability: the Social Security disability insurance program (title II of the Social Security Act) and the supplemental security income (SSI) program (title XVI of the Act).

Title II provides for payment of disability benefits to individuals who are insured under the Act by virtue of their contributions to the Social Security trust fund through the Social Security tax on their earnings, as well as to certain disabled dependents of insured individuals. Title

XVI provides for SSI payments to individuals (including children under age 18) who are disabled and have limited income and resources.

The Act and SSA's implementing regulations prescribe rules for deciding if an individual is disabled. SSA's criteria for deciding if someone is disabled are not necessarily the same as the criteria applied in other government and private disability programs.

Definition of Disability

For all individuals applying for disability benefits under title II, and for adults applying under title XVI, the definition of disability is the same. The law defines disability as the inability to engage in any substantial gainful activity by reason of any medically determinable physical or mental impairment(s) which can be expected to result in death or which has lasted or can be expected to last for a continuous period of not less than 12 months.

Disability in Children

Under title XVI, a child under age 18 will be considered disabled if he or she has a medically determinable physical or mental impairment or combination of impairments that causes marked and severe functional limitations, and that can be expected to cause death or that has lasted or can be expected to last for a continuous period of not less than 12 months.

What is a "Medically Determinable Impairment"?

A medically determinable physical or mental impairment is an impairment that results from anatomical, physiological, or psychological abnormalities which can be shown by medically acceptable clinical and laboratory diagnostic techniques. A physical or mental impairment must be established by medical evidence consisting of signs, symptoms, and laboratory findings—not only by the individual's statement of symptoms.

The Disability Determination Process

Most disability claims are initially processed through a network of local Social Security field offices and State agencies (usually called disability determination services, or DDS). Subsequent appeals of unfavorable determinations may be decided in the DDS or by administrative law judges in SSA's Office of Hearings and Appeals.

Social Security Field Offices

SSA representatives in the field offices usually obtain applications for disability benefits, either in person, by telephone, or by mail. The application and related forms ask for a description of the claimant's impairment(s), names, addresses, and telephone numbers of treatment sources, and other information that relates to the alleged disability. (The claimant is the person who is requesting disability benefits.)

The field office is responsible for verifying nonmedical eligibility requirements, which may include age, employment, marital status, or Social Security coverage information. The field office sends the case to a DDS for evaluation of disability.

State Disability Determination Services

The DDS, which are fully funded by the Federal Government, are State agencies responsible for developing medical evidence and rendering the initial determination on whether the claimant is or is not disabled or blind under the law.

Usually, the DDS tries to obtain evidence from the claimant's own medical sources first. If that evidence is unavailable or insufficient to make a determination, the DDS will arrange for a consultative examination (CE) in order to obtain the additional information needed. The claimant's treating source is the preferred source for the CE; however, the DDS may also obtain the CE from an independent source.

After completing its initial development, the DDS makes the disability determination. The determination is made by a two-person adjudicative team consisting of a medical or psychological consultant and a disability examiner. If the adjudicative team finds that additional evidence is still needed, the consultant or examiner may recontact a medical source(s) and ask for supplemental information.

The DDS also makes a determination whether the claimant is a candidate for vocational rehabilitation (VR). If so, the DDS makes a referral to the State VR agency.

After the DDS makes the disability determination, it returns the case to the field office for appropriate action depending on whether the claim is allowed or denied. If the DDS finds the claimant disabled, SSA will complete any outstanding non-disability development, compute the benefit amount, and begin paying benefits. If the claimant is found not disabled, the file is retained in the field office in case the claimant decides to appeal the determination.

If the claimant files an appeal of an initial unfavorable determination, the appeal is usually handled much the same as the initial claim, except that the disability determination is made by a different adjudicative team in the DDS than the one that handled the original case.

Office of Hearings and Appeals

Claimants dissatisfied with the first appeal of a determination may file subsequent appeals. The second appeal is processed by a Hearing Office within SSA's Office of Hearings and Appeals. An administrative law judge makes the second appeal decision, usually after conducting a hearing and receiving any additional evidence from the claimant's medical sources or other sources.

Medical development by the Office of Hearings and Appeals is frequently conducted through the DDS. However, hearing offices may also contact medical sources directly. In rare circumstances, an administrative law judge may issue a subpoena requiring production of evidence or testimony at a hearing.

Treating Sources

A treating source is a claimant's own physician, psychologist, or other acceptable medical source that has provided the claimant with medical treatment or evaluation and has or has had an ongoing treatment relationship with the claimant. The treating source is usually the best source of medical evidence about the nature and severity of an individual's impairment(s). If an additional examination or testing is needed, SSA usually considers a treating source to be the preferred source for performing the examination or test for his or her own patient.

The treating source is neither asked nor expected to make a decision whether the claimant is disabled. However, a treating source will usually be asked to provide a statement about an adult claimant's ability, despite his or her impairments, to do work-related physical or mental activities or a child's functional limitations compared to children the child's age who do not have impairments.

Consultative Examiners for the DDS

In the absence of sufficient medical evidence from a claimant's own medical sources, SSA, through the State DDS, may request an additional examination(s). This CE is performed by physicians (medical or osteopathic physicians), psychologists or, in certain circumstances, other health professionals. All CE sources must be currently licensed in the State and have the training and experience to perform the type of examination or test SSA requests.

Confidentiality of Records

Two separate laws, the Freedom of Information Act and the Privacy Act, have special significance for Federal agencies. Under the Freedom of Information Act, Federal agencies are required to provide the public with access to their files and records. This means the public has the right, with certain exceptions, to examine records pertaining to the functions, procedures, final opinions, and policy of these Federal agencies.

The Privacy Act permits an individual or his or her authorized representative to examine records pertaining to him or her in a Federal agency. For disability applicants, this means that an individual may request to see the medical or other evidence used to evaluate his or her application for disability benefits under the Social Security or the SSI programs. (This evidence, however, is not available to the general public.)

SSA screens all requests to see medical evidence in a claim file to determine if release of the evidence directly to the individual might have an adverse effect on that individual. If so, the report will be released only to an authorized representative designated by the individual.

Who can get disability benefits under Social Security?

Under the Social Security disability insurance program (title II of the Act), there are three basic categories of individuals who can qualify for benefits on the basis of disability:

- a disabled insured worker under 65;

- a person disabled since childhood (before age 22) who is a dependent of a deceased insured parent or a parent entitled to title II disability or retirement benefits;

- a disabled widow or widower, age 50–60 if the deceased spouse was insured under Social Security.

Under title XVI, or SSI, there are two basic categories under which a financially needy person can get payments on the basis of disability:

- an adult age 18 or over who is disabled;

- a child (under age 18) who is disabled.

How is the disability determination made?

SSA's regulations provide for disability evaluation under a procedure known as the "sequential evaluation process." For adults, this process requires sequential review of the claimant's current work activity, the severity of his or her impairment(s), the claimant's residual functional capacity, his or her past work, and his or her age, education, and work experience. For children applying for SSI, the process requires sequential review of the child's current work activity (if any), the severity of his or her impairment(s), and an assessment of whether his or her impairment(s) results in marked and severe functional limitations. If an adult or child is found disabled or not disabled at any point in the evaluation, the evaluation does not continue.

When do disability benefits start?

The law provides that, under the Social Security disability program, disability benefits for workers and widows usually cannot begin for five months after the established onset of the disability. Therefore, Social Security disability benefits will be paid for the sixth full month after the date the disability began. The five-month waiting period does not apply to individuals filing as children of workers. Under SSI, disability payments may begin as early as the first full month after the individual applied or became eligible for SSI.

In addition, under the SSI disability program, an applicant may be found "presumptively disabled or blind," and receive cash payments for up to six months while the formal disability determination is made. The presumptive payment is designed to allow a needy individual to meet his or her basic living expenses during the time it takes to process the application. If it is finally determined that the individual is not disabled, he or she is not required to refund the payments. There is no provision for a finding of presumptive disability or blindness under the Title II program.

What can an individual do if he or she disagrees with the determination?

If an individual disagrees with the initial determination in the case, he or she may appeal it. The first administrative appeal is reconsideration, which is generally a case review at the State level by an adjudicative team that was not involved in the original determination.

If dissatisfied with the reconsideration determination, the individual may request a hearing before an administrative law judge. If he or she is dissatisfied with the hearing decision, the final administrative appeal is for review by the Appeals Council. In general, a claimant has 60 days to appeal an unfavorable determination or decision. Appeals must be filed in writing and may be submitted by mail or in person to any Social Security office. If the individual exhausts all administrative appeals, but wishes to continue pursuing the case, he or she may file a civil suit in Federal District Court and eventually appeal all the way to the United States Supreme Court.

Can individuals receiving disability benefits or payments get Medicare or Medicaid coverage?

Medicare helps pay hospital and doctor bills of disabled or retired people who have worked long enough under Social Security to be insured for Social Security benefits. It generally covers people who are 65 and over; people who have been determined to be disabled and have been receiving benefits for at least 24 months or have amyotrophic lateral sclerosis; and people who need long-term dialysis treatment for chronic kidney disease or require a kidney transplant. In general, Medicare pays 80 percent of reasonable charges.

In most States, individuals who qualify for SSI disability payments also qualify for Medicaid. (The name varies in some States—the term Medicaid is not used everywhere.) The program covers all of the approved charges of the Medicaid patient. Medicaid is financed by Federal and State matching funds, but eligibility rules may vary from State to State.

Can someone work and still receive disability benefits?

Social Security rules make it possible for people to test their ability to work without losing their rights to cash benefits and Medicare or Medicaid. These rules are called work incentives. The rules are different for title II and title XVI, but under both programs they may provide:

- continued cash benefits;
- continued help with medical bills;
- help with work expenses or;
- vocational training.

Listing of Impairments

The Listing of Impairments describes, for each major body system, impairments that are considered severe enough to prevent a person from doing any gainful activity (or in the case of children under age 18 applying for SSI, cause marked and severe functional limitations). Most of the listed impairments are permanent or expected to result in death, or a specific statement of duration is made. For all others, the evidence must show that the impairment has lasted or is expected to last for a continuous period of at least 12 months. The criteria in the Listing of Impairments are applicable to evaluation of claims for disability benefits or payments under both the Social Security disability insurance and SSI programs.

Part A of the Listing of Impairments contains medical criteria that apply to adults age 18 and over. The medical criteria in Part A may also be applied in evaluating impairments in persons under age 18 if the disease processes have a similar effect on adults and younger persons.

Part A: Multiple Sclerosis

11.09 Multiple sclerosis. With:

A. Disorganization of motor function as described in 11.04B; or

B. Visual or mental impairment as described under the criteria in 2.02, 2.03, 2.04, or 12.02; or

C. Significant, reproducible fatigue of motor function with substantial muscle weakness on repetitive activity, demonstrated on physical examination, resulting from neurological dysfunction in areas of the central nervous system known to be pathologically involved by the multiple sclerosis process.

The major criteria for evaluating impairment caused by multiple sclerosis are discussed in Listing 11.09. Paragraph A provides criteria for evaluating disorganization of motor function and gives reference to 11.04B (11.04 B then refers to 11.09C). Paragraph B provides references to other listings for evaluating visual or mental impairments caused by multiple sclerosis. Paragraph C provides criteria for evaluating the impairment of individuals who do not have muscle weakness or other significant disorganization of motor function at rest, but who do develop muscle weakness on activity as a result of fatigue.

Use of the criteria in 11.09C is dependent upon:

- documenting a diagnosis of multiple sclerosis;
- obtaining a description of fatigue considered to be characteristic of multiple sclerosis; and
- obtaining evidence that the system has actually become fatigued.

The evaluation of the magnitude of the impairment must consider the degree of exercise and the severity of the resulting muscle weakness.

The criteria in 11.09C deal with motor abnormalities which occur on activity. If the disorganization of motor function is present at rest, paragraph A must be used, taking into account any further increase in muscle weakness resulting from activity.

Sensory abnormalities may occur, particularly involving central visual acuity. The decrease in visual acuity may occur after brief attempts at activity involving near vision, such as reading. This decrease in visual acuity may not persist when the specific activity is terminated, as with rest, but is predictably reproduced with resumption of the activity. The impairment of central visual acuity in these cases should be evaluated under the criteria in Listing 2.02, taking into account the fact that the decrease in visual acuity will wax and wane.

Clarification of the evidence regarding central nervous system dysfunction responsible for the symptoms may require supporting technical evidence of functional impairment such as evoked response tests during exercise.

Additional Information

Social Security Administration
Office of Public Inquiries
Windsor Park Building
6401 Security Blvd.
Baltimore, MD 21235
Toll-Free: 800-772-1213
Toll-Free TTY: 800-325-0778
Website: http://www.socialsecurity.gov

Chapter 51

Financial Planning: Security for the Years Ahead

Attaining financial security is a goal that everyone shares. This goal is particularly important for families whose financial obligations include caring for one or more members who are unable to work, and who may be sick or disabled. Having adequate funds available, as well as money held in a trust with very specific instructions, are just two of several strategies that can help to ensure financial protection and security for your family in the years ahead.

Achieving such a goal, however, requires important decisions, sound investments, and informed planning for the future. Insurance, investments, trusts, and wills have become far more complicated than just a generation ago, when our parents were planning for their own futures.

Legal battles and the resultant changes in government laws over the years have led to the need for specific wording in all financial and health-related documents. New laws have added many restrictions. Without such important documents in place, you and your family may not necessarily have the opportunity to decide how one will be cared for, how the money will be distributed, and who will represent a family member if he or she cannot make decisions on his or her own.

According to Thomas D. Foy, Jr. of Foy Financial Services in Mount Laurel, New Jersey, specific language within a document is crucial for how things will be handled when the time comes to put these plans into action. While the expert Multiple Sclerosis Association of America

(MSAA) consulted for the cover story, "Planning for the Future" (in MSAA's Fall 2005 issue of *The Motivator*), holds the opinion that most legal documents may be completed using standard forms without a lawyer, Mr. Foy strongly defends the need for a lawyer when creating documents such as wills and trusts. He also encourages seeking professional help when purchasing insurance and making investment decisions, all of which can have an enormous impact on a family's financial future and healthcare choices.

What is the advantage of professional input? According to Mr. Foy, "Specific language is needed to follow HIPAA (Health Insurance Portability and Accountability Act) laws, which became effective in 1996. The legal forms found online probably do not cover all of the issues. Even with a durable power of attorney, you need to have specific language to allow doctors to discuss personal information with the selected individual; otherwise, such forms are useless."

This information has been written under the professional guidance of Mr. Foy. As an experienced financial advisor, he has seen first-hand the advantages of planning for one's future with the help of informed legal and financial experts. He has also seen the pitfalls of handling such plans improperly, as well as not having any plans in place.

The Basics, Part I: Income Replacement Strategies, Medical Insurance, and Estate Documents

The basics of any financial plan include income replacement strategies, adequate medical insurance coverage, carefully worded estate documents, and investment planning. The importance of having these plans, documents, and savings in place cannot be understated. These four areas of financial planning will protect and support you and your loved ones when employment and/or health situations change.

Income replacement strategies, medical insurance, and estate documents are described in this first section on the basics of financial planning. Part II provides an overview of investment planning.

Income Replacement Strategies

The following four types of insurance plans provide income when someone becomes sick or hurt and is unable to work, or when this person dies. If you are eligible for these different types of insurance, having adequate coverage in these four areas will ensure that you and your family receive the necessary financial support when an income-earner in the household is no longer able to work. These include:

- disability insurance;

- long-term care insurance;

- life insurance;

- critical illness insurance (new).

The latter type of insurance, "critical illness insurance," is new and is quickly gaining popularity. This works by paying a lump sum to the policy holder if and when he or she is diagnosed with an illness that is listed as one of several predetermined "critical illnesses" (as specified in the policy). This provides the policy holder with a large amount of money in one payment, which can be used to take care of extra medical bills, as well as household and family expenses while unable to work.

Medical Insurance

Whenever possible, having adequate medical insurance coverage in place for each member of the family will not only allow for adequate medical care, but will also protect the family's financial security. Whether being treated for a medical condition, long-term illness, or an unexpected injury, medical bills can add up fast and quickly deplete a family's savings.

Opportunities for medical insurance coverage vary between the states. New Jersey has a "no pre-existing conditions" clause, so no one may be excluded due to a condition when starting with a new policy. While this means higher premiums because the insurance companies are forced to cover existing conditions, it also means that you won't be left without coverage should you or a family member encounter a health problem while making a change with a policy.

Estate Documents

A durable power of attorney, advanced medical directive (living will), wills, and trusts are all different types of estate documents. According to Mr. Foy, "Today, every individual needs to have at least a durable power of attorney, a living will, and a will, all in place and up-to-date. These documents are crucial to your future as well as that of your family."

Mr. Foy continues, "I also strongly recommend that individuals seek the advice of a legal professional when creating these documents. You can't afford not to seek professional advice, especially in today's highly scrutinized legal environment. If these documents are not worded correctly, you cannot be guaranteed that health care and financial instructions will be carried out according to your wishes. Additionally, government programs and medical assistance may be affected for a loved one if the money in a will or trust is not handled correctly."

A durable power of attorney and a living will are examples of "living documents," which means that they are in effect while one is still living; after death, these are no longer active. Wills take over after one dies; and the different types of trusts may be active during one's lifetime as well as afterward.

Durable power of attorney (DPOA): This gives someone else the authority to act on your behalf and make decisions for you. It includes the ability to make medical decisions (durable adds the medical capacity). This document needs to be worded so that all rights are passed along should you become ill or injured and unable to make and communicate your own decisions. A good idea is to prepare this document in multiples, as you may need to surrender copies to the different professionals or institutions involved. Most people typically name a significant other and their children as choices for DPOA.

Living will: This document is used to dictate how to be cared for in your final days. For example, it may include which life-prolonging procedures you may or may not choose to have, such as tube feeding or a respirator. Among other points, it also may state your preference as to where you would like to spend your final days (in a medical facility or at home).

Advanced medical directive: Also known as a "healthcare power," this document combines a DPOA with a living will—either in one document or in two separate ones.

Will: Also known as a testament, a will takes over after death and explains how one's property is distributed. The contents of a will become public information, accessible to anyone after you die. A will can also leave everything to a living trust, which has certain advantages, including confidentiality, even after you are gone.

Trust: This is a legal arrangement in which an individual gives legal control of property to a person or institute (the trustee), for the benefit of the trust's beneficiaries—who will ultimately receive the property in the trust. A trustor is the individual who sets up a trust, also known as the grantor. The trustee is an individual or organization which holds or manages and invests assets for the benefit of another, often with the legal authority and duty to make decisions regarding financial matters.

As an addition to these documents, individuals may find that they have a need for other types of supporting documents. These may include a living trust, a special needs trust, or a testamentary trust.

Living trust: This trust may be a substitute for a will, but is frequently an entity within the will, giving instructions that could replace all the other documents; it is perpetual and private. You can have the will (which is public information) leave everything to the living trust (which remains confidential).

Special needs trust: This takes care of the special needs of someone who may be physically and/or mentally impaired. This trust allows someone to be creative within the will or trust, but may also be done separately. The trustor who creates the special needs trust can distribute funds as needed before his or her death. Afterward, the appointed trustee or committee of trustees takes over how the funds are managed. Sometimes a life insurance policy will be used as a funding vehicle for a special needs trust (so that after the trustor has died, his or her life insurance benefits are added into the trust).

A carefully structured and adequately funded trust can ensure that a spouse, child, or other family members with special needs are cared for throughout their years, even after the person supporting them is no longer living. Some individuals set-up a charity that may continue after the beneficiaries have also passed away.

Mr. Foy notes, "Any family who cares for a loved one with special needs should seriously consider seeking legal advice to create a special needs trust. It should include language focused on the needs of the family member with physical or mental limitations. When drafted by a qualified attorney, the language should be specific enough to maximize state and federal benefits."

Testamentary trust: This is a trust that is created within a will and it does not take effect until the trustor's death. Someone may want to set-up a testamentary trust when specific instructions are needed for how the funds and/or property are to be distributed. A series of instructions lists specific conditions for the beneficiary.

For instance, a testamentary trust may be advisable when the beneficiary is under 18 and you are concerned about the responsibility of the child; when the beneficiary is a spendthrift; or if the beneficiary may be facing financial problems—such as bankruptcy or divorce. This type of trust can include spendthrift language to provide a level of liability, creditor, and bankruptcy protection.

Mr. Foy explains, "The funds are not easily accessible and this trust protects the beneficiary from his or her own poor money management, as well as losing money to an ex-spouse during a divorce. A trustee has full power of discretion at the time of legal trouble, having the authority not to disperse any funding at that particular time. In order for this type of trust to work in this capacity, it must be worded correctly by a lawyer."

Part II: Investment Planning

The first advice given by Mr. Foy is to assume that the government won't provide assistance. To be safe, he recommends that a person assumes complete and total responsibility, not depending on any family entitlements. The best way to ensure one's future financially is to save through the following two methods:

- Maximize saving through one's employer, using a retirement plan such as a 401K.

- Create a portfolio of investments—whether for a retirement fund or other accumulated assets. Individuals may wish to seek investment advice to help determine their tolerance for risk and the appropriate investment selection designed to meet their identified investment goals.

For example, young families may be more growth oriented with their financial investments (high risk, high potential), and may choose to purchase company stocks. When people purchase mutual funds, they are investing in company stocks, but they reduce some of their risk because this includes stocks in several companies—so one's success does not depend on the performance of a single company.

Older families, whose objective may be focused on conserving the principle of present investments, also known as preservation of capital, may stay with more conservative, less vulnerable investments (low-risk, consistent potential). Examples of such investments include cash equivalents (bank accounts, certificates of deposit) and money market funds.

Opportunities are available for individuals who feel compelled to invest on their own, however, if someone has resources for investment and qualifies, then he or she may be well advised to seek professional advice. An excellent how-to guide on investing is a book by Peter Navarro titled, *If It's Raining in Brazil, Buy Starbucks* (published by McGraw-Hill Companies; first edition, 2004).

Mr. Foy points out, "Various financial publications, such as *Money Magazine*, *Fortune*, *Wall Street Journal*, and *Barron's*, may be recommended as resources for individuals to learn terminology and to find out about some general investing tips, but newcomers need to be skeptical of financial advice within these types of publications. Advice should be taken with a grain of salt, as financial editors are not the same as financial planners. Additionally, some may find that the financial advice in certain publications relates directly to the advertisers within the magazine."

To follow are various types of investments, beginning with the most conservative, having the least risk and lowest potential for a high rate of return. As the list continues, it moves onto the least conservative investments, which have the greatest risk but also the best potential for a high rate of return.

More Conservative Investments with Less Risk

Cash Equivalents

- savings accounts
- checking accounts
- bank certificates of deposit (CDs)

Sometimes cash equivalents are insured by the Federal Deposit Insurance Corporation (FDIC). Most investments in general are not insured, because little money can be made if insured. These three types of investments are all handled through a bank.

According to Investorwords.com, a certificate of deposit is a short or medium-term, interest-bearing, FDIC-insured debt instrument offered by banks as well as savings and loans. CDs offer higher rates of return than most comparable investments, in exchange for tying up invested money for the duration of the certificate's maturity. Money removed before maturity is subject to a penalty. CDs are low-risk, low-return investments, and are also known as time deposits, because the account holder has agreed to keep the money in the account for a specified amount of time, anywhere from three months to six years.

485

Money Market Funds

- Money market funds are the safest form of mutual funds, although money markets are not insured. Money market funds are usually purchased at an investment firm. Investing money in cash equivalents through the bank (savings, checking, or CD) or through money market funds, may not bring a high rate of return, but does provide a good deal of security, knowing that these types of investments carry the least amount of risk.

- Investorwords.com defines a money market fund as an open-ended mutual fund which invests only in money markets. These funds invest in short-term (one day to one year) debt obligations such as treasury bills, certificates of deposit, and commercial paper (which is an unsecured obligation issued by a corporation or bank to finance its short-term credit needs). The main goal is the preservation of principal, accompanied by modest dividends. The fund's net asset value remains a constant $1.00 per share to simplify accounting, but the interest rate does fluctuate.

- Investorwords.com continues by noting that money market funds are very liquid investments, and therefore, are often used by financial institutions to store money that is not currently invested. Although money market mutual funds are among the safest types of mutual funds, it still is possible for money market funds to fail, but it is unlikely. In fact, the biggest risk involved in investing in money market funds is the risk that inflation will outpace the funds' returns, thereby eroding the purchasing power of the investor's money.

Bonds

- These are fixed-income investments. If held until maturity, the rate of return is guaranteed, as well as the return of the original investment. Purchasing bonds involves going through a professional such as a broker. Although not recommended, bonds may also be purchased through an internet trading company. Bonds in general have a relatively low risk for loss of investment. Examples of bonds include:
  - municipal bonds (issued by a legislative body);
  - corporate bonds (issued by a privately owned company);
  - government bonds (issued by the United States Treasury Department).

Investorwords.com defines a bond as a debt instrument issued for a period of more than one year with the purpose of raising capital by borrowing. The Federal government, states, cities, corporations, and many other types of institutions sell bonds. Generally, a bond is a promise to repay the principal along with interest (coupons) on a specified date (maturity). Some bonds do not pay interest, but all bonds require a repayment of principal. When an investor buys a bond, he or she becomes a creditor of the issuer, although the buyer does not gain any kind of ownership rights to the issuer.

Bonds are often divided into different categories based on tax status, credit quality, issuer type, maturity, and whether secured or unsecured (and there are several other ways to classify bonds as well). United States Treasury bonds are generally considered the safest unsecured bonds, since the possibility of the Treasury defaulting on payments is almost zero. The yield from a bond is made up of three components: coupon interest, capital gains, and interest on interest (if a bond pays no coupon interest, the only yield will be capital gains).

A riskier bond has to provide a higher payout to compensate for that additional risk. Some bonds are tax-exempt, and these are typically issued by municipal, county, or state governments, whose interest payments are not subject to federal income tax, and sometimes also state or local income tax.

Less Conservative Investments with Greater Risk

Mutual Funds

These are a safer way to invest in a corporation. The sole objective is for the portfolio manager to buy, sell, or hold securities (which include stocks and bonds) for all those who are investing. Mutual funds may be just stocks, or they may include government bonds, real estate, or almost any other investment—even stock in oil futures. The purpose is to be diversified, providing a "basket of securities" for the investors. The portfolio manager oversees the entire "basket" of investments, enabling investors to each purchase a portion of the basket (holding several investments), so separate purchases of individual securities are not needed.

Investorwords.com defines a mutual fund as an open-ended fund operated by an investment company, which raises money from shareholders and invests in a group of assets, in accordance with a stated set of objectives. Mutual funds raise money by selling shares of the fund to the public, much like any other type of company can sell stock in itself to the public. Mutual funds then take the money they receive from the sale of their shares (along with any money made from previous investments) and use it to purchase various investment vehicles, such as stocks, bonds, and money market instruments.

In return for the money they give to the fund when purchasing shares, shareholders receive an equity position in the fund and, in effect, in each of its underlying securities. For most mutual funds, shareholders are free to sell their shares at any time, although the price of a share in a mutual fund will fluctuate daily, depending upon the performance of the securities held by the fund. Benefits of mutual funds include diversification and professional money management. Mutual funds offer choice, liquidity, and convenience, but charge fees and often require a minimum investment.

Mr. Foy notes that some individuals may consider using insurance company annuities as a means of not outliving their income. These serve a valuable function in certain financial plans, but they are highly complicated and can be very expensive. If structured correctly, annuities can hold investments similar to mutual funds. Individuals should not just buy any annuity; they need to use the right one from the right company, so again, Mr. Foy recommends seeking the advice of a professional.

Investorwords.com defines an annuity as a contract sold by an insurance company, designed to provide payments to the holder at specified intervals, usually after retirement. The holder is taxed only when he or she starts taking distributions or if funds from the account are withdrawn.

All annuities are tax-deferred, meaning that the earnings from investments in these accounts grow tax-deferred until withdrawal. Annuity earnings are also tax-deferred so they cannot be withdrawn without penalty until a certain specified age. Fixed annuities guarantee a certain payment amount, while variable annuities do not, but do have the potential for greater returns. Both are relatively safe, low-yielding investments.

Stocks

Stocks are usually purchased through an investment professional. Stocks may be from small companies, or they may be from large companies, which are known as blue chip stocks.

- Individuals investing in small companies are looking for a total return of investment, known as "capital appreciation."

- Individuals investing in blue chip stocks are investing in big companies and are looking to receive periodic dividends.

As described by Investorwords.com, a stock is an instrument that signifies an ownership position (called equity) in a corporation, and represents a claim on its proportional share in the corporation's assets and profits. Ownership in the company is determined by the number of shares a person owns divided by the total number of shares outstanding. For example, if a company has 1000 shares of stock outstanding and a person owns 50 of them, then he or she owns five percent of the company. Most stock also provides voting rights, which give shareholders a proportional vote in certain corporate decisions. Only a certain type of company called a corporation has stock; other types of companies such as sole proprietorships and limited partnerships do not issue stock.

Investing for the Future

Many individuals are on fixed incomes and have little extra cash for investments. Readers should note, however, that even a small amount of money saved or invested each month can add up over the years. Financial calculators are available on many financial websites. With these, individuals may look into various levels of investment and rate of return to determine how their financial investments may grow.

For example, if someone is able to find $100 per month (about $25 extra per week) to invest in a low-risk, fixed-interest type of account, and estimate the rate interest to be at two percent, the savings become significant after several years. Before tax and inflation (BTI) factors are figured in, saving $100 monthly at two percent interest will yield more than $13,000 after 10 years, and nearly $30,000 after 20 years. If the interest is at five percent, $100 monthly would grow to nearly $15,500 after 10 years and more than $40,000 after 20 years (BTI).

Of course, bigger investments into stocks can yield even greater profits—provided they perform well. Stocks are high-risk but have the potential for high interest and a strong return on investment.

For More Information

For assistance with insurance options, readers may contact their local insurance agent, or they may also visit insurance company websites on the internet. Readers are cautioned to look into their options and compare costs, benefits, and the reputation of the insurance company before signing for an insurance policy designed to protect you and your family's future.

Regarding investments, Mr. Foy points out that many mutual fund companies have websites that provide a wealth of information. Often, these resources offer general investing information which is not necessarily designed to encourage selling their own products.

- Infoplease™ offers a listing of personal financial websites which may be found at http://www.infoplease.com/ipa/A0001507.html.

Chapter 52

Health Care Options: Home Care, Assisted Living, Skilled Nursing Care

Home Health Care: A Guide for Families

As with any important purchase, it is always a good idea to talk with friends, neighbors, and your local area agency on aging to learn more about the home health care agencies in your community.

In looking for a home health care agency, the following 20 questions can be used to help guide your search:

1. How long has the agency been serving this community?

2. Does the agency have any printed brochures describing the services it offers and how much they cost? If so, get one.

3. Is the agency an approved Medicare provider?

4. Is the quality of care certified by a national accrediting body such as the Joint Commission for the Accreditation of Healthcare Organizations?

5. Does the agency have a current license to practice (if required in the state where you live)?

This chapter includes: "Home Health Care: A Guide for Families," U.S. Department of Health and Human Services (HHS) Administration on Aging, updated August 27, 2003; "Fact Sheets: Assisted Living," HHS, updated July 6, 2005; and, "Nursing Homes: Making the Right Choice," National Institute on Aging (NIA), January 2007.

6. Does the agency offer seniors a "Patients' Bill of Rights" that describes the rights and responsibilities of both the agency and the senior being cared for?

7. Does the agency write a plan of care for the patient (with input from the patient, his or her doctor and family), and update the plan as necessary?

8. Does the care plan outline the patient's course of treatment, describing the specific tasks to be performed by each caregiver?

9. How closely do supervisors oversee care to ensure quality?

10. Will agency caregivers keep family members informed about the kind of care their loved one is getting?

11. Are agency staff members available around the clock, seven days a week, if necessary?

12. Does the agency have a nursing supervisor available to provide on-call assistance 24 hours a day?

13. How does the agency ensure patient confidentiality?

14. How are agency caregivers hired and trained?

15. What is the procedure for resolving problems when they occur, and who can I call with questions or complaints?

16. How does the agency handle billing?

17. Is there a sliding fee schedule based on ability to pay, and is financial assistance available to pay for services?

18. Will the agency provide a list of references for its caregivers?

19. Who does the agency call if the home health care worker cannot come when scheduled?

20. What type of employee screening is done?

What is involved in the screening process?

When purchasing home health care directly from an individual provider (instead of through an agency), it is even more important to screen the person thoroughly. This should include an interview with the home health caregiver to make sure that he or she is qualified for the job. You should request references. Also, prepare for the interview by making a list if any special needs the patient might have. For example, you would want to note whether the patient needs help getting into or out of a wheelchair. Clearly, if this is the case, the home health caregiver must be able to provide that assistance. The screening process will go easier if you have a better idea of what you are looking for first.

Another thing to remember is that it always helps to look ahead, anticipate changing needs, and have a backup plan for special situations. Since every employee occasionally needs time off (or a vacation), it is unrealistic to assume that one home health care worker will always be around to provide care. Family members who hire home health workers directly may want to consider interviewing a second part-time or on-call person who can be available when the primary caregiver cannot be. Calling an agency for temporary respite care also may help to solve this problem.

In any event, whether you arrange for home health care through an agency or hire an independent home health care aide on an individual basis, it helps to spend some time preparing for the person who will be doing the work. Ideally, you could spend a day with him or her, before the job formally begins, to discuss what will be involved in the daily routine. If nothing else, tell the home health care provider (both verbally and in writing) the following things that he or she should know about the care recipient:

- illnesses, injuries, and signs of an emergency medical situation;
- likes and dislikes;
- medications, and how and when they should be taken;
- need for dentures, eyeglasses, canes, walkers, etc.;
- possible behavior problems and how best to deal with them;
- problems getting around (in or out of a wheelchair, for example, or trouble walking);
- special diets or nutritional needs;
- therapeutic exercises.

In addition, you should give the home health care provider more information about:

- clothing the patient may need (when it gets too hot or too cold);
- how you can be contacted (and who else should be contacted in an emergency);

- how to find and use medical supplies and medications;

- when to lock up the apartment or house and where to find the keys;

- where to find food, cooking utensils, and serving items;

- where to find cleaning supplies;

- where to find light bulbs and flash lights, and where the fuse box is located (in case of a power failure);

- where to find the washer, dryer, and other household appliances (as well as instructions for how to use them).

A word of caution: Although most states require that home health care agencies perform criminal background checks on their workers and carefully screen job applicants for these positions, the actual regulations will vary depending on where you live. Therefore, before contacting a home health care agency, you may want to call your local area agency on aging or department of public health to learn what laws apply in your state.

How can I pay for home health care?

The cost of home health care varies across states and within states. In addition, costs will fluctuate depending on the type of health care professional required. Home care services can be paid for directly by the patient and his or her family members, or through a variety of public and private sources. Sources for home health care funding include Medicare, Medicaid, the Older Americans Act, the Veterans' Administration, and private insurance. Medicare is the largest single payer of home care services. The Medicare program will pay for home health care if all of the following conditions are met:

- The patient must be homebound and under a doctor's care.

- The patient must need skilled nursing care, or occupational, physical, or speech therapy, on at least an intermittent basis (that is, regularly but not continuously).

- The services provided must be under a doctor's supervision and performed as part of a home health care plan written specifically for that patient.

- The patient must be eligible for the Medicare program and the services ordered must be medically reasonable and necessary.

- The home health care agency providing the services must be certified by the Medicare program.

Assisted Living

Assisted living facilities offer a housing alternative for adults who may need help with dressing, bathing, eating, and toileting, but do not require the intensive medical and nursing care provided in nursing homes. Assisted living facilities may be part of a retirement community, nursing home, senior housing complex, or may stand alone. Licensing requirements for assisted living facilities vary by state and can be known by as many as 26 different names including: residential care, board and care, congregate care, and personal care.

What services are provided in assisted living?

Residents of assisted living facilities usually have their own units or apartment. In addition to having a support staff and providing meals, most assisted living facilities also offer at least some of the following services:

- health care management and monitoring;
- help with activities of daily living such as bathing, dressing, and eating;
- housekeeping and laundry;
- medication reminders or help with medications;
- recreational activities;
- security;
- transportation.

What should be considered when choosing an assisted living facility?

A good match between a facility and a resident's needs depends as much on the philosophy and services of the assisted living facility as it does on the quality of care. The following suggestions can help you get started in your search for a safe, comfortable, and appropriate assisted living facility:

- Think ahead. What will the resident's future needs be and how will the facility meet those needs?

- Is the facility close to family and friends? Are there any shopping centers or other businesses nearby (within walking distance)?

- Do admission and retention policies exclude people with severe cognitive impairments or severe physical disabilities?

- Does the facility provide a written statement of the philosophy of care?

- Visit each facility more than once, sometimes unannounced.

- Visit at meal times, sample the food, and observe the quality of mealtime and the service.

- Observe interactions among residents and staff.

- Check to see if the facility offers social, recreational, and spiritual activities.

- Talk to residents.

- Learn what types of training staff receive and how frequently they receive training.

- Review state licensing reports.

The following steps should also be considered:

- Contact your state's long-term care ombudsman to see if any complaints have recently been filed against the assisted living facility you are interested in. In many states, the ombudsman checks on conditions at assisted living units as well as nursing homes.

- Contact the local Better Business Bureau to see if that agency has received any complaints about the assisted living facility.

- If the assisted living facility is connected to a nursing home, ask for information about it, too. (Information on nursing homes can be found on the Medicare website at http://www.medicare.gov/nhcompare/home.asp).

What is the cost for assisted living?

Although assisted living costs less than nursing home care, it is still fairly expensive. Depending on the kind of assisted living facility and type of services an older person chooses, the price costs can range from less than $10,000 a year to more than $50,000 a year.

Across the U.S., monthly rates average $1,800 per month. Because there can be extra fees for additional services, it is very important for to find out what is included in the basic rate and how much other services will cost.

Primarily, the individual or their families pay the cost of assisted living. Some health and long-term care insurance policies may cover some of the costs associated with assisted living. In addition, some residences have their own financial assistance programs.

The federal Medicare program does not cover the costs of assisted living facilities or the care they provide. In some states, Medicaid may pay for the service component of assisted living. Medicaid is the joint federal and state program that helps older people and those with disabilities pay for health care when they are not able to afford the expenses themselves.

Nursing Homes: Making the Right Choice

A nursing home is a place for people who don't need to be in a hospital but can no longer be cared for at home. Most nursing homes have nursing aides and skilled nurses on hand 24-hours a day. Sometimes a nursing home is the best choice for people who need personal and medical care.

Nursing homes can be:

Hospital-like. This type of nursing home is often set up like a hospital. Staff give medical care, as well as physical, speech, and occupational therapy. There can be a nurses' station on each floor. As a rule, one or two people live in a room. A number of nursing homes will let couples live together. Things that make a room special, like family photos, are often welcome.

Household-like. These facilities are designed to be more like homes and the day-to-day routine isn't fixed. Teams of staff and residents try to create a neighborhood feel. Kitchens are often open to residents, decorations give a sense of home, and the staff is encouraged to develop relationships with residents.

Some nursing homes have visiting doctors who see their patients on site. Other nursing homes have patients visit the doctor's office. Nursing homes sometimes have separate areas called Special Care Units for people with serious memory problems, often called dementia. When looking for a nursing home, it's important for families to think about these special needs.

How do you choose?

If you are looking for a nursing home here are some things to keep in mind:

- **Look:** What choices are in your area? Is there a place close to family and friends? What's important to you—nursing care, meals, a religious connection, hospice care, or Special Care Units for dementia care?

- **Ask:** Talk with friends, relatives, social workers, and religious groups to find out what places they suggest. Ask doctors which nursing homes they feel provide good care?

- **Call:** Get in touch with each place on your list. Ask questions about how many people live there and what it costs. Find out about waiting lists.

- **Visit:** Make plans to meet with the director and the nursing director. Some things to look for:

  - Medicare and Medicaid certification

  - handicap access

  - strong odors (either bad or good)

  - many food choices

  - residents who look well cared for

  - enough staff for the number of patients

- **Talk:** Don't be afraid to ask questions. Ask how long the director and department heads (nursing, food, and social services) have worked at the nursing home. If key staff changes a lot, that could mean there is a problem.

- **Visit again:** Make a second visit without first calling. Try another day of the week or time of day so you will meet other staff members and see other activities. Stop by at mealtime. Do people seem to be enjoying their food?

- **Understand:** Once you choose, carefully read the contract. Check with your State Ombudsman for help making sense of the contract.

Do nursing homes have to meet standards?

The Centers for Medicare and Medicaid Services (CMS) asks each State to inspect any nursing home that gets money from the government. Homes that don't pass inspection are not certified. Ask to see the current inspection report and certification of homes you are thinking about. Visit www.medicare.gov for more information.

How do you pay for nursing home care?

People pay for nursing home care in many ways:

- **Private pay:** Some people pay for long-term care with their own savings for as long as possible. When that is no longer possible, they may get help from Medicaid. If you think you may need to apply for Medicaid at some point, make sure the nursing home accepts it. Not all homes do.

- **Medicaid:** This is a State program for people with low incomes. Each State decides who qualifies. Contact your State government to learn if you qualify. Keep in mind that getting approved for Medicaid can take three or more months.

- **Long-term care insurance:** Some people buy private long-term care insurance. It can pay part of the costs for a nursing home or other long-term care. This type of insurance is sold by many different companies and benefits vary widely. Look carefully at several policies before making a choice.

Many people believe Medicare will pay for long stays in a nursing home, but it doesn't. It is important to check with Medicare and private Medigap (Medicare add-on) insurance to find out the current rules. For example, Medicare may only cover the first 100 days in a skilled nursing home for people needing special care after leaving the hospital.

When thinking about costs, keep in mind that there can be extra out-of-pocket charges for some supplies, personal care like hair appointments, laundry, and services that are outside routine care.

What resources can help?

The rules about programs and benefits for nursing homes can change. Medicare has some helpful resources online. Visit www.medicare.gov for information about different care options. You can find nursing homes in your area that are approved by CMS by visiting the Medicare website.

You can also see summaries of recent inspection reports. Visit Nursing Home Compare at www.medicare.gov/NHCompare. The Nursing Home Checklist at the same website is a good guide to use when thinking about nursing homes.

Many States have State Health Insurance Counseling and Assistance Programs (SHIP). These programs can help you choose the health insurance that is right for you and your family.

Each State also has a Long-Term Care Ombudsman office that helps people learn about long-term care. Your local office may be able to answer general questions about a specific nursing home. Also, once you are living in a nursing home, the Ombudsman can help solve problems you may have with a facility. The National Long-Term Care Ombudsman Resource Center has more information. Visit http://www.ltcombudsman.org.

A veteran in need of long-term care might be able to get help through the Department of Veterans Affairs programs. Visit http://www.va.gov or call VA Health Care Benefits toll-free at 877-222-8387. You can also contact a VA medical center near you.

Additional Information

Assisted Living Federation of America
1650 King St. Suite 602
Alexandria, VA 22314-2747
Phone: 703-894-1805
Fax: 703-894-1831
Website: http://www.alfa.org
E-mail: info@alfa.org

Centers for Medicare and Medicaid Services (CMS)
7500 Security Blvd.
Baltimore, MD 21244-1850
Toll-Free: 877-267-2323
Toll-Free TTY: 866-226-1819
Phone: 410-786-3000
TTY: 410-786-0727
Website: http://cms.hhs.gov

Department of Veterans Affairs
Toll-Free Health Care Benefits: 877-222-8387
Toll-Free TTY: 800-829-4833
Website: http://www.va.gov

National Association for Home Care
228 7th Street, S.E.
Washington, DC 20003
Phone: 202-547-7424
Fax: 202-547-3540
Website: http://www.nahc.org

National Center for Assisted Living
1201 L Street, N.W.
Washington, DC 20005
Phone: 202-842-4444
Website: http://www.ncal.org
E-mail: webmaster@ahca.org

Visiting Nurse Associations of America
99 Summer St., Suite 1700
Boston, MA 02110
Phone: 617-737-3200
Fax: 617-737-1144
Website: http://www.vnaa.org
E-mail: vnaa@vnaa.org

Chapter 53

Put It In Writing: Questions and Answers on Advance Directives

Many people today are worried about the medical care they would be given if they should become terminally ill and unable to communicate their wishes. They don't want to spend months or years dependent on life-support machines, and they don't want to cause unnecessary emotional or financial distress for their loved ones.

That's why a growing number of people are taking an active role in their care before they become seriously ill. They are stating their health care preferences in writing, while they are still healthy and able to make such decisions, through legal documents called advance directives.

Before deciding what choices about your care at the end of life are best, you should talk over the issues involved with your family and your physician. Find out about the laws and forms that apply in your state. Decide whether advance directives are right for you. This chapter will give you some basic facts about advance directives to get you started on this process.

What are advance directives?

Formal advance directives are documents written in advance of serious illness that state your choices for health care, or name someone to make those choices, if you become unable to make decisions.

Through advance directives, such as living wills and durable powers of attorney for health care, you can make legally valid decisions about your future medical treatment.

Why is there so much interest in advance directives now?

Questions about medical care at the end of life are of great concern today, partly because of the growing ability of medical technology to prolong life and partly because of highly publicized legal cases involving comatose patients whose families wanted to withdraw treatment. Many people want to avoid extending personal and family suffering by artificial prolongation of life if they are in a vegetative state or when there is no hope of recovery. The best way for you to retain control in such a situation is to record your preferences for medical care in advance, and share your decisions with your physician, loved ones, and clergyman.

What does the law say about this issue?

Laws differ somewhat from state to state, but in general a patient's expressed wishes will be honored. No law or court has invalidated the concept of advance directives, and an increasing number of statutes and court decisions support it. In 1990, the U.S. Supreme Court found in the case of Nancy Cruzan that the state of Missouri could require "clear and convincing" evidence of a patient's wishes in order to remove life supports. Formal advance directives can be critical to establishing such clear and convincing evidence of a patient's wishes. The Patient Self-Determination Act of 1990 requires hospitals to inform their patients about advance directives.

What is a living will?

A living will is a document in which you can stipulate the kind of life-prolonging medical care you want if you become terminally ill, permanently unconscious, or in a vegetative state and unable to make your own decisions. Many states have their own living-will forms, each with somewhat different requirements. It is also possible to complete and sign a standard form from a stationery store, draw up your own form, or simply write a statement of your preferences for treatment, as long as you follow the state's witnessing requirements.

A living will should be signed, dated, and witnessed by two people, preferably individuals who know you well but are not related to you and are not your potential heirs or your health care providers. A number of states require a notary, or permit a notary, in lieu of two witnesses. The living will should be discussed and shared with your physician, family, and clergy, and you should ask your physician to make it a part of your permanent medical record. Verify that the living will is indeed in your medical record, including your hospital chart. Although you do not need a lawyer to draw up a living will, you may wish to discuss it with a lawyer and leave a copy with the family lawyer.

What is a durable power of attorney for health care?

A durable power of attorney for health care is another kind of advance directive: a signed, dated, and witnessed document naming another person to make medical decisions for you if you are unable to make them for yourself at any time, not just at the end of life. You can include instructions about any treatment you want or wish to avoid, such as surgery or artificial nutrition and hydration. The majority of states have specific laws allowing a health care power of attorney, and provide suggested forms. You can draw up a durable power of attorney for health care with or without the advice of a lawyer; however most states do not allow the appointed agent to act as a witness.

Which is better—a living will or a durable power of attorney for health care?

Historically, living wills were developed first, and health care powers of attorney were designed later to be more flexible and apply to more situations. Today the distinction between the two types of documents is becoming blurred. It is possible to have both a living will and a durable power of attorney for health care. Some states combine them in a single document that both describes one's treatment preferences in a variety of situations and names a proxy.

How can I know in advance which procedures I would want or not want to prolong my life?

Although it isn't possible to specify every possible procedure under every possible circumstance, it is possible to decide what kind of treatment you would want in most situations. There are certain common conditions (terminal, irreversible brain damage, and dementing illnesses) and treatments commonly used in end-of-life situations (cardiopulmonary resuscitation [CPR], ventilators, artificial nutrition and hydration, dialysis, and antibiotics) that can be discussed in advance.

Preferences can be clarified by thinking about and discussing with your family, friends, and others your views about death, being totally dependent on the care of others, the role of family finances, the conditions that would make life intolerable to you, and how artificial life-support would affect the dying process. If you have questions about the kinds of procedures that are often used when illness is severe and recovery unlikely, ask your physician. It is never too early to start this decision-making process, and you should not postpone it until you face serious illness. Patients need to play an active role in determining their own health care decisions.

What is the legal status of advance directives?

All states legally recognize some form of advance medical directive. Even if a particular instruction in an advance directive might not be enforceable under some circumstances, it is better to express your wishes and intent in some kind of written document than not to express them at all.

What if I draw up a living will or health care power of attorney and then change my mind?

You may change or revoke these documents at any time. Any alterations and any written revocation should be signed and dated, and copies should be given to your family, physician, and other appropriate people. (For substantial changes, a new living will should be written and witnessed.) Even without an official written change, your orally expressed direction to your physician generally has priority over any statement made in a living will or power of attorney as long as you are able to decide for yourself and can communicate your wishes. If you wish to revoke an advance directive at any time, you should notify your primary physician, family, clergyman, and others who might need to know. If you consulted an attorney in drawing up your document, you should also notify him or her.

What if I fill out an advance directive in one state and am hospitalized in a different state?

The majority of states have reciprocity provisions. Even in those states that do not explicitly address the issue, there is a common law and constitutional right to accept or refuse treatment that may be broader than the rights identified under the state law. Because an advance directive is an expression of your intent regarding your medical care, it will influence that care no matter where you are hospitalized. However, if you spend a great deal of time in more than one state you might wish to consider executing an advance directive in those states.

If a comatose or mentally incompetent patient doesn't have a living will or durable power of attorney, who decides whether to withdraw treatment?

If there is no advance directive by the patient, the decision is left to the patient's family, physician, and hospital, and ultimately a judge. Usually the family, physician, and hospital can reach an agreement without resorting to the courts, often with the help of a hospital ethics committee. However, many times the individual who has the authority to make the decision is not the person the patient would have chosen. There also may be more restrictions on a surrogate than an appointed agent.

What will the hospital do to help if I or my family member should be in this situation?

Many hospitals have ethics committees or ethics consultation services, one of whose functions is to help in decision making about the end of life. Physicians, nurses, social workers, lawyers, clergy, patient representatives, and sometimes professional bioethicists discuss issues, advise on hospital policy, and review cases if there is a conflict or lack of clarity. Although they will often counsel a patient's family and make a recommendation, the final decision is still up to the patient, the family, and the physician.

Glossary

advance directive: A document in which a person either states choices for medical treatment or designates who should make treatment choices if the person should lose decision-making capacity. The term can also include oral statements by the patient.

artificial nutrition and hydration: A method of delivering a chemically-balanced mix of nutrients and fluids when a patient is unable to eat or drink. The patient may be fed through a tube inserted directly into the stomach, a tube put through the nose and throat into the stomach, or an intravenous tube.

cardiopulmonary resuscitation (CPR): A medical procedure, often involving external chest compression, administration of drugs, and electric shock, used to restore the heartbeat at the time of a cardiac arrest.

decision-making capacity: The ability to make choices that reflect an understanding and appreciation of the nature and consequences of one's actions.

declaration: One type of advance directive, commonly referred to as a living will.

do not resuscitate (DNR): A medical order to refrain from cardiopulmonary resuscitation if a patient's heart stops beating.

durable power of attorney for health care (DPOA): An advance directive in which an individual names someone else (the agent or proxy) to make health care decisions in the event the individual becomes unable to make them. The DPOA can also include instructions about specific possible choices to be made.

hospice: A program that provides care for the terminally ill in the form of pain relief, counseling, and custodial care, either at home or in a facility.

legal guardian: A person charged (usually by court appointment) with the power and duty of taking care of and managing the property and rights of another person who is considered incapable of administering his or her own affairs.

life-sustaining treatment: A medical intervention administered to a patient that prolongs life and delays death.

palliative care: Medical interventions intended to alleviate suffering, discomfort, and dysfunction but not to cure (such as pain medication or treatment of an annoying infection).

persistent vegetative state: As defined by the American Academy of Neurology, "a form of eyes-open permanent unconsciousness in which the patient has periods of wakefulness and physiologic sleep and wake cycles but at no time is aware of himself or his environment."

proxy: A person appointed to make decisions for someone else, as in a durable power of attorney for health care (also called a surrogate or agent).

terminal condition: In most states, a status that is incurable or irreversible and in which death will occur within a short time. There is no precise, universally accepted definition of' "a short time," but in general it is considered to be less than one year.

ventilator: A machine that moves air into the lungs for a patient who is unable to breathe naturally.

For More Information

Information is available from the following organizations and your state or local Office on Aging, your local bar association, and many local civic and service organizations.

American Hospital Association
One N. Franklin
Chicago, IL 60606-3421
Phone: 312-422-3000
Website: http://www.putitinwriting.org

AARP (formerly the American Association of Retired Persons)
601 E Street N.W.
Washington, DC 20049
Toll-Free: 888-687-2277
Website: http://www.aarp.org/families/end_life

National Hospice and Palliative Care Organization
1700 Diagonal Road, Suite 625
Alexandria, VA 22314
Toll-Free: 800-658-8898
Phone: 703-837-1500
Fax: 703-837-1233
Website: http://www.nhpco.org
E-mail: info@nhpco.org

Through their website, the National Hospice and Palliative Care Organization (NHPCO) offers free, state specific advance directives and advice for communicating wishes to family and close friends. The site is focused around learning, implementing, voicing, and engaging in the care you receive at the end-of-life.

Part Six

Additional Help and Information

Chapter 54

Glossary of Terms Related to MS

antibodies: Proteins made by the immune system that bind to structures (antigens) they recognize as foreign to the body.

antigen: A structure foreign to the body, such as a virus. The body usually responds to antigens by producing antibodies.

ataxia: A condition in which the muscles fail to function in a coordinated manner.

autoimmune disease: A disease in which the body's defense system malfunctions and attacks a part of the body itself rather than foreign matter.

axon: The long, thin extension of a nerve cell that conducts impulses away from the cell body.[1]

blood-brain barrier: A membrane that controls the passage of substances from the blood into the central nervous system.

Definitions in this chapter are excerpted from "Multiple Sclerosis: Hope Through Research," National Institute of Neurological Disorders and Stroke (NINDS), NIH Publication No. 96–75, updated April 16, 2007. Additional terms marked [1] are reprinted from "Spinal Cord Injury: Hope Through Research," National Institute of Neurological Disorders and Stroke (NINDS), NIH Publication No. 03–160, updated May 21, 2007, and other terms marked [2] are reprinted from "Medicare Coverage of Durable Medical Equipment," Centers for Medicare and Medicaid Services (CMS), Publication No. CMS–11045, February 2004.

cerebrospinal fluid: The colorless liquid, consisting partially of substances filtered from blood and partially by secretions released by brain cells, that circulates around and through the cavities of the brain and spinal cord. Physicians use a variety of tests—electrophoresis, isoelectric focusing, capillary isotachophoresis, and radioimmunoassay—to study cerebrospinal fluid for abnormalities often associated with multiple sclerosis (MS).

Certificate of Medical Necessity: A form required by Medicare that allows you to use certain durable medical equipment prescribed by your doctor or one of the doctor's office staff. [2]

cervical: The part of the spine in the neck region. [1]

coccygeal: The part of the spine at the bottom of the spinal column, above the buttocks. [1]

cytokines: Powerful chemical substances secreted by T cells. Cytokines are an important factor in the production of inflammation and show promise as treatments for MS.

deductible: The amount you must pay for health care before Medicare begins to pay, either each benefit period for Part A, or each year for Part B. These amounts can change every year. [2]

demyelination: Damage caused to myelin by recurrent attacks of inflammation. Demyelination ultimately results in nervous system scars, called plaques, which interrupt communications between the nerves and the rest of the body.

dendrite: A short arm-like protuberance from a neuron. Dendrite is from the Greek for "branched like a tree." [1]

disc: Shortened terminology for an intervertebral disc, a disc-shaped piece of specialized tissue that separates the bones of the spinal column. [1]

durable medical equipment: Medical equipment that is ordered by a doctor (or, if Medicare allows, a nurse practitioner, physician assistant, or clinical nurse specialist) for use in the home. A hospital or nursing home that mostly provides skilled care can't qualify as a home in this situation. These items must be reusable, such as walkers, wheelchairs, or hospital beds. [2]

experimental allergic encephalomyelitis (EAE): A chronic brain and spinal cord disease similar to MS which is induced by injecting myelin basic protein into laboratory animals.

fatigue: Tiredness that may accompany activity or may persist even without exertion.

functional electrical stimulation (FES): The therapeutic use of low-level electrical current to stimulate muscle movement and restore useful movements such as standing or stepping; also called functional neuromuscular stimulation. [1]

gadolinium: A chemical compound given during magnetic resonance imaging (MRI) scans that helps distinguish new lesions from old.

glia: Supportive cells in the brain and spinal cord. Glial cells are the most abundant cell types in the central nervous system. There are three types: astrocytes, oligodendrocytes, and microglia. [1]

glutamate: An excitatory neurotransmitter. [1]

human leukocyte antigens (HLA): Antigens, tolerated by the body, that correspond to genes that govern immune responses. Also known as major histocompatibility complex.

immunoglobulin G (IgG): An antibody-containing substance produced by human plasma cells in diseased central nervous system plaques. Levels of IgG are increased in the cerebrospinal fluid of most MS patients.

immunosuppression: Suppression of immune system functions. Many medications under investigation for the treatment of MS are immunosuppressants.

interferons: Cytokines belonging to a family of antiviral proteins that occur naturally in the body. Gamma interferon is produced by immune system cells, enhances T-cell recognition of antigens, and causes worsening of MS symptoms. Alpha and beta interferon probably exert a suppressive effect on the immune system and may be beneficial in the treatment of MS.

lesion: An abnormal change in the structure of an organ due to disease or injury.

lumbar: The part of the spine in the middle back, below the thoracic vertebrae and above the sacral vertebrae. [1]

macrophage: A type of white blood cell that engulfs foreign material. Macrophages are key players in the immune response to foreign invaders such as infectious microorganisms. Macrophages also release substances that stimulate other cells of the immune system. [1]

magnetic resonance imaging (MRI): A non-invasive scanning technique that enables investigators to see and track MS lesions as they evolve.

medically necessary: Services or supplies that:

- are proper and needed for the diagnosis or treatment of your medical condition;
- are provided for the diagnosis, direct care, and treatment of your medical condition;
- meet the standards of good medical practice in the local area; and
- are not mainly for the convenience of you or your doctor. [2]

methylprednisolone: A steroid drug used to improve recovery from spinal cord injury. [1]

microglia: Glial cells that function as part of the immune system in the brain and spinal cord.

myelin: A fatty covering insulating nerve cell fibers in the brain and spinal cord, myelin facilitates the smooth, high-speed transmission of electrochemical messages between these components of the central nervous system and the rest of the body. In MS, myelin is damaged through a process known as demyelination, which results in distorted or blocked signals.

myelin basic protein (MBP): A major component of myelin. When myelin breakdown occurs (as in MS), MBP can often be found in abnormally high levels in the patient's cerebrospinal fluid. When injected into laboratory animals, MBP induces experimental allergic encephalomyelitis, a chronic brain and spinal cord disease similar to MS.

neurogenic pain: Generalized pain that results from nervous system malfunction. [1]

neuromodulation: A series of techniques employing electrical stimulation or the administration of medication by means of devices implanted in the body. These techniques allow the treatment of a range of disorders including certain forms of pain, spasticity, tremor, and urinary problems. [1]

neuron: Also known as a nerve cell; the structural and functional unit of the nervous system. A neuron consists of a cell body and its processes: an axon and one or more dendrites. [1]

neurostimulation: The act of stimulating neurons with electrical impulses delivered via electrodes attached to the brain. [1]

neurotransmitter: A chemical released from neurons that transmits an impulse to another neuron, muscle, organ, or other tissue. [1]

oligodendrocytes: Cells that make and maintain myelin.

optic neuritis: An inflammatory disorder of the optic nerve that usually occurs in only one eye and causes visual loss and sometimes blindness. It is generally temporary.

paralysis: The inability to control movement of a part of the body. [1]

paresthesias: Abnormal sensations such as numbness, prickling, or "pins and needles."

patient lifts: Equipment to move a patient from a bed or wheelchair using your strength or a motor. [2]

plaques: Patchy areas of inflammation and demyelination typical of MS, plaques disrupt or block nerve signals that would normally pass through the regions affected by the plaques.

pressure sore (also known as a pressure ulcer or bed sore): A reddened area or open sore caused by unrelieved pressure on the skin over bony areas such as the hipbone or tailbone. [1]

receptor: A protein on a cell's surface that allows the cell to identify antigens.

regeneration: Repair, regrowth, or restoration of tissues; opposite of degeneration. [1]

retrobulbar neuritis: An inflammatory disorder of the optic nerve that is usually temporary. It causes rapid loss of vision and may cause pain upon moving the eye.

rhizotomy: An operation to disconnect specific nerve roots in order to stop severe spasticity. [1]

sacral: Refers to the part of the spine in the hip area. [1]

Schwann cell: The cell of the peripheral nervous system that forms the myelin sheath. [1]

spasticity: Involuntary muscle contractions leading to spasms and stiffness or rigidity. In MS, this condition primarily affects the lower limbs.

stem cell: Special cells that have the ability to grow into any one of the body's more than 200 cell types. Unlike mature cells, which are permanently committed to their fate, stem cells can both renew themselves and create cells of other tissues. [1]

synapse: A specialized junction between two nerve cells. At the synapse, a neuron releases neurotransmitters that diffuse across the gap and activate receptors situated on the target cell. [1]

T cells: Immune system cells that develop in the thymus gland. Findings suggest that T cells are implicated in myelin destruction.

thoracic: The part of the spine at the upper-back to mid-back level. [1]

transverse myelitis: An acute spinal cord disorder causing sudden low back pain and muscle weakness and abnormal sensory sensations in the lower extremities. Transverse myelitis often remits spontaneously; however, severe or long-lasting cases may lead to permanent disability.

vertebrae: The 33 hollow bones that make up the spine. [1]

white matter: Nerve fibers that are the site of MS lesions and underlie the gray matter of the brain and spinal cord.

Chapter 55

Organizations with Additional Information about MS

Government Organizations That Provide Additional Information about Multiple Sclerosis

Administration on Aging
Washington, DC 20201
Phone: 202-619-0724
Fax: 202-357-3556
Website: http://www.aoa.gov
E-mail: aoainfo@aoa.gov

Brain Resources and Information Network (BRAIN)
P.O. Box 5801
Bethesda, MD 20824
Toll-Free: 800-352-9424
Website: http://www.ninds.nih.gov
E-mail: braininfo@ninds.nih.gov

Centers for Medicare and Medicaid Services (CMS)
7500 Security Blvd.
Baltimore, MD 21244-1850
Toll-Free: 877-267-2323
Toll-Free TTY: 866-226-1819
Phone: 410-786-3000
TTY: 410-786-0727
Website: http://cms.hhs.gov

ClinicalTrials.gov
Toll-Free: 800-411-1222
Toll-Free TTY: 866-411-1010
Website: http://clinicaltrials.gov
E-mail: prpl@mail.cc.nih.gov

Resources in this chapter were compiled from several sources deemed reliable; all contact information was verified and updated in July 2007.

Department of Veterans Affairs

Toll-Free Health Care Benefits:
877-222-8387
Toll-Free TTY: 800-829-4833
Website: http://www.va.gov

National Institute of Arthritis and Musculoskeletal and Skin Diseases (NIAMS)

1 AMS Circle
Bethesda, MD 20892-3675
Toll-Free: 877-22-NIAMS (64267)
Phone: 301-495-4484
TTY: 301-565-2966
Fax: 301-718-6366
Website: http://www.niams.nih.gov
E-mail: niamsinfo@mail.nih.gov

National Institute of Neurological Disorders and Stroke (NINDS)

P.O. Box 5801
Bethesda, MD 20824
Toll-Free: 800-352-9424
Phone: 301-496-5751
Fax: 301-402-2186
Website: http://www.ninds.nih.gov
E-mail: braininfo@ninds.nih.gov

National Kidney and Urologic Diseases Information Clearinghouse

3 Information Way
Bethesda, MD 20892-3580
Toll-Free: 800-891-5390
Fax: 703-738-4929
Website: http://kidney.niddk.nih.gov
E-mail: nkudic@info.niddk.nih.gov

National Women's Health Information Center

200 Independence Ave., S.W., Rm. 712 E
Washington, DC 20201
Toll-Free: 800-994-9662
Phone: 703-289-7923
Fax: 703-663-6942
Website: http://www.womenshealth.gov

Social Security Administration (SSA)

Office of Public Inquiries
Windsor Park Building
6401 Security Blvd.
Baltimore, MD 21235
Toll-Free: 800-772-1213
Toll-Free TTY: 800-325-0778
Website: http://www.socialsecurity.gov

U.S. Dept. of Housing and Urban Development (HUD)

451 7th Street S.W.
Washington, DC 20410
Phone: 202-708-1112
TTY: 202-708-1455
Website: http://www.hud.gov

U.S. Department of Justice

950 Pennsylvania Ave., N.W.
Civil Rights Division
Disability Rights Section–NYA
Washington, DC 20530
Toll-Free: 800-514-0301
Toll-Free TTY: 800-514-0383
Fax: 202-307-1198
Website: http://www.usdoj.gov/crt/ada/adahom1.htm

Private Organizations That Provide Information about Multiple Sclerosis and Related Issues

AARP (formerly the American Association of Retired Persons)
601 E Street N.W.
Washington, DC 20049
Toll-Free: 888-687-2277
Website: http://www.aarp.org

Accelerated Cure Project, Inc.
300 Fifth Ave.
Waltham, MA 02451
Phone: 781-487-0008
Fax: 781-487-0009
Website: http://
www.acceleratedcure.org
E-mail: info-web0107
@acceleratedcure.org

Accessible Space, Inc. (ASI)
2550 University Ave., Suite 330N
St. Paul, MN 55114
Toll-Free: 800-466-7722
Phone: 651-645-7271
Website: http://
www.accessiblespace.org
E-mail: info@accessiblespace.org

American Autoimmune Related Diseases Association
22100 Gratiot Ave., Eastpointe
East Detroit, MI 48021-2227
Toll-Free: 800-598-4668
Phone: 586-776-3900
Fax: 586-776-3903
Website: http://www.aarda.org
E-mail: aarda@aarda.org

American Hospital Association
One N. Franklin
Chicago, IL 60606-3421
Phone: 312-422-3000
Website: http://www.aha.org

American Institute of Stress
124 Park Ave.
Yonkers, NY 10703
Phone: 914-963-1200
Fax: 914-965-6267
Website: http://www.stress.org
E-mail: stress125@optonline.net

American Urological Association Foundation
1000 Corporate Blvd.
Linthicum, MD 21090
Toll-Free: 866-RING-AUA
(746-4282)
Phone: 410-689-3990
Fax: 410-689-3800
Website: http://
www.urologyhealth.org

Anxiety Disorders Association of America
8730 Georgia Ave., Suite 600
Silver Spring, MD 20910
Phone: 240-485-1001
Fax: 240-485-1035
Website: http://www.adaa.org

Assisted Living Federation of America

1650 King St., Suite 602
Alexandria, VA 22314-2747
Phone: 703-894-1805
Fax: 703-894-1831
Website: http://www.alfa.org
E-mail: info@alfa.org

Center for Universal Design

College of Design
North Carolina State University
Campus Box 8613
Raleigh, NC 27695-8613
Toll-Free: 800-647-6777
Phone: 919-515-3082
Fax: 919-515-8951
Website: http://
www.centerforuniversaldesign.org

Consortium of MS Centers

c/o Gimbel MS Center
718 Teaneck Road
Teaneck, NJ 07666
Phone: 201-837-0727
Fax: 201-837-9414
E-mail: info@mscare.org
Website: http://www.mscare.org

Family Caregiver Alliance

180 Montgomery St., Suite 1100
San Francisco, CA 94104
Toll-Free: 800-445-8106
Phone: 415-434-3388
Fax: 415-434-3508
Website: http://
www.caregiver.org
E-mail: info@caregiver.org

Human Brain and Spinal Fluid Resource Center

W. LA Healthcare Center
Bldg. 212, Rm. 16
11301 Wilshire Blvd. (127A)
Los Angeles, CA 90073
Phone: 310-268-3536
Fax: 310-268-4768
24-hour pager: 310-636-5199
Website: http://
www.loni.ucla.edu/
uclabrainbank
E-mail: RMNbbank@ucla.edu

International Essential Tremor Foundation

P.O. Box 14005
Lenexa, KS 66285-4005
Toll-Free: 888-387-3667
Phone: 913-341-3880
Fax: 913-341-1296
http://www.essentialtremor.org
E-mail:
staff@essentialtremor.org

Mental Health America (formerly known as National Mental Health Association)

2000 N. Beauregard St., 6th Floor
Alexandria, VA 22311
Toll-Free: 800-969-6642
Toll-Free TTY: 800-433-5959
Phone: 703-684-7722
Fax: 703-684-5968
Website: http://
www.mentalhealthamerica.net

Multiple Sclerosis Association of America
706 Haddonfield Road
Cherry Hill, NJ 08002
Toll-Free: 800-532-7667
Phone: 856-488-4500
Fax: 856-661-9797
Website: http://
www.msassociation.org
E-mail: msaa@msaa.com

Multiple Sclerosis Foundation
6350 N. Andrews Ave.
Ft. Lauderdale, FL 33309-2130
Toll-Free: 888-MSFOCUS
(673-6287)
Phone: 954-776-6805
Fax: 954-351-0630
Website: http://www.msfocus.org
E-mail: support@msfocus.org

National Association for Continence
P.O. Box 1019
Charleston, SC 29402-1019
Toll-Free: 800-BLADDER
(252-3337)
Phone: 843-377-0900
Fax: 843-377-0905
Website: http://www.nafc.org
E-mail:
memberservices@nafc.org

National Association for Home Care
228 7th St., S.E.
Washington, DC 20003
Phone: 202-547-7424
Fax: 202-547-3540
Website: http://www.nahc.org

National Ataxia Foundation (NAF)
2600 Fernbrook Lane N
Suite 119
Minneapolis, MN 55447-4752
Phone: 763-553-0020
Fax: 763-553-0167
Website: http://www.ataxia.org
E-mail: naf@ataxia.org

National Center for Assisted Living
1201 L St., N.W.
Washington, DC 20005
Phone: 202-842-4444
Website: http://www.ncal.org
E-mail: webmaster@ahca.org

National Center on Physical Activity and Disability
1640 W. Roosevelt Rd.
Suite 711
Chicago, IL 60608-6904
Toll-Free Voice/TTY: 800-900-8086
Fax: 312-355-4058
Website: http://www.ncpad.org
E-mail: ncpad@uic.edu

National Hospice and Palliative Care Organization
1700 Diagonal Road
Suite 625
Alexandria, VA 22314
Toll-Free: 800-658-8898
Phone: 703-837-1500
Fax: 703-837-1233
Website: http://www.nhpco.org
E-mail: info@nhpco.org

National Mental Health Consumers' Self-Help Clearinghouse
1211 Chestnut St., Suite 1207
Philadelphia, PA 19107
Toll-Free: 800-553-4539
Phone: 215-751-1810
Fax: 215-636-6312
Website: http://
www.mhselfhelp.org
E-mail: info@mhselfhelp.org

National Mental Health Information Center
P.O. Box 42557
Washington, DC 20015
Toll-Free: 800-789-2647
Toll-Free TDD: 866-889-2647
International Calls: 240-221-4021
Fax: 240-747-5470
Website: http://
www.mentalhealth.org
E-mail: info@mentalhealth.org

National Multiple Sclerosis Society
733 Third Ave., 6th Fl.
New York, NY 10017-3288
Toll-Free: 800-344-4867
(FIGHTMS)
Phone: 212-986-3240
Fax: 212-986-7981
Website: http://
www.nationalmssociety.org
E-mail: nat@nmss.org

National Organization for Rare Disorders (NORD)
P.O. Box 1968
Danbury, CT 06813-1968
Toll-Free: 800-999-NORD (6673)
Phone: 203-744-0100
Fax: 203-798-2291
Website: http://
www.rarediseases.org
E-mail:
orphan@rarediseases.org

National Tay-Sachs and Allied Diseases Association
2001 Beacon Street, Suite 204
Brighton, MA 02135
Toll-Free: 800-90-NTSAD
(906-8723)
Phone: 617-277-4463
Fax: 617-277-0134
Website: http://www.ntsad.org
E-mail: info@ntsad.org

Neuropathy Association
60 East 42nd Street, Suite 942
New York, NY 10165-0999
Phone: 212-692-0662
Fax: 212-692-0668
Website: http://
www.neuropathy.org
E-mail: info@neuropathy.org

Tremor Action Network
P.O. Box 5013
Pleasanton, CA 94566-5013
Phone: 925-462-0111
Fax: 925-369-0485
Website: http://
www.tremoraction.org
E-mail:
tremor@tremoraction.org

United Leukodystrophy Foundation
2304 Highland Drive
Sycamore, IL 60178
Toll-Free: 800-728-5483
Phone: 815-895-3211
Fax: 815-895-2432
Website: http://www.ulf.org
E-mail: office@ulf.org

Visiting Nurse Associations of America
99 Summer St., Suite 1700
Boston, MA 02110
Phone: 617-737-3200
Fax: 617-737-1144
Website: http://www.vnaa.org
E-mail: vnaa@vnaa.org

WE MOVE (Worldwide Education and Awareness for Movement Disorders)
204 West 84th Street
New York, NY 10024
Phone: 212-875-8312
Fax: 212-875-8389
Website: http://www.wemove.org
E-mail: wemove@wemove.org

Well Spouse Association
63 W. Main St., Suite H
Freehold, NJ 07728
Toll-Free: 800-838-0879
Phone: 732-577-8899
Website: http://www.wellspouse.org
E-mail: info@wellspouse.org

Index

Index

Page numbers followed by 'n' indicate a footnote. Page numbers in *italics* indicate a table or illustration.

529

D

Dantrium (dantrolene) 168, *170*, 198, 317
dantrolene 168, *170*, 198, 317
darifenacin 237
DBS *see* deep brain stimulation
decision-making capacity, defined 508
declaration, defined 508
deductible, defined 514
deep brain stimulation (DBS)
    overview 319–23
    tremor 189
"Deep Brain Stimulation for Multiple Sclerosis" (Cleveland Clinic) 319n
DeLange, Lindsey 243n
demyelination
    children 74
    defined 514
    described 46, 50
    exacerbations 137
    potassium 15
    vitamin B12 deficiency 100
dendrites
    defined 514
    described 42
    spinal cord 40
dental amalgams
    immune system 93
    multiple sclerosis 88, 91
dental filling removal 18
Department of Health and Human Services (DHHS; HHS) *see* US Department of Health and Human Services
Department of Housing and Urban Development (HUD) *see* US Department of Housing and Urban Development
Department of Justice (DOJ) *see* US Department of Justice
Department of Labor (DOL) *see* US Department of Labor
Department of Veterans Affairs (VA), contact information 500, 520
depression
    cognitive impairments 245–46
    described 166
    overview 251–54

desipramine 306
Detrol (tolterodine) 236–37
Devic disease 148–49
dexamethasone 13, 286
DHHS *see* US Department of Health and Human Services
diazepam 10, 168, *170*, 198, 238, 317
Dieruf, Kathy 178
diet and nutrition
    autoimmune diseases 27
    caregivers 416–17
    multiple sclerosis 97
    multiple sclerosis treatment 17–18
    multiple sclerosis triggers 84
    overview 98–122, 369–73
    swallowing disorders 218–19
dietary fats, described 338
dietitians, described 275
diffusion tensor magnetic resonance imaging (DT-MRI) 11
digestion, described 114
Dilaudid (hydromorphone) 308
disability
    chronic conditions 363–68
    employment support 460–67
disc, defined 514
"Diseases that Mimic MS" (Ratliff) 147n
Ditropan (oxybutynin chloride) 236–37
DNA (deoxyribonucleic acid)
    heredity 59
    radiation damage 81
DNR *see* do not resuscitate
DOJ *see* US Department of Justice
DOL *see* US Department of Labor
Dolophine HCl (methadone) 308
do not resuscitate (DNR), defined 508
dopamine, Parkinson disease 45
Doskoch, Peter 335n
double-blind studies, described 353
doxazosin 238
DPOA *see* durable power of attorney for health care
dressing assistance 434–36
"Dressing with Ease, Style, and Comfort" (Cazzolli) 434n
DT-MRI *see* diffusion tensor magnetic resonance imaging

immune system, continued
 myelin 46
 pregnancy 9–10
 toxic agents 92–93
immunoglobulin G (IgG)
 cerebrospinal fluid 11
 defined 515
immunoglobulin therapy,
 Guillain-Barré syndrome 159
immunosuppression
 defined 515
 infections 16
immunotherapy, research 13–15
"Improved Employment
 Opportunities for People with
 Disabilities" (Kaye) 460n
Imuran (azathioprine) 14
incontinence, exercise 376
Indocin (indomethacin) 288
indomethacin 288
infant formula, research 111
infants, leukodystrophy 160
infections
 Guillain-Barré syndrome 157
 multiple sclerosis 7, 12, 82, 96
infectious diseases, overview 123–35
inheritance *see* heredity
inhibitory neurotransmitter,
 described 45
inner brain
 depicted *37*
 described 37–38
interaction, toxic agents 90–91
interferon gamma, exacerbations 53
interferons
 African Americans 70
 defined 515
 described 53, 292–93
 research 13
interleukin 4 (IL-4)
 demyelination 17
 lesions 53
interleukin 12 (IL-12)
 autoimmune diseases 29–30
 exacerbations 53
interleukins, described 53
International Essential Tremor
 Foundation, contact information
 190, 522

"Intimacy and Sexuality with
 Multiple Sclerosis" (Foley) 395n
intrathecal contrast enhanced CT
 scan 266–67
intravenous immunoglobulin (IVIG)
 17, 156
investment planning, described
 484–85
iodine 101
iron 101, 102, 115, 116
IVIG *see* intravenous
 immunoglobulin

J

Jacobs, Cindy 382n
JC virus, described 129
jejunum, described 114
Joffe, Rosalind 446n, 452n, 458n
Jones-London, Michelle D. 23n

K

Kadian (morphine) 308
Kailes, June Isaacson 368
Kalb, Rosalind 256, 258
Kaye, H. Stephen 460n
Kegel exercises, bladder
 disorders 237–38
Keppra (levetiracetam) 306
ketoprofen 288
killer T cells
 described 52–53
 immune system 6
 plaques 56
Klonopin (clonazepam) 168, *170*
Kos, Daphne 329n
Krabbe disease 160
Kushner, Sue 175–76, 180

L

Lamictal (lamotrigine) 306
lamotrigine 306
LaRocca, Nicholas 252
LD *see* Lyme disease

540

OxyContin (oxycodone) 308
oxytocin 390
Oxytrol (oxybutynin) 237

P

"Pain in Multiple Sclerosis"
(Maloni) 193n, 303n
pain management
autoimmune diseases 28
medications 169
overview 193–98, 303–8
physical therapy 328
palliative care, defined 508
Pamelor (nortriptyline) 306
papaverine *170*, 398
parainfluenza, described 130–31
paralysis, defined 517
paramyxoviruses, described 130–31
paresthesias
defined 517
described 166
parietal lobes, described 36
Parkinsonian tremor, described 185
paroxysmal attacks, relapses 142–43
paroxysmal pain syndromes,
described 195–96
"Part I: General Information,
Disability Evaluation under
Social Security" (SSA) 469n
"Patient Information Sheet for
Natalizumab" (FDA) 299n
patient lifts, defined 517
pediatric multiple sclerosis,
overview 73–77
PEG *see* percutaneous
endoscopic gastrostomy
Pelizaeus-Merzbacher disease 160
pemoline 169
peptide therapy, described 15–16
percutaneous endoscopic
gastrostomy (PEG),
described 220
pergolide mesylate 188
peripheral nervous system (PNS)
described 41–42
Guillain-Barré syndrome 156
myelin 45–46, 54

persistent vegetative state,
defined 508
PET scan *see* positron emission
tomography
Petter, R. 332n
pharmacodynamics, research 116–18
pharmacogenetics, multiple sclerosis
57
pharmacokinetics
multiple sclerosis 89–92
nutrients 114–16
phenol 168, 318
phenylbutazone 288
phenytoin, pregnancy 10
phospholipids, research 105
phosphorus 101
physical therapists
caregivers 411
described 29, 274
dressing assistance 435
physical therapy
overview 326–29
spasticity 314
tremor 188
physiologic tremor, described 186
"Physiotherapy: Its Role in
Rehabilitation" (Prasad) 326n
phytochemicals, research 106
phytoestrogens, research 106
Pittock, Sean J. 277–80
placebo, described 352
placebo effect, described 352
plant toxins, multiple sclerosis 82
plaques
defined 517
demyelination 50
described 3, 55–56
magnetic resonance imaging 10
plasma cells, described 53
plasmapheresis
chronic inflammatory demyelinating
polyneuropathy 156
described 14
exacerbations 288
Guillain-Barré syndrome 158
overview 343–45
"Plasmapheresis (Plasma Exchange)"
(National Multiple Sclerosis
Society) 343n

receptors, defined 517
Refsum disease 160
regeneration, defined 517
relapse rate
  copolymer I 15
  prognosis *144*
relapses
  described 142–45
  treatment 282–89
  see also exacerbations
relapsing remitting multiple
  sclerosis (RRMS)
  children 73
  described 8–9, 140, 143
  myelin 51
  treatment 282
  women 61
remission, described 138
remyelination
  animal studies 17
  described 54
research
  bladder disorders 240
  brain 34
  gait problems 181
  multiple sclerosis 18–19
  myelin 51
  neural injury 46–47
  tremor 189–90
respiratory conditions, multiple
  sclerosis 229–31
rest, autoimmune diseases 28
resting tremor, described 184
retrobulbar neuritis, defined 517
rheumatologists, described 28
rhizotomy, defined 517
risk factors, autoimmune
  diseases 23–24
Rogers, Judith 258
"The Role of Counseling in
  Rehabilitation" (Tromp; Petter)
  332n
rolipram 17
ropinirole 188
RRMS *see* relapsing remitting
  multiple sclerosis
rubella (German measles),
  described 131
rural areas, multiple sclerosis 86

S

sacral, defined 517
sacral spinal nerves, described 39
sacral vertebrae, described 39
safety considerations
  caregivers 415–16
  clinical studies 353–54
  complementary and alternative
    medicine 336–37, 339–41
  plasmapheresis 343–45
St. John's wort 338
Sanctura (trospium chloride) 237
Sandimmune (cyclosporine) 14
sarcoidosis, described 150
saturated fats
  blood-brain barrier 118
  limitations 370
  research 104, 109
saw palmetto 341
scavenger cells
  see macrophages
Schapiro, Randall 176
Schilder disease, described 161
"Schilder's Disease Information
  Page" (NINDS) 155n
Schwann cells
  defined 517
  myelin 46
  remyelination 54
Schwid, S. 347n
sclerosis, described 4
secondary progressive
  multiple sclerosis (SPMS)
  described 8–9, 141
  plaques 56
Segal, Benjamin 30
selenium 101, 102
self cells, described 6
Sendai virus 130–31
serotonins, described 45
"7 Habits for Regaining Power
  in the Workplace with Chronic
  Illness" (Joffe) 458n
sexual dysfunction
  multiple sclerosis 166
  overview 395–401
  treatment 64, 169–70
Shevach, Ethan 30

Health Reference Series
COMPLETE CATALOG
List price $87 per volume. **School and library price $78 per volume.**

Adolescent Health Sourcebook, 2nd Edition

Basic Consumer Health Information about the Physical, Mental, and Emotional Growth and Development of Adolescents, Including Medical Care, Nutritional and Physical Activity Requirements, Puberty, Sexual Activity, Acne, Tanning, Body Piercing, Common Physical Illnesses and Disorders, Eating Disorders, Attention Deficit Hyperactivity Disorder, Depression, Bullying, Hazing, and Adolescent Injuries Related to Sports, Driving, and Work

Along with Substance Abuse Information about Nicotine, Alcohol, and Drug Use, a Glossary, and Directory of Additional Resources

Edited by Joyce Brennfleck Shannon. 683 pages. 2006. 978-0-7808-0943-7.

"It is written in clear, nontechnical language aimed at general readers. . . . Recommended for public libraries, community colleges, and other agencies serving health care consumers."
—*American Reference Books Annual, 2003*

"Recommended for school and public libraries. Parents and professionals dealing with teens will appreciate the easy-to-follow format and the clearly written text. This could become a 'must have' for every high school teacher." —*E-Streams, Jan '03*

"A good starting point for information related to common medical, mental, and emotional concerns of adolescents." —*School Library Journal, Nov '02*

"This book provides accurate information in an easy to access format. It addresses topics that parents and caregivers might not be aware of and provides practical, useable information."
—*Doody's Health Sciences Book Review Journal, Sep-Oct '02*

"Recommended reference source."
—*Booklist, American Library Association, Sep '02*

AIDS Sourcebook, 3rd Edition

Basic Consumer Health Information about Acquired Immune Deficiency Syndrome (AIDS) and Human Immunodeficiency Virus (HIV) Infection, Including Facts about Transmission, Prevention, Diagnosis, Treatment, Opportunistic Infections, and Other Complications, with a Section for Women and Children, Including Details about Associated Gynecological Concerns, Pregnancy, and Pediatric Care

Along with Updated Statistical Information, Reports on Current Research Initiatives, a Glossary, and Directories of Internet, Hotline, and Other Resources

Edited by Dawn D. Matthews. 664 pages. 2003. 978-0-7808-0631-3.

"The 3rd edition of the *AIDS Sourcebook*, part of Omnigraphics' *Health Reference Series*, is a welcome update. . . . This resource is highly recommended for academic and public libraries."
—*American Reference Books Annual, 2004*

"Excellent sourcebook. This continues to be a highly recommended book. There is no other book that provides as much information as this book provides."
—*AIDS Book Review Journal, Dec-Jan '00*

"Recommended reference source."
—*Booklist, American Library Association, Dec '99*

Alcoholism Sourcebook, 2nd Edition

Basic Consumer Health Information about Alcohol Use, Abuse, and Dependence, Featuring Facts about the Physical, Mental, and Social Health Effects of Alcohol Addiction, Including Alcoholic Liver Disease, Pancreatic Disease, Cardiovascular Disease, Neurological Disorders, and the Effects of Drinking during Pregnancy

Along with Information about Alcohol Treatment, Medications, and Recovery Programs, in Addition to Tips for Reducing the Prevalence of Underage Drinking, Statistics about Alcohol Use, a Glossary of Related Terms, and Directories of Resources for More Help and Information

Edited by Amy L. Sutton. 653 pages. 2006. 978-0-7808-0942-0.

"This title is one of the few reference works on alcoholism for general readers. For some readers this will be a welcome complement to the many self-help books on the market. Recommended for collections serving general readers and consumer health collections."
—*E-Streams, Mar '01*

"This book is an excellent choice for public and academic libraries."
—*American Reference Books Annual, 2001*

"Recommended reference source."
—*Booklist, American Library Association, Dec '00*

"Presents a wealth of information on alcohol use and abuse and its effects on the body and mind, treatment, and prevention." —*SciTech Book News, Dec '00*

"Important new health guide which packs in the latest consumer information about the problems of alcoholism." —*Reviewer's Bookwatch, Nov '00*

SEE ALSO *Drug Abuse Sourcebook*

Allergies Sourcebook, 3rd Edition

Basic Consumer Health Information about Allergic Disorders, Such as Anaphylaxis, Hives, Eczema, Rhinitis, Sinusitis, and Conjunctivitis, and Their Triggers, Including Pollen, Mold, Dust Mites, Animal Dander, Insects, Chemicals, Food, Food Additives, and Medications;

Along with Advice about the Diagnosis and Treatment of Allergy Symptoms, a Glossary of Related Terms, a Directory of Resources for Help and Information, and Suggestions for Additional Reading

Edited by Amy L. Sutton. 598 pages. 2007. 978-0-7808-0950-5.

"This book brings a great deal of useful material together. . . . This is an excellent addition to public and consumer health library collections."
— *American Reference Books Annual, 2003*

"This second edition would be useful to laypersons with little or advanced knowledge of the subject matter. This book would also serve as a resource for nursing and other health care professions students. It would be useful in public, academic, and hospital libraries with consumer health collections." — *E-Streams, Jul '02*

Alternative Medicine Sourcebook

SEE Complementary & Alternative Medicine Sourcebook

Alzheimer's Disease Sourcebook, 3rd Edition

Basic Consumer Health Information about Alzheimer's Disease, Other Dementias, and Related Disorders, Including Multi-Infarct Dementia, AIDS Dementia Complex, Dementia with Lewy Bodies, Huntington's Disease, Wernicke-Korsakoff Syndrome (Alcohol-Related Dementia), Delirium, and Confusional States

Along with Information for People Newly Diagnosed with Alzheimer's Disease and Caregivers, Reports Detailing Current Research Efforts in Prevention, Diagnosis, and Treatment, Facts about Long-Term Care Issues, and Listings of Sources for Additional Information

Edited by Karen Bellenir. 645 pages. 2003. 978-0-7808-0666-5.

"This very informative and valuable tool will be a great addition to any library serving consumers, students and health care workers."
— *American Reference Books Annual, 2004*

"This is a valuable resource for people affected by dementias such as Alzheimer's. It is easy to navigate and includes important information and resources."
— *Doody's Review Service, Feb '04*

"Recommended reference source."
— *Booklist, American Library Association, Oct '99*

SEE ALSO *Brain Disorders Sourcebook*

Arthritis Sourcebook, 2nd Edition

Basic Consumer Health Information about Osteoarthritis, Rheumatoid Arthritis, Other Rheumatic Disorders, Infectious Forms of Arthritis, and Diseases with Symptoms Linked to Arthritis, Featuring Facts about Diagnosis, Pain Management, and Surgical Therapies

Along with Coping Strategies, Research Updates, a Glossary, and Resources for Additional Help and Information

Edited by Amy L. Sutton. 593 pages. 2004. 978-0-7808-0667-2.

"This easy-to-read volume is recommended for consumer health collections within public or academic libraries." — *E-Streams, May '05*

"As expected, this updated edition continues the excellent reputation of this series in providing sound, usable health information. . . . Highly recommended."
— *American Reference Books Annual, 2005*

"Excellent reference." — *The Bookwatch, Jan '05*

Asthma Sourcebook, 2nd Edition

Basic Consumer Health Information about the Causes, Symptoms, Diagnosis, and Treatment of Asthma in Infants, Children, Teenagers, and Adults, Including Facts about Different Types of Asthma, Common Co-Occurring Conditions, Asthma Management Plans, Triggers, Medications, and Medication Delivery Devices

Along with Asthma Statistics, Research Updates, a Glossary, a Directory of Asthma-Related Resources, and More

Edited by Karen Bellenir. 609 pages. 2006. 978-0-7808-0866-9.

"A worthwhile reference acquisition for public libraries and academic medical libraries whose readers desire a quick introduction to the wide range of asthma information." — *Choice, Association of College & Research Libraries, Jun '01*

"Recommended reference source."
— *Booklist, American Library Association, Feb '01*

"Highly recommended." — *The Bookwatch, Jan '01*

"There is much good information for patients and their families who deal with asthma daily."
— *American Medical Writers Association Journal, Winter '01*

"This informative text is recommended for consumer health collections in public, secondary school, and community college libraries and the libraries of universities with a large undergraduate population."
— *American Reference Books Annual, 2001*

Attention Deficit Disorder Sourcebook

Basic Consumer Health Information about Attention Deficit/Hyperactivity Disorder in Children and Adults,

Including Facts about Causes, Symptoms, Diagnostic Criteria, and Treatment Options Such as Medications, Behavior Therapy, Coaching, and Homeopathy

Along with Reports on Current Research Initiatives, Legal Issues, and Government Regulations, and Featuring a Glossary of Related Terms, Internet Resources, and a List of Additional Reading Material

Edited by Dawn D. Matthews. 470 pages. 2002. 978-0-7808-0624-5.

"Recommended reference source."
— *Booklist, American Library Association, Jan '03*

"This book is recommended for all school libraries and the reference or consumer health sections of public libraries." — *American Reference Books Annual, 2003*

■

Back & Neck Sourcebook, 2nd Edition

Basic Consumer Health Information about Spinal Pain, Spinal Cord Injuries, and Related Disorders, Such as Degenerative Disk Disease, Osteoarthritis, Scoliosis, Sciatica, Spina Bifida, and Spinal Stenosis, and Featuring Facts about Maintaining Spinal Health, Self-Care, Pain Management, Rehabilitative Care, Chiropractic Care, Spinal Surgeries, and Complementary Therapies

Along with Suggestions for Preventing Back and Neck Pain, a Glossary of Related Terms, and a Directory of Resources

Edited by Amy L. Sutton. 633 pages. 2004. 978-0-7808-0738-9.

"Recommended . . . an easy to use, comprehensive medical reference book." — *E-Streams, Sep '05*

"The strength of this work is its basic, easy-to-read format. Recommended." — *Reference and User Services Quarterly, American Library Association, Winter '97*

■

Blood & Circulatory Disorders Sourcebook, 2nd Edition

Basic Consumer Health Information about the Blood and Circulatory System and Related Disorders, Such as Anemia and Other Hemoglobin Diseases, Cancer of the Blood and Associated Bone Marrow Disorders, Clotting and Bleeding Problems, and Conditions That Affect the Veins, Blood Vessels, and Arteries, Including Facts about the Donation and Transplantation of Bone Marrow, Stem Cells, and Blood and Tips for Keeping the Blood and Circulatory System Healthy

Along with a Glossary of Related Terms and Resources for Additional Help and Information

Edited by Amy L. Sutton. 659 pages. 2005. 978-0-7808-0746-4.

"Highly recommended pick for basic consumer health reference holdings at all levels." — *The Bookwatch, Aug '05*

"Recommended reference source."
— *Booklist, American Library Association, Feb '99*

"An important reference sourcebook written in simple language for everyday, non-technical users. " — *Reviewer's Bookwatch, Jan '99*

■

Brain Disorders Sourcebook, 2nd Edition

Basic Consumer Health Information about Acquired and Traumatic Brain Injuries, Infections of the Brain, Epilepsy and Seizure Disorders, Cerebral Palsy, and Degenerative Neurological Disorders, Including Amyotrophic Lateral Sclerosis (ALS), Dementias, Multiple Sclerosis, and More

Along with Information on the Brain's Structure and Function, Treatment and Rehabilitation Options, Reports on Current Research Initiatives, a Glossary of Terms Related to Brain Disorders and Injuries, and a Directory of Sources for Further Help and Information

Edited by Sandra J. Judd. 625 pages. 2005. 978-0-7808-0744-0.

"Highly recommended pick for basic consumer health reference holdings at all levels."
— *The Bookwatch, Aug '05*

"Belongs on the shelves of any library with a consumer health collection." — *E-Streams, Mar '00*

"Recommended reference source."
— *Booklist, American Library Association, Oct '99*

SEE ALSO *Alzheimer's Disease Sourcebook*

■

Breast Cancer Sourcebook, 2nd Edition

Basic Consumer Health Information about Breast Cancer, Including Facts about Risk Factors, Prevention, Screening and Diagnostic Methods, Treatment Options, Complementary and Alternative Therapies, Post-Treatment Concerns, Clinical Trials, Special Risk Populations, and New Developments in Breast Cancer Research

Along with Breast Cancer Statistics, a Glossary of Related Terms, and a Directory of Resources for Additional Help and Information

Edited by Sandra J. Judd. 595 pages. 2004. 978-0-7808-0668-9.

"This book will be an excellent addition to public, community college, medical, and academic libraries."
— *American Reference Books Annual, 2006*

"It would be a useful reference book in a library or on loan to women in a support group."
— *Cancer Forum, Mar '03*

"Recommended reference source."
— *Booklist, American Library Association, Jan '02*

"This reference source is highly recommended. It is quite informative, comprehensive and detailed in nature, and yet it offers practical advice in easy-to-read language. It could be thought of as the 'bible' of breast cancer for the consumer." —*E-Streams, Jan '02*

"From the pros and cons of different screening methods and results to treatment options, *Breast Cancer Sourcebook* provides the latest information on the subject." —*Library Bookwatch, Dec '01*

"This thoroughgoing, very readable reference covers all aspects of breast health and cancer. . . . Readers will find much to consider here. Recommended for all public and patient health collections." —*Library Journal, Sep '01*

SEE ALSO *Cancer Sourcebook for Women, Women's Health Concerns Sourcebook*

Breastfeeding Sourcebook

Basic Consumer Health Information about the Benefits of Breastmilk, Preparing to Breastfeed, Breastfeeding as a Baby Grows, Nutrition, and More, Including Information on Special Situations and Concerns Such as Mastitis, Illness, Medications, Allergies, Multiple Births, Prematurity, Special Needs, and Adoption

Along with a Glossary and Resources for Additional Help and Information

Edited by Jenni Lynn Colson. 388 pages. 2002. 978-0-7808-0332-9.

"Particularly useful is the information about professional lactation services and chapters on breastfeeding when returning to work. . . . *Breastfeeding Sourcebook* will be useful for public libraries, consumer health libraries, and technical schools offering nurse assistant training, especially in areas where Internet access is problematic." —*American Reference Books Annual, 2003*

SEE ALSO *Pregnancy & Birth Sourcebook*

Burns Sourcebook

Basic Consumer Health Information about Various Types of Burns and Scalds, Including Flame, Heat, Cold, Electrical, Chemical, and Sun Burns

Along with Information on Short-Term and Long-Term Treatments, Tissue Reconstruction, Plastic Surgery, Prevention Suggestions, and First Aid

Edited by Allan R. Cook. 604 pages. 1999. 978-0-7808-0204-9.

"This is an exceptional addition to the series and is highly recommended for all consumer health collections, hospital libraries, and academic medical centers." —*E-Streams, Mar '00*

"This key reference guide is an invaluable addition to all health care and public libraries in confronting this ongoing health issue." —*American Reference Books Annual, 2000*

"Recommended reference source." · —*Booklist, American Library Association, Dec '99*

SEE ALSO *Dermatological Disorders Sourcebook*

Cancer Sourcebook, 5th Edition

Basic Consumer Health Information about Major Forms and Stages of Cancer, Featuring Facts about Head and Neck Cancers, Lung Cancers, Gastrointestinal Cancers, Genitourinary Cancers, Lymphomas, Blood Cell Cancers, Endocrine Cancers, Skin Cancers, Bone Cancers, Metastatic Cancers, and More

Along with Facts about Cancer Treatments, Cancer Risks and Prevention, a Glossary of Related Terms, Statistical Data, and a Directory of Resources for Additional Information

Edited by Karen Bellenir. 1,133 pages. 2007. 978-0-7808-0947-5.

"With cancer being the second leading cause of death for Americans, a prodigious work such as this one, which locates centrally so much cancer-related information, is clearly an asset to this nation's citizens and others." —*Journal of the National Medical Association, 2004*

"This title is recommended for health sciences and public libraries with consumer health collections." —*E-Streams, Feb '01*

". . . can be effectively used by cancer patients and their families who are looking for answers in a language they can understand. Public and hospital libraries should have it on their shelves." —*American Reference Books Annual, 2001*

"Recommended reference source." —*Booklist, American Library Association, Dec '00*

SEE ALSO *Breast Cancer Sourcebook, Cancer Sourcebook for Women, Pediatric Cancer Sourcebook, Prostate Cancer Sourcebook*

Cancer Sourcebook for Women, 3rd Edition

Basic Consumer Health Information about Leading Causes of Cancer in Women, Featuring Facts about Gynecologic Cancers and Related Concerns, Such as Breast Cancer, Cervical Cancer, Endometrial Cancer, Uterine Sarcoma, Vaginal Cancer, Vulvar Cancer, and Common Non-Cancerous Gynecologic Conditions, in Addition to Facts about Lung Cancer, Colorectal Cancer, and Thyroid Cancer in Women

Along with Information about Cancer Risk Factors, Screening and Prevention, Treatment Options, and Tips on Coping with Life after Cancer Treatment, a Glossary of Cancer Terms, and a Directory of Resources for Additional Help and Information

Edited by Amy L. Sutton. 715 pages. 2006. 978-0-7808-0867-6.

"An excellent addition to collections in public, consumer health, and women's health libraries." —*American Reference Books Annual, 2003*

"Overall, the information is excellent, and complex topics are clearly explained. As a reference book for the consumer it is a valuable resource to assist them to make informed decisions about cancer and its treatments." —*Cancer Forum, Nov '02*

"Highly recommended for academic and medical reference collections." — *Library Bookwatch, Sep '02*

"This is a highly recommended book for any public or consumer library, being reader friendly and containing accurate and helpful information." — *E-Streams, Aug '02*

"Recommended reference source." — *Booklist, American Library Association, Jul '02*

SEE ALSO *Breast Cancer Sourcebook, Women's Health Concerns Sourcebook*

■

Cancer Survivorship Sourcebook

Basic Consumer Health Information about the Physical, Educational, Emotional, Social, and Financial Needs of Cancer Patients from Diagnosis, through Cancer Treatment, and Beyond, Including Facts about Researching Specific Types of Cancer and Learning about Clinical Trials and Treatment Options, and Featuring Tips for Coping with the Side Effects of Cancer Treatments and Adjusting to Life after Cancer Treatment Concludes

Along with Suggestions for Caregivers, Friends, and Family Members of Cancer Patients, a Glossary of Cancer Care Terms, and Directories of Related Resources

Edited by Karen Bellenir. 6561 pages. 2007. 978-0-7808-0985-7.

■

Cardiovascular Diseases & Disorders Sourcebook, 3rd Edition

Basic Consumer Health Information about Heart and Vascular Diseases and Disorders, Such as Angina, Heart Attacks, Arrhythmias, Cardiomyopathy, Valve Disease, Atherosclerosis, and Aneurysms, with Information about Managing Cardiovascular Risk Factors and Maintaining Heart Health, Medications and Procedures Used to Treat Cardiovascular Disorders, and Concerns of Special Significance to Women

Along with Reports on Current Research Initiatives, a Glossary of Related Medical Terms, and a Directory of Sources for Further Help and Information

Edited by Sandra J. Judd. 713 pages. 2005. 978-0-7808-0739-6.

"This updated sourcebook is still the best first stop for comprehensive introductory information on cardiovascular diseases." — *American Reference Books Annual, 2006*

"Recommended for public libraries and libraries supporting health care professionals." — *E-Streams, Sep '05*

"This should be a standard health library reference." — *The Bookwatch, Jun '05*

"Recommended reference source." — *Booklist, American Library Association, Dec '00*

"... comprehensive format provides an extensive overview on this subject." — *Choice, Association of College & Research Libraries*

■

Caregiving Sourcebook

Basic Consumer Health Information for Caregivers, Including a Profile of Caregivers, Caregiving Responsibilities and Concerns, Tips for Specific Conditions, Care Environments, and the Effects of Caregiving

Along with Facts about Legal Issues, Financial Information, and Future Planning, a Glossary, and a Listing of Additional Resources

Edited by Joyce Brennfleck Shannon. 600 pages. 2001. 978-0-7808-0331-2.

"Essential for most collections." — *Library Journal, Apr 1, 2002*

"An ideal addition to the reference collection of any public library. Health sciences information professionals may also want to acquire the *Caregiving Sourcebook* for their hospital or academic library for use as a ready reference tool by health care workers interested in aging and caregiving." — *E-Streams, Jan '02*

"Recommended reference source." — *Booklist, American Library Association, Oct '01*

■

Child Abuse Sourcebook

Basic Consumer Health Information about the Physical, Sexual, and Emotional Abuse of Children, with Additional Facts about Neglect, Munchausen Syndrome by Proxy (MSBP), Shaken Baby Syndrome, and Controversial Issues Related to Child Abuse, Such as Withholding Medical Care, Corporal Punishment, and Child Maltreatment in Youth Sports, and Featuring Facts about Child Protective Services, Foster Care, Adoption, Parenting Challenges, and Other Abuse Prevention Efforts

Along with a Glossary of Related Terms and Resources for Additional Help and Information

Edited by Dawn D. Matthews. 620 pages. 2004. 978-0-7808-0705-1.

"A valuable and highly recommended resource for school, academic and public libraries whether used on its own or as a starting point for more in-depth research." — *E-Streams, Apr '05*

"Every week the news brings cases of child abuse or neglect, so it is useful to have a source that supplies so much helpful information. . . . Recommended. Public and academic libraries, and child welfare offices." — *Choice, Association of College & Research Libraries, Mar '05*

"Packed with insights on all kinds of issues, from foster care and adoption to parenting and abuse prevention." — *The Bookwatch, Nov '04*

SEE ALSO: *Domestic Violence Sourcebook*

Childhood Diseases & Disorders Sourcebook

Basic Consumer Health Information about Medical Problems Often Encountered in Pre-Adolescent Children, Including Respiratory Tract Ailments, Ear Infections, Sore Throats, Disorders of the Skin and Scalp, Digestive and Genitourinary Diseases, Infectious Diseases, Inflammatory Disorders, Chronic Physical and Developmental Disorders, Allergies, and More

Along with Information about Diagnostic Tests, Common Childhood Surgeries, and Frequently Used Medications, with a Glossary of Important Terms and Resource Directory

Edited by Chad T. Kimball. 662 pages. 2003. 978-0-7808-0458-6.

"This is an excellent book for new parents and should be included in all health care and public libraries."
—*American Reference Books Annual, 2004*

SEE ALSO: *Healthy Children Sourcebook*

Colds, Flu & Other Common Ailments Sourcebook

Basic Consumer Health Information about Common Ailments and Injuries, Including Colds, Coughs, the Flu, Sinus Problems, Headaches, Fever, Nausea and Vomiting, Menstrual Cramps, Diarrhea, Constipation, Hemorrhoids, Back Pain, Dandruff, Dry and Itchy Skin, Cuts, Scrapes, Sprains, Bruises, and More

Along with Information about Prevention, Self-Care, Choosing a Doctor, Over-the-Counter Medications, Folk Remedies, and Alternative Therapies, and Including a Glossary of Important Terms and a Directory of Resources for Further Help and Information

Edited by Chad T. Kimball. 638 pages. 2001. 978-0-7808-0435-7.

"A good starting point for research on common illnesses. It will be a useful addition to public and consumer health library collections."
—*American Reference Books Annual, 2002*

"Will prove valuable to any library seeking to maintain a current, comprehensive reference collection of health resources. . . . Excellent reference."
—*The Bookwatch, Aug '01*

"Recommended reference source."
—*Booklist, American Library Association, Jul '01*

Communication Disorders Sourcebook

Basic Information about Deafness and Hearing Loss, Speech and Language Disorders, Voice Disorders, Balance and Vestibular Disorders, and Disorders of Smell, Taste, and Touch

Edited by Linda M. Ross. 533 pages. 1996. 978-0-7808-0077-9.

"This is skillfully edited and is a welcome resource for the layperson. It should be found in every public and medical library."
—*Booklist Health Sciences Supplement, American Library Association, Oct '97*

Complementary & Alternative Medicine Sourcebook, 3rd Edition

Basic Consumer Health Information about Complementary and Alternative Medical Therapies, Including Acupuncture, Ayurveda, Traditional Chinese Medicine, Herbal Medicine, Homeopathy, Naturopathy, Biofeedback, Hypnotherapy, Yoga, Art Therapy, Aromatherapy, Clinical Nutrition, Vitamin and Mineral Supplements, Chiropractic, Massage, Reflexology, Crystal Therapy, Therapeutic Touch, and More

Along with Facts about Alternative and Complementary Treatments for Specific Conditions Such as Cancer, Diabetes, Osteoarthritis, Chronic Pain, Menopause, Gastrointestinal Disorders, Headaches, and Mental Illness, a Glossary, and a Resource List for Additional Help and Information

Edited by Sandra J. Judd. 657 pages. 2006. 978-0-7808-0864-5.

"Recommended for public, high school, and academic libraries that have consumer health collections. Hospital libraries that also serve the public will find this to be a useful resource." —*E-Streams, Feb '03*

"Recommended reference source."
—*Booklist, American Library Association, Jan '03*

"An important alternate health reference."
—*MBR Bookwatch, Oct '02*

"A great addition to the reference collection of every type of library." —*American Reference Books Annual, 2000*

Congenital Disorders Sourcebook, 2nd Edition

Basic Consumer Health Information about Nonhereditary Birth Defects and Disorders Related to Prematurity, Gestational Injuries, Congenital Infections, and Birth Complications, Including Heart Defects, Hydrocephalus, Spina Bifida, Cleft Lip and Palate, Cerebral Palsy, and More

Along with Facts about the Prevention of Birth Defects, Fetal Surgery and Other Treatment Options, Research Initiatives, a Glossary of Related Terms, and Resources for Additional Information and Support

Edited by Sandra J. Judd. 647 pages. 2006. 978-0-7808-0945-1.

"Recommended reference source."
—*Booklist, American Library Association, Oct '97*

SEE ALSO *Pregnancy & Birth Sourcebook*

Contagious Diseases Sourcebook

Basic Consumer Health Information about Infectious Diseases Spread by Person-to-Person Contact through

Direct Touch, Airborne Transmission, Sexual Contact, or Contact with Blood or Other Body Fluids, Including Hepatitis, Herpes, Influenza, Lice, Measles, Mumps, Pinworm, Ringworm, Severe Acute Respiratory Syndrome (SARS), Streptococcal Infections, Tuberculosis, and Others

Along with Facts about Disease Transmission, Antimicrobial Resistance, and Vaccines, with a Glossary and Directories of Resources for More Information

Edited by Karen Bellenir. 643 pages. 2004. 978-0-7808-0736-5.

"This easy-to-read volume is recommended for consumer health collections within public or academic libraries." —E-Streams, May '05

"This informative book is highly recommended for public libraries, consumer health collections, and secondary schools and undergraduate libraries." —American Reference Books Annual, 2005

"Excellent reference." —The Bookwatch, Jan '05

■

Death & Dying Sourcebook, 2nd Edition

Basic Consumer Health Information about End-of-Life Care and Related Perspectives and Ethical Issues, Including End-of-Life Symptoms and Treatments, Pain Management, Quality-of-Life Concerns, the Use of Life Support, Patients' Rights and Privacy Issues, Advance Directives, Physician-Assisted Suicide, Caregiving, Organ and Tissue Donation, Autopsies, Funeral Arrangements, and Grief

Along with Statistical Data, Information about the Leading Causes of Death, a Glossary, and Directories of Support Groups and Other Resources

Edited by Joyce Brennfleck Shannon. 653 pages. 2006. 978-0-7808-0871-3.

"Public libraries, medical libraries, and academic libraries will all find this sourcebook a useful addition to their collections." —American Reference Books Annual, 2001

"An extremely useful resource for those concerned with death and dying in the United States." —Respiratory Care, Nov '00

"Recommended reference source." —Booklist, American Library Association, Aug '00

"This book is a definite must for all those involved in end-of-life care." —Doody's Review Service, 2000

■

Dental Care & Oral Health Sourcebook, 2nd Edition

Basic Consumer Health Information about Dental Care, Including Oral Hygiene, Dental Visits, Pain Management, Cavities, Crowns, Bridges, Dental Implants, and Fillings, and Other Oral Health Concerns, Such as Gum Disease, Bad Breath, Dry Mouth, Genetic and Developmental Abnormalities, Oral Cancers, Orthodontics, and Temporomandibular Disorders

Along with Updates on Current Research in Oral Health, a Glossary, a Directory of Dental and Oral Health Organizations, and Resources for People with Dental and Oral Health Disorders

Edited by Amy L. Sutton. 609 pages. 2003. 978-0-7808-0634-4.

"This book could serve as a turning point in the battle to educate consumers in issues concerning oral health." —American Reference Books Annual, 2004

"Unique source which will fill a gap in dental sources for patients and the lay public. A valuable reference tool even in a library with thousands of books on dentistry. Comprehensive, clear, inexpensive, and easy to read and use. It fills an enormous gap in the health care literature." —Reference & User Services Quarterly, American Library Association, Summer '98

"Recommended reference source." —Booklist, American Library Association, Dec '97

■

Depression Sourcebook

Basic Consumer Health Information about Unipolar Depression, Bipolar Disorder, Postpartum Depression, Seasonal Affective Disorder, and Other Types of Depression in Children, Adolescents, Women, Men, the Elderly, and Other Selected Populations

Along with Facts about Causes, Risk Factors, Diagnostic Criteria, Treatment Options, Coping Strategies, Suicide Prevention, a Glossary, and a Directory of Sources for Additional Help and Information

Edited by Karen Bellenir. 602 pages. 2002. 978-0-7808-0611-5.

"Depression Sourcebook is of a very high standard. Its purpose, which is to serve as a reference source to the lay reader, is very well served." —Journal of the National Medical Association, 2004

"Invaluable reference for public and school library collections alike." —Library Bookwatch, Apr '03

"Recommended for purchase." —American Reference Books Annual, 2003

■

Dermatological Disorders Sourcebook, 2nd Edition

Basic Consumer Health Information about Conditions and Disorders Affecting the Skin, Hair, and Nails, Such as Acne, Rosacea, Rashes, Dermatitis, Pigmentation Disorders, Birthmarks, Skin Cancer, Skin Injuries, Psoriasis, Scleroderma, and Hair Loss, Including Facts about Medications and Treatments for Dermatological Disorders and Tips for Maintaining Healthy Skin, Hair, and Nails

Along with Information about How Aging Affects the Skin, a Glossary of Related Terms, and a Directory of Resources for Additional Help and Information

Edited by Amy L. Sutton. 645 pages. 2005. 978-0-7808-0795-2.

■

Diabetes Sourcebook, 3rd Edition

Basic Consumer Health Information about Type 1 Diabetes (Insulin-Dependent or Juvenile-Onset Diabetes), Type 2 Diabetes (Noninsulin-Dependent or Adult-Onset Diabetes), Gestational Diabetes, Impaired Glucose Tolerance (IGT), and Related Complications, Such as Amputation, Eye Disease, Gum Disease, Nerve Damage, and End-Stage Renal Disease, Including Facts about Insulin, Oral Diabetes Medications, Blood Sugar Testing, and the Role of Exercise and Nutrition in the Control of Diabetes

Along with a Glossary and Resources for Further Help and Information

Edited by Dawn D. Matthews. 622 pages. 2003. 978-0-7808-0629-0.

■

Diet & Nutrition Sourcebook, 3rd Edition

Basic Consumer Health Information about Dietary Guidelines and the Food Guidance System, Recommended Daily Nutrient Intakes, Serving Proportions, Weight Control, Vitamins and Supplements, Nutrition Issues for Different Life Stages and Lifestyles, and the Needs of People with Specific Medical Concerns, Including Cancer, Celiac Disease, Diabetes, Eating Disorders, Food Allergies, and Cardiovascular Disease

Along with Facts about Federal Nutrition Support Programs, a Glossary of Nutrition and Dietary Terms, and Directories of Additional Resources for More Information about Nutrition

Edited by Joyce Brennfleck Shannon. 633 pages. 2006. 978-0-7808-0800-3.

SEE ALSO *Digestive Diseases & Disorders Sourcebook, Eating Disorders Sourcebook, Gastrointestinal Diseases & Disorders Sourcebook, Vegetarian Sourcebook*

■

Digestive Diseases & Disorders Sourcebook

Basic Consumer Health Information about Diseases and Disorders that Impact the Upper and Lower Digestive System, Including Celiac Disease, Constipation, Crohn's Disease, Cyclic Vomiting Syndrome, Diarrhea, Diverticulosis and Diverticulitis, Gallstones, Heartburn, Hemorrhoids, Hernias, Indigestion (Dyspepsia), Irritable Bowel Syndrome, Lactose Intolerance, Ulcers, and More

Along with Information about Medications and Other Treatments, Tips for Maintaining a Healthy Digestive Tract, a Glossary, and Directory of Digestive Diseases Organizations

Edited by Karen Bellenir. 335 pages. 2000. 978-0-7808-0327-5.

SEE ALSO *Eating Disorders Sourcebook, Gastrointestinal Diseases & Disorders Sourcebook*

■

Disabilities Sourcebook

Basic Consumer Health Information about Physical and Psychiatric Disabilities, Including Descriptions of Major Causes of Disability, Assistive and Adaptive Aids, Workplace Issues, and Accessibility Concerns

Along with Information about the Americans with Disabilities Act, a Glossary, and Resources for Additional Help and Information

Edited by Dawn D. Matthews. 616 pages. 2000. 978-0-7808-0389-3.

"A much needed addition to the Omnigraphics *Health Reference Series*. A current reference work to provide people with disabilities, their families, caregivers or those who work with them, a broad range of information in one volume, has not been available until now. . . . It is recommended for all public and academic library reference collections." — *E-Streams, May '01*

"An excellent source book in easy-to-read format covering many current topics; highly recommended for all libraries." — *Choice, Association of College & Research Libraries, Jan '01*

"Recommended reference source."
— *Booklist, American Library Association, Jul '00*

■

Domestic Violence Sourcebook, 2nd Edition

Basic Consumer Health Information about the Causes and Consequences of Abusive Relationships, Including Physical Violence, Sexual Assault, Battery, Stalking, and Emotional Abuse, and Facts about the Effects of Violence on Women, Men, Young Adults, and the Elderly, with Reports about Domestic Violence in Selected Populations, and Featuring Facts about Medical Care, Victim Assistance and Protection, Prevention Strategies, Mental Health Services, and Legal Issues

Along with a Glossary of Related Terms and Resources for Additional Help and Information

Edited by Dawn D. Matthews. 628 pages. 2004. 978-0-7808-0669-6.

"Educators, clergy, medical professionals, police, and victims and their families will benefit from this realistic and easy-to-understand resource."
— *American Reference Books Annual, 2005*

"Recommended for all collections supporting consumer health information. It should also be considered for any collection needing general, readable information on domestic violence." — *E-Streams, Jan '05*

"This sourcebook complements other books in its field, providing a one-stop resource . . . Recommended."
— *Choice, Association of College & Research Libraries, Jan '05*

"Interested lay persons should find the book extremely beneficial. . . . A copy of *Domestic Violence and Child Abuse Sourcebook* should be in every public library in the United States."
— *Social Science & Medicine, No. 56, 2003*

"This is important information. The Web has many resources but this sourcebook fills an important societal need. I am not aware of any other resources of this type." — *Doody's Review Service, Sep '01*

"Recommended reference source."
— *Booklist, American Library Association, Apr '01*

"Important pick for college-level health reference libraries." — *The Bookwatch, Mar '01*

"Because this problem is so widespread and because this book includes a lot of issues within one volume, this work is recommended for all public libraries."
— *American Reference Books Annual, 2001*

SEE ALSO Child Abuse Sourcebook

■

Drug Abuse Sourcebook, 2nd Edition

Basic Consumer Health Information about Illicit Substances of Abuse and the Misuse of Prescription and Over-the-Counter Medications, Including Depressants, Hallucinogens, Inhalants, Marijuana, Stimulants, and Anabolic Steroids

Along with Facts about Related Health Risks, Treatment Programs, Prevention Programs, a Glossary of Abuse and Addiction Terms, a Glossary of Drug-Related Street Terms, and a Directory of Resources for More Information

Edited by Catherine Ginther. 607 pages. 2004. 978-0-7808-0740-2.

"Commendable for organizing useful, normally scattered government and association-produced data into a logical sequence."
— *American Reference Books Annual, 2006*

"This easy-to-read volume is recommended for consumer health collections within public or academic libraries." — *E-Streams, Sep '05*

"An excellent library reference."
— *The Bookwatch, May '05*

"Containing a wealth of information, this book will be useful to the college student just beginning to explore the topic of substance abuse. This resource belongs in libraries that serve a lower-division undergraduate or community college clientele as well as the general public." — *Choice, Association of College & Research Libraries, Jun '01*

"Recommended reference source."
— *Booklist, American Library Association, Feb '01*

SEE ALSO Alcoholism Sourcebook

■

Ear, Nose & Throat Disorders Sourcebook, 2nd Edition

Basic Consumer Health Information about Disorders of the Ears, Hearing Loss, Vestibular Disorders, Nasal and Sinus Problems, Throat and Vocal Cord Disorders, and Otolaryngologic Cancers, Including Facts about Ear Infections and Injuries, Genetic and Congenital Deafness, Sensorineural Hearing Disorders, Tinnitus, Vertigo, Ménière Disease, Rhinitis, Sinusitis, Snoring, Sore Throats, Hoarseness, and More

Along with Reports on Current Research Initiatives, a Glossary of Related Medical Terms, and a Directory of Sources for Further Help and Information

Edited by Sandra J. Judd. 659 pages. 2006. 978-0-7808-0872-0.

"Overall, this sourcebook is helpful for the consumer seeking information on ENT issues. It is recommended for public libraries."
— American Reference Books Annual, 1999

"Recommended reference source."
— Booklist, American Library Association, Dec '98

Eating Disorders Sourcebook, 2nd Edition

Basic Consumer Health Information about Anorexia Nervosa, Bulimia Nervosa, Binge Eating, Compulsive Exercise, Female Athlete Triad, and Other Eating Disorders, Including Facts about Body Image and Other Cultural and Age-Related Risk Factors, Prevention Efforts, Adverse Health Effects, Treatment Options, and the Recovery Process

Along with Guidelines for Healthy Weight Control, a Glossary, and Directories of Additional Resources

Edited by Joyce Brennfleck Shannon. 585 pages. 2007. 978-0-7808-0948-2.

"Recommended for health science libraries that are open to the public, as well as hospital libraries. This book is a good resource for the consumer who is concerned about eating disorders." — E-Streams, Mar '02

"This volume is another convenient collection of excerpted articles. Recommended for school and public library patrons; lower-division undergraduates; and two-year technical program students."
— Choice, Association of College & Research Libraries, Jan '02

"Recommended reference source."
— Booklist, American Library Association, Oct '01

SEE ALSO Diet & Nutrition Sourcebook, Digestive Diseases & Disorders Sourcebook, Gastrointestinal Diseases & Disorders Sourcebook

---

Emergency Medical Services Sourcebook

Basic Consumer Health Information about Preventing, Preparing for, and Managing Emergency Situations, When and Who to Call for Help, What to Expect in the Emergency Room, the Emergency Medical Team, Patient Issues, and Current Topics in Emergency Medicine

Along with Statistical Data, a Glossary, and Sources of Additional Help and Information

Edited by Jenni Lynn Colson. 494 pages. 2002. 978-0-7808-0420-3.

"Handy and convenient for home, public, school, and college libraries. Recommended."
— Choice, Association of College & Research Libraries, Apr '03

"This reference can provide the consumer with answers to most questions about emergency care in the United States, or it will direct them to a resource where the answer can be found."
— American Reference Books Annual, 2003

"Recommended reference source."
— Booklist, American Library Association, Feb '03

Endocrine & Metabolic Disorders Sourcebook

Basic Information for the Layperson about Pancreatic and Insulin-Related Disorders Such as Pancreatitis, Diabetes, and Hypoglycemia; Adrenal Gland Disorders Such as Cushing's Syndrome, Addison's Disease, and Congenital Adrenal Hyperplasia; Pituitary Gland Disorders Such as Growth Hormone Deficiency, Acromegaly, and Pituitary Tumors; Thyroid Disorders Such as Hypothyroidism, Graves' Disease, Hashimoto's Disease, and Goiter; Hyperparathyroidism; and Other Diseases and Syndromes of Hormone Imbalance or Metabolic Dysfunction

Along with Reports on Current Research Initiatives

Edited by Linda M. Shin. 574 pages. 1998. 978-0-7808-0207-0.

"Omnigraphics has produced another needed resource for health information consumers."
— American Reference Books Annual, 2000

"Recommended reference source."
— Booklist, American Library Association, Dec '98

Environmental Health Sourcebook, 2nd Edition

Basic Consumer Health Information about the Environment and Its Effect on Human Health, Including the Effects of Air Pollution, Water Pollution, Hazardous Chemicals, Food Hazards, Radiation Hazards, Biological Agents, Household Hazards, Such as Radon, Asbestos, Carbon Monoxide, and Mold, and Information about Associated Diseases and Disorders, Including Cancer, Allergies, Respiratory Problems, and Skin Disorders

Along with Information about Environmental Concerns for Specific Populations, a Glossary of Related Terms, and Resources for Further Help and Information

Edited by Dawn D. Matthews. 673 pages. 2003. 978-0-7808-0632-0.

"This recently updated edition continues the level of quality and the reputation of the numerous other volumes in Omnigraphics' Health Reference Series."
— American Reference Books Annual, 2004

"An excellent updated edition."
— The Bookwatch, Oct '03

"Recommended reference source."
— Booklist, American Library Association, Sep '98

"This book will be a useful addition to anyone's library." — Choice Health Sciences Supplement, Association of College & Research Libraries, May '98

". . . a good survey of numerous environmentally induced physical disorders . . . a useful addition to anyone's library."
— Doody's Health Sciences Book Reviews, Jan '98

Ethnic Diseases Sourcebook

Basic Consumer Health Information for Ethnic and Racial Minority Groups in the United States, Including General Health Indicators and Behaviors, Ethnic Diseases, Genetic Testing, the Impact of Chronic Diseases, Women's Health, Mental Health Issues, and Preventive Health Care Services

Along with a Glossary and a Listing of Additional Resources

Edited by Joyce Brennfleck Shannon. 664 pages. 2001. 978-0-7808-0336-7.

"Recommended for health sciences libraries where public health programs are a priority."
— *E-Streams, Jan '02*

"Not many books have been written on this topic to date, and the *Ethnic Diseases Sourcebook* is a strong addition to the list. It will be an important introductory resource for health consumers, students, health care personnel, and social scientists. It is recommended for public, academic, and large hospital libraries."
— *American Reference Books Annual, 2002*

"Recommended reference source."
— *Booklist, American Library Association, Oct '01*

"Will prove valuable to any library seeking to maintain a current, comprehensive reference collection of health resources. . . . An excellent source of health information about genetic disorders which affect particular ethnic and racial minorities in the U.S."
— *The Bookwatch, Aug '01*

Eye Care Sourcebook, 2nd Edition

Basic Consumer Health Information about Eye Care and Eye Disorders, Including Facts about the Diagnosis, Prevention, and Treatment of Common Refractive Problems Such as Myopia, Hyperopia, Astigmatism, and Presbyopia, and Eye Diseases, Including Glaucoma, Cataract, Age-Related Macular Degeneration, and Diabetic Retinopathy

Along with a Section on Vision Correction and Refractive Surgeries, Including LASIK and LASEK, a Glossary, and Directories of Resources for Additional Help and Information

Edited by Amy L. Sutton. 543 pages. 2003. 978-0-7808-0635-1.

". . . a solid reference tool for eye care and a valuable addition to a collection."
— *American Reference Books Annual, 2004*

Family Planning Sourcebook

Basic Consumer Health Information about Planning for Pregnancy and Contraception, Including Traditional Methods, Barrier Methods, Hormonal Methods, Permanent Methods, Future Methods, Emergency Contraception, and Birth Control Choices for Women at Each Stage of Life

Along with Statistics, a Glossary, and Sources of Additional Information

Edited by Amy Marcaccio Keyzer. 520 pages. 2001. 978-0-7808-0379-4.

"Recommended for public, health, and undergraduate libraries as part of the circulating collection."
— *E-Streams, Mar '02*

"Information is presented in an unbiased, readable manner, and the sourcebook will certainly be a necessary addition to those public and high school libraries where Internet access is restricted or otherwise problematic." — *American Reference Books Annual, 2002*

"Recommended reference source."
— *Booklist, American Library Association, Oct '01*

"Will prove valuable to any library seeking to maintain a current, comprehensive reference collection of health resources. . . . Excellent reference."
— *The Bookwatch, Aug '01*

SEE ALSO *Pregnancy & Birth Sourcebook*

Fitness & Exercise Sourcebook, 3rd Edition

Basic Consumer Health Information about the Physical and Mental Benefits of Fitness, Including Cardiorespiratory Endurance, Muscular Strength, Muscular Endurance, and Flexibility, with Facts about Sports Nutrition and Exercise-Related Injuries and Tips about Physical Activity and Exercises for People of All Ages and for People with Health Concerns

Along with Advice on Selecting and Using Exercise Equipment, Maintaining Exercise Motivation, a Glossary of Related Terms, and a Directory of Resources for More Help and Information

Edited by Amy L. Sutton. 663 pages. 2007. 978-0-7808-0946-8.

"This work is recommended for all general reference collections."
— *American Reference Books Annual, 2002*

"Highly recommended for public, consumer, and school grades fourth through college." — *E-Streams, Nov '01*

"Recommended reference source."
— *Booklist, American Library Association, Oct '01*

"The information appears quite comprehensive and is considered reliable. . . . This second edition is a welcomed addition to the series."
— *Doody's Review Service, Sep '01*

Food Safety Sourcebook

Basic Consumer Health Information about the Safe Handling of Meat, Poultry, Seafood, Eggs, Fruit Juices, and Other Food Items, and Facts about Pesticides, Drinking Water, Food Safety Overseas, and the Onset, Duration, and Symptoms of Foodborne Illnesses, Including Types of Pathogenic Bacteria, Parasitic Protozoa, Worms, Viruses, and Natural Toxins

Along with the Role of the Consumer, the Food Handler, and the Government in Food Safety; a Glossary, and Resources for Additional Help and Information

Edited by Dawn D. Matthews. 339 pages. 1999. 978-0-7808-0326-8.

"This book is recommended for public libraries and universities with home economic and food science programs."
— E-Streams, Nov '00

"Recommended reference source."
— Booklist, American Library Association, May '00

"This book takes the complex issues of food safety and foodborne pathogens and presents them in an easily understood manner. [It does] an excellent job of covering a large and often confusing topic."
— American Reference Books Annual, 2000

■

Forensic Medicine Sourcebook

Basic Consumer Information for the Layperson about Forensic Medicine, Including Crime Scene Investigation, Evidence Collection and Analysis, Expert Testimony, Computer-Aided Criminal Identification, Digital Imaging in the Courtroom, DNA Profiling, Accident Reconstruction, Autopsies, Ballistics, Drugs and Explosives Detection, Latent Fingerprints, Product Tampering, and Questioned Document Examination

Along with Statistical Data, a Glossary of Forensics Terminology, and Listings of Sources for Further Help and Information

Edited by Annemarie S. Muth. 574 pages. 1999. 978-0-7808-0232-2.

"Given the expected widespread interest in its content and its easy to read style, this book is recommended for most public and all college and university libraries."
— E-Streams, Feb '01

"Recommended for public libraries."
— Reference & User Services Quarterly, American Library Association, Spring 2000

"Recommended reference source."
— Booklist, American Library Association, Feb '00

"A wealth of information, useful statistics, references are up-to-date and extremely complete. This wonderful collection of data will help students who are interested in a career in any type of forensic field. It is a great resource for attorneys who need information about types of expert witnesses needed in a particular case. It also offers useful information for fiction and nonfiction writers whose work involves a crime. A fascinating compilation. All levels."
— Choice, Association of College & Research Libraries, Jan '00

"There are several items that make this book attractive to consumers who are seeking certain forensic data. . . . This is a useful current source for those seeking general forensic medical answers."
— American Reference Books Annual, 2000

Gastrointestinal Diseases & Disorders Sourcebook, 2nd Edition

Basic Consumer Health Information about the Upper and Lower Gastrointestinal (GI) Tract, Including the Esophagus, Stomach, Intestines, Rectum, Liver, and Pancreas, with Facts about Gastroesophageal Reflux Disease, Gastritis, Hernias, Ulcers, Celiac Disease, Diverticulitis, Irritable Bowel Syndrome, Hemorrhoids, Gastrointestinal Cancers, and Other Diseases and Disorders Related to the Digestive Process

Along with Information about Commonly Used Diagnostic and Surgical Procedures, Statistics, Reports on Current Research Initiatives and Clinical Trials, a Glossary, and Resources for Additional Help and Information

Edited by Sandra J. Judd. 681 pages. 2006. 978-0-7808-0798-3.

". . . very readable form. The successful editorial work that brought this material together into a useful and understandable reference makes accessible to all readers information that can help them more effectively understand and obtain help for digestive tract problems."
— Choice, Association of College & Research Libraries, Feb '97

SEE ALSO Diet & Nutrition Sourcebook, Digestive Diseases & Disorders Sourcebook, Eating Disorders Sourcebook

■

Genetic Disorders Sourcebook, 3rd Edition

Basic Consumer Health Information about Hereditary Diseases and Disorders, Including Facts about the Human Genome, Genetic Inheritance Patterns, Disorders Associated with Specific Genes, Such as Sickle Cell Disease, Hemophilia, and Cystic Fibrosis, Chromosome Disorders, Such as Down Syndrome, Fragile X Syndrome, and Turner Syndrome, and Complex Diseases and Disorders Resulting from the Interaction of Environmental and Genetic Factors, Such as Allergies, Cancer, and Obesity

Along with Facts about Genetic Testing, Suggestions for Parents of Children with Special Needs, Reports on Current Research Initiatives, a Glossary of Genetic Terminology, and Resources for Additional Help and Information

Edited by Karen Bellenir. 777 pages. 2004. 978-0-7808-0742-6.

"This text is recommended for any library with an interest in providing consumer health resources."
— E-Streams, Aug '05

"This is a valuable resource for anyone wishing to have an understandable description of any of the topics or disorders included. The editor succeeds in making complex genetic issues understandable."
— Doody's Book Review Service, May '05

"A good acquisition for public libraries."
— American Reference Books Annual, 2005

"Excellent reference." — *The Bookwatch, Jan '05*

"Recommended reference source."
— *Booklist, American Library Association, Apr '01*

"Important pick for college-level health reference libraries." — *The Bookwatch, Mar '01*

Head Trauma Sourcebook

Basic Information for the Layperson about Open-Head and Closed-Head Injuries, Treatment Advances, Recovery, and Rehabilitation

Along with Reports on Current Research Initiatives

Edited by Karen Bellenir. 414 pages. 1997. 978-0-7808-0208-7.

Headache Sourcebook

Basic Consumer Health Information about Migraine, Tension, Cluster, Rebound and Other Types of Headaches, with Facts about the Cause and Prevention of Headaches, the Effects of Stress and the Environment, Headaches during Pregnancy and Menopause, and Childhood Headaches

Along with a Glossary and Other Resources for Additional Help and Information

Edited by Dawn D. Matthews. 362 pages. 2002. 978-0-7808-0337-4.

"Highly recommended for academic and medical reference collections." — *Library Bookwatch, Sep '02*

Healthy Aging Sourcebook

Basic Consumer Health Information about Maintaining Health through the Aging Process, Including Advice on Nutrition, Exercise, and Sleep, Help in Making Decisions about Midlife Issues and Retirement, and Guidance Concerning Practical and Informed Choices in Health Consumerism

Along with Data Concerning the Theories of Aging, Different Experiences in Aging by Minority Groups, and Facts about Aging Now and Aging in the Future; and Featuring a Glossary, a Guide to Consumer Help, Additional Suggested Reading, and Practical Resource Directory

Edited by Jenifer Swanson. 536 pages. 1999. 978-0-7808-0390-9.

"Recommended reference source."
— *Booklist, American Library Association, Feb '00*

SEE ALSO *Physical & Mental Issues in Aging Sourcebook*

Healthy Children Sourcebook

Basic Consumer Health Information about the Physical and Mental Development of Children between the Ages of 3 and 12, Including Routine Health Care, Preventative Health Services, Safety and First Aid,

Healthy Sleep, Dental Care, Nutrition, and Fitness, and Featuring Parenting Tips on Such Topics as Bedwetting, Choosing Day Care, Monitoring TV and Other Media, and Establishing a Foundation for Substance Abuse Prevention

Along with a Glossary of Commonly Used Pediatric Terms and Resources for Additional Help and Information.

Edited by Chad T. Kimball. 647 pages. 2003. 978-0-7808-0247-6.

"It is hard to imagine that any other single resource exists that would provide such a comprehensive guide of timely information on health promotion and disease prevention for children aged 3 to 12."
— *American Reference Books Annual, 2004*

"The strengths of this book are many. It is clearly written, presented and structured."
— *Journal of the National Medical Association, 2004*

SEE ALSO *Childhood Diseases & Disorders Sourcebook*

Healthy Heart Sourcebook for Women

Basic Consumer Health Information about Cardiac Issues Specific to Women, Including Facts about Major Risk Factors and Prevention, Treatment and Control Strategies, and Important Dietary Issues

Along with a Special Section Regarding the Pros and Cons of Hormone Replacement Therapy and Its Impact on Heart Health, and Additional Help, Including Recipes, a Glossary, and a Directory of Resources

Edited by Dawn D. Matthews. 336 pages. 2000. 978-0-7808-0329-9.

"A good reference source and recommended for all public, academic, medical, and hospital libraries."
— *Medical Reference Services Quarterly, Summer '01*

"Because of the lack of information specific to women on this topic, this book is recommended for public libraries and consumer libraries."
— *American Reference Books Annual, 2001*

"Contains very important information about coronary artery disease that all women should know. The information is current and presented in an easy-to-read format. The book will make a good addition to any library." — *American Medical Writers Association Journal, Summer '00*

"Important, basic reference."
— *Reviewer's Bookwatch, Jul '00*

SEE ALSO *Cardiovascular Diseases & Disorders Sourcebook, Women's Health Concerns Sourcebook*

Hepatitis Sourcebook

Basic Consumer Health Information about Hepatitis A, Hepatitis B, Hepatitis C, and Other Forms of Hepatitis, Including Autoimmune Hepatitis, Alcoholic Hepatitis, Nonalcoholic Steatohepatitis, and Toxic Hepatitis, with

Facts about Risk Factors, Screening Methods, Diagnostic Tests, and Treatment Options

Along with Information on Liver Health, Tips for People Living with Chronic Hepatitis, Reports on Current Research Initiatives, a Glossary of Terms Related to Hepatitis, and a Directory of Sources for Further Help and Information

Edited by Sandra J. Judd. 597 pages. 2005. 978-0-7808-0749-5.

"Highly recommended."
— *American Reference Books Annual, 2006*

■

Household Safety Sourcebook

Basic Consumer Health Information about Household Safety, Including Information about Poisons, Chemicals, Fire, and Water Hazards in the Home

Along with Advice about the Safe Use of Home Maintenance Equipment, Choosing Toys and Nursery Furniture, Holiday and Recreation Safety, a Glossary, and Resources for Further Help and Information

Edited by Dawn D. Matthews. 606 pages. 2002. 978-0-7808-0338-1.

"This work will be useful in public libraries with large consumer health and wellness departments."
— *American Reference Books Annual, 2003*

"As a sourcebook on household safety this book meets its mark. It is encyclopedic in scope and covers a wide range of safety issues that are commonly seen in the home." — *E-Streams, Jul '02*

■

Hypertension Sourcebook

Basic Consumer Health Information about the Causes, Diagnosis, and Treatment of High Blood Pressure, with Facts about Consequences, Complications, and Co-Occurring Disorders, Such as Coronary Heart Disease, Diabetes, Stroke, Kidney Disease, and Hypertensive Retinopathy, and Issues in Blood Pressure Control, Including Dietary Choices, Stress Management, and Medications

Along with Reports on Current Research Initiatives and Clinical Trials, a Glossary, and Resources for Additional Help and Information

Edited by Dawn D. Matthews and Karen Bellenir. 613 pages. 2004. 978-0-7808-0674-0.

"Academic, public, and medical libraries will want to add the *Hypertension Sourcebook* to their collections." — *E-Streams, Aug '05*

"The strength of this source is the wide range of information given about hypertension."
— *American Reference Books Annual, 2005*

■

Immune System Disorders Sourcebook, 2nd Edition

Basic Consumer Health Information about Disorders of the Immune System, Including Immune System Function and Response, Diagnosis of Immune Disorders, Information about Inherited Immune Disease, Acquired Immune Disease, and Autoimmune Diseases, Including Primary Immune Deficiency, Acquired Immunodeficiency Syndrome (AIDS), Lupus, Multiple Sclerosis, Type 1 Diabetes, Rheumatoid Arthritis, and Graves' Disease

Along with Treatments, Tips for Coping with Immune Disorders, a Glossary, and a Directory of Additional Resources.

Edited by Joyce Brennfleck Shannon. 671 pages. 2005. 978-0-7808-0748-8.

"Highly recommended for academic and public libraries." — *American Reference Books Annual, 2006*

"The updated second edition is a 'must' for any consumer health library seeking a solid resource covering the treatments, symptoms, and options for immune disorder sufferers. . . . An excellent guide."
— *MBR Bookwatch, Jan '06*

■

Infant & Toddler Health Sourcebook

Basic Consumer Health Information about the Physical and Mental Development of Newborns, Infants, and Toddlers, Including Neonatal Concerns, Nutrition Recommendations, Immunization Schedules, Common Pediatric Disorders, Assessments and Milestones, Safety Tips, and Advice for Parents and Other Caregivers

Along with a Glossary of Terms and Resource Listings for Additional Help

Edited by Jenifer Swanson. 585 pages. 2000. 978-0-7808-0246-9.

"As a reference for the general public, this would be useful in any library." — *E-Streams, May '01*

"Recommended reference source."
— *Booklist, American Library Association, Feb '01*

"This is a good source for general use."
— *American Reference Books Annual, 2001*

■

Infectious Diseases Sourcebook

Basic Consumer Health Information about Non-Contagious Bacterial, Viral, Prion, Fungal, and Parasitic Diseases Spread by Food and Water, Insects and Animals, or Environmental Contact, Including Botulism, E. Coli, Encephalitis, Legionnaires' Disease, Lyme Disease, Malaria, Plague, Rabies, Salmonella, Tetanus, and Others, and Facts about Newly Emerging Diseases, Such as Hantavirus, Mad Cow Disease, Monkeypox, and West Nile Virus

Along with Information about Preventing Disease Transmission, the Threat of Bioterrorism, and Current Research Initiatives, with a Glossary and Directory of Resources for More Information

Edited by Karen Bellenir. 634 pages. 2004. 978-0-7808-0675-7.

"This reference continues the excellent tradition of the *Health Reference Series* in consolidating a wealth of information on a selected topic into a format that is easy to use and accessible to the general public."
— *American Reference Books Annual, 2005*

"Recommended for public and academic libraries."
— *E-Streams, Jan '05*

Injury & Trauma Sourcebook

Basic Consumer Health Information about the Impact of Injury, the Diagnosis and Treatment of Common and Traumatic Injuries, Emergency Care, and Specific Injuries Related to Home, Community, Workplace, Transportation, and Recreation

Along with Guidelines for Injury Prevention, a Glossary, and a Directory of Additional Resources

Edited by Joyce Brennfleck Shannon. 696 pages. 2002. 978-0-7808-0421-0.

"This publication is the most comprehensive work of its kind about injury and trauma."
— *American Reference Books Annual, 2003*

"This sourcebook provides concise, easily readable, basic health information about injuries. . . . This book is well organized and an easy to use reference resource suitable for hospital, health sciences and public libraries with consumer health collections."
— *E-Streams, Nov '02*

"Practitioners should be aware of guides such as this in order to facilitate their use by patients and their families."
— *Doody's Health Sciences Book Review Journal, Sep-Oct '02*

"Recommended reference source."
— *Booklist, American Library Association, Sep '02*

"Highly recommended for academic and medical reference collections." — *Library Bookwatch, Sep '02*

Kidney & Urinary Tract Diseases & Disorders Sourcebook

SEE Urinary Tract & Kidney Diseases & Disorders Sourcebook

Learning Disabilities Sourcebook, 2nd Edition

Basic Consumer Health Information about Learning Disabilities, Including Dyslexia, Developmental Speech and Language Disabilities, Non-Verbal Learning Disorders, Developmental Arithmetic Disorder, Developmental Writing Disorder, and Other Conditions That Impede Learning Such as Attention Deficit/Hyperactivity Disorder, Brain Injury, Hearing Impairment, Klinefelter Syndrome, Dyspraxia, and Tourette's Syndrome

Along with Facts about Educational Issues and Assistive Technology, Coping Strategies, a Glossary of Related Terms, and Resources for Further Help and Information

Edited by Dawn D. Matthews. 621 pages. 2003. 978-0-7808-0626-9.

"The second edition of Learning Disabilities Sourcebook far surpasses the earlier edition in that it is more focused on information that will be useful as a consumer health resource."
— *American Reference Books Annual, 2004*

"Teachers as well as consumers will find this an essential guide to understanding various syndromes and their latest treatments. [An] invaluable reference for public and school library collections alike."
— *Library Bookwatch, Apr '03*

Named "Outstanding Reference Book of 1999."
— *New York Public Library, Feb '00*

"An excellent candidate for inclusion in a public library reference section. It's a great source of information. Teachers will also find the book useful. Definitely worth reading."
— *Journal of Adolescent & Adult Literacy, Feb 2000*

"Readable . . . provides a solid base of information regarding successful techniques used with individuals who have learning disabilities, as well as practical suggestions for educators and family members. Clear language, concise descriptions, and pertinent information for contacting multiple resources add to the strength of this book as a useful tool." — *Choice, Association of College & Research Libraries, Feb '99*

"Recommended reference source."
— *Booklist, American Library Association, Sep '98*

"A useful resource for libraries and for those who don't have the time to identify and locate the individual publications." — *Disability Resources Monthly, Sep '98*

Leukemia Sourcebook

Basic Consumer Health Information about Adult and Childhood Leukemias, Including Acute Lymphocytic Leukemia (ALL), Chronic Lymphocytic Leukemia (CLL), Acute Myelogenous Leukemia (AML), Chronic Myelogenous Leukemia (CML), and Hairy Cell Leukemia, and Treatments Such as Chemotherapy, Radiation Therapy, Peripheral Blood Stem Cell and Marrow Transplantation, and Immunotherapy

Along with Tips for Life During and After Treatment, a Glossary, and Directories of Additional Resources

Edited by Joyce Brennfleck Shannon. 587 pages. 2003. 978-0-7808-0627-6.

"Unlike other medical books for the layperson, . . . the language does not talk down to the reader. . . . This volume is highly recommended for all libraries."
— *American Reference Books Annual, 2004*

". . . a fine title which ranges from diagnosis to alternative treatments, staging, and tips for life during and after diagnosis." — *The Bookwatch, Dec '03*

Liver Disorders Sourcebook

Basic Consumer Health Information about the Liver and How It Works; Liver Diseases, Including Cancer, Cirrhosis, Hepatitis, and Toxic and Drug Related Diseases; Tips for Maintaining a Healthy Liver; Laboratory Tests, Radiology Tests, and Facts about Liver Transplantation

Along with a Section on Support Groups, a Glossary, and Resource Listings

Edited by Joyce Brennfleck Shannon. 591 pages. 2000. 978-0-7808-0383-1.

"A valuable resource."
—American Reference Books Annual, 2001

"This title is recommended for health sciences and public libraries with consumer health collections."
— E-Streams, Oct '00

"Recommended reference source."
—Booklist, American Library Association, Jun '00

■

Lung Disorders Sourcebook

Basic Consumer Health Information about Emphysema, Pneumonia, Tuberculosis, Asthma, Cystic Fibrosis, and Other Lung Disorders, Including Facts about Diagnostic Procedures, Treatment Strategies, Disease Prevention Efforts, and Such Risk Factors as Smoking, Air Pollution, and Exposure to Asbestos, Radon, and Other Agents

Along with a Glossary and Resources for Additional Help and Information

Edited by Dawn D. Matthews. 678 pages. 2002. 978-0-7808-0339-8.

"This title is a great addition for public and school libraries because it provides concise health information on the lungs."
— American Reference Books Annual, 2003

"Highly recommended for academic and medical reference collections." *— Library Bookwatch, Sep '02*

SEE ALSO Respiratory Diseases & Disorders Sourcebook

■

Medical Tests Sourcebook, 2nd Edition

Basic Consumer Health Information about Medical Tests, Including Age-Specific Health Tests, Important Health Screenings and Exams, Home-Use Tests, Blood and Specimen Tests, Electrical Tests, Scope Tests, Genetic Testing, and Imaging Tests, Such as X-Rays, Ultrasound, Computed Tomography, Magnetic Resonance Imaging, Angiography, and Nuclear Medicine

Along with a Glossary and Directory of Additional Resources

Edited by Joyce Brennfleck Shannon. 654 pages. 2004. 978-0-7808-0670-2.

"Recommended for hospital and health sciences

libraries with consumer health collections."
—E-Streams, Mar '00

"This is an overall excellent reference with a wealth of general knowledge that may aid those who are reluctant to get vital tests performed."
—Today's Librarian, Jan '00

"A valuable reference guide."
—American Reference Books Annual, 2000

■

Men's Health Concerns Sourcebook, 2nd Edition

Basic Consumer Health Information about the Medical and Mental Concerns of Men, Including Theories about the Shorter Male Lifespan, the Leading Causes of Death and Disability, Physical Concerns of Special Significance to Men, Reproductive and Sexual Concerns, Sexually Transmitted Diseases, Men's Mental and Emotional Health, and Lifestyle Choices That Affect Wellness, Such as Nutrition, Fitness, and Substance Use

Along with a Glossary of Related Terms and a Directory of Organizational Resources in Men's Health

Edited by Robert Aquinas McNally. 644 pages. 2004. 978-0-7808-0671-9.

"A very accessible reference for non-specialist general readers and consumers." *— The Bookwatch, Jun '04*

"This comprehensive resource and the series are highly recommended."
—American Reference Books Annual, 2000

"Recommended reference source."
— Booklist, American Library Association, Dec '98

■

Mental Health Disorders Sourcebook, 3rd Edition

Basic Consumer Health Information about Mental and Emotional Health and Mental Illness, Including Facts about Depression, Bipolar Disorder, and Other Mood Disorders, Phobias, Post-Traumatic Stress Disorder (PTSD), Obsessive-Compulsive Disorder, and Other Anxiety Disorders, Impulse Control Disorders, Eating Disorders, Personality Disorders, and Psychotic Disorders, Including Schizophrenia and Dissociative Disorders

Along with Statistical Information, a Special Section Concerning Mental Health Issues in Children and Adolescents, a Glossary, and Directories of Resources for Additional Help and Information

Edited by Karen Bellenir. 661 pages. 2005. 978-0-7808-0747-1.

"Recommended for public libraries and academic libraries with an undergraduate program in psychology."
—American Reference Books Annual, 2006

"Recommended reference source."
—Booklist, American Library Association, Jun '00

Mental Retardation Sourcebook

Basic Consumer Health Information about Mental Retardation and Its Causes, Including Down Syndrome, Fetal Alcohol Syndrome, Fragile X Syndrome, Genetic Conditions, Injury, and Environmental Sources

Along with Preventive Strategies, Parenting Issues, Educational Implications, Health Care Needs, Employment and Economic Matters, Legal Issues, a Glossary, and a Resource Listing for Additional Help and Information

Edited by Joyce Brennfleck Shannon. 642 pages. 2000. 978-0-7808-0377-0.

"Public libraries will find the book useful for reference and as a beginning research point for students, parents, and caregivers."
— American Reference Books Annual, 2001

"The strength of this work is that it compiles many basic fact sheets and addresses for further information in one volume. It is intended and suitable for the general public. This sourcebook is relevant to any collection providing health information to the general public."
— E-Streams, Nov '00

"From preventing retardation to parenting and family challenges, this covers health, social and legal issues and will prove an invaluable overview."
— Reviewer's Bookwatch, Jul '00

Movement Disorders Sourcebook

Basic Consumer Health Information about Neurological Movement Disorders, Including Essential Tremor, Parkinson's Disease, Dystonia, Cerebral Palsy, Huntington's Disease, Myasthenia Gravis, Multiple Sclerosis, and Other Early-Onset and Adult-Onset Movement Disorders, Their Symptoms and Causes, Diagnostic Tests, and Treatments

Along with Mobility and Assistive Technology Information, a Glossary, and a Directory of Additional Resources

Edited by Joyce Brennfleck Shannon. 655 pages. 2003. 978-0-7808-0628-3.

". . . a good resource for consumers and recommended for public, community college and undergraduate libraries." *— American Reference Books Annual, 2004*

Muscular Dystrophy Sourcebook

Basic Consumer Health Information about Congenital, Childhood-Onset, and Adult-Onset Forms of Muscular Dystrophy, Such as Duchenne, Becker, Emery-Dreifuss, Distal, Limb-Girdle, Facioscapulohumeral (FSHD), Myotonic, and Ophthalmoplegic Muscular Dystrophies, Including Facts about Diagnostic Tests, Medical and Physical Therapies, Management of Co-Occurring Conditions, and Parenting Guidelines

Along with Practical Tips for Home Care, a Glossary, and Directories of Additional Resources

Edited by Joyce Brennfleck Shannon. 577 pages. 2004. 978-0-7808-0676-4.

"This book is highly recommended for public and academic libraries as well as health care offices that support the information needs of patients and their families."
— E-Streams, Apr '05

"Excellent reference." *— The Bookwatch, Jan '05*

Obesity Sourcebook

Basic Consumer Health Information about Diseases and Other Problems Associated with Obesity, and Including Facts about Risk Factors, Prevention Issues, and Management Approaches

Along with Statistical and Demographic Data, Information about Special Populations, Research Updates, a Glossary, and Source Listings for Further Help and Information

Edited by Wilma Caldwell and Chad T. Kimball. 376 pages. 2001. 978-0-7808-0333-6.

"The book synthesizes the reliable medical literature on obesity into one easy-to-read and useful resource for the general public."
— American Reference Books Annual, 2002

"This is a very useful resource book for the lay public."
— Doody's Review Service, Nov '01

"Well suited for the health reference collection of a public library or an academic health science library that serves the general population." *— E-Streams, Sep '01*

"Recommended reference source."
— Booklist, American Library Association, Apr '01

"Recommended pick both for specialty health library collections and any general consumer health reference collection." *— The Bookwatch, Apr '01*

Oral Health Sourcebook

SEE *Dental Care & Oral Health Sourcebook*

Osteoporosis Sourcebook

Basic Consumer Health Information about Primary and Secondary Osteoporosis and Juvenile Osteoporosis and Related Conditions, Including Fibrous Dysplasia, Gaucher Disease, Hyperthyroidism, Hypophosphatasia, Myeloma, Osteopetrosis, Osteogenesis Imperfecta, and Paget's Disease

Along with Information about Risk Factors, Treatments, Traditional and Non-Traditional Pain Management, a Glossary of Related Terms, and a Directory of Resources

Edited by Allan R. Cook. 584 pages. 2001. 978-0-7808-0239-1.

"This would be a book to be kept in a staff or patient library. The targeted audience is the layperson, but the therapist who needs a quick bit of information on a particular topic will also find the book useful."
— Physical Therapy, Jan '02

"This resource is recommended as a great reference source for public, health, and academic libraries, and is another triumph for the editors of Omnigraphics."
— *American Reference Books Annual, 2002*

"Recommended for all public libraries and general health collections, especially those supporting patient education or consumer health programs."
— *E-Streams, Nov '01*

"Will prove valuable to any library seeking to maintain a current, comprehensive reference collection of health resources. . . . From prevention to treatment and associated conditions, this provides an excellent survey."
— *The Bookwatch, Aug '01*

"Recommended reference source."
— *Booklist, American Library Association, Jul '01*

SEE ALSO *Healthy Aging Sourcebook, Physical & Mental Issues in Aging Sourcebook, Women's Health Concerns Sourcebook*

■

Pain Sourcebook, 2nd Edition

Basic Consumer Health Information about Specific Forms of Acute and Chronic Pain, Including Muscle and Skeletal Pain, Nerve Pain, Cancer Pain, and Disorders Characterized by Pain, Such as Fibromyalgia, Shingles, Angina, Arthritis, and Headaches

Along with Information about Pain Medications and Management Techniques, Complementary and Alternative Pain Relief Options, Tips for People Living with Chronic Pain, a Glossary, and a Directory of Sources for Further Information

Edited by Karen Bellenir. 670 pages. 2002. 978-0-7808-0612-2.

"A source of valuable information. . . . This book offers help to nonmedical people who need information about pain and pain management. It is also an excellent reference for those who participate in patient education."
— *Doody's Review Service, Sep '02*

"Highly recommended for academic and medical reference collections." — *Library Bookwatch, Sep '02*

"The text is readable, easily understood, and well indexed. This excellent volume belongs in all patient education libraries, consumer health sections of public libraries, and many personal collections."
— *American Reference Books Annual, 1999*

"The information is basic in terms of scholarship and is appropriate for general readers. Written in journalistic style . . . intended for non-professionals. Quite thorough in its coverage of different pain conditions and summarizes the latest clinical information regarding pain treatment." — *Choice, Association of College and Research Libraries, Jun '98*

"Recommended reference source."
— *Booklist, American Library Association, Mar '98*

■

Pediatric Cancer Sourcebook

Basic Consumer Health Information about Leukemias, Brain Tumors, Sarcomas, Lymphomas, and Other Cancers in Infants, Children, and Adolescents, Including Descriptions of Cancers, Treatments, and Coping Strategies

Along with Suggestions for Parents, Caregivers, and Concerned Relatives, a Glossary of Cancer Terms, and Resource Listings

Edited by Edward J. Prucha. 587 pages. 1999. 978-0-7808-0245-2.

"An excellent source of information. Recommended for public, hospital, and health science libraries with consumer health collections." — *E-Streams, Jun '00*

"Recommended reference source."
— *Booklist, American Library Association, Feb '00*

"A valuable addition to all libraries specializing in health services and many public libraries."
— *American Reference Books Annual, 2000*

SEE ALSO *Childhood Diseases & Disorders Sourcebook, Healthy Children Sourcebook*

■

Physical & Mental Issues in Aging Sourcebook

Basic Consumer Health Information on Physical and Mental Disorders Associated with the Aging Process, Including Concerns about Cardiovascular Disease, Pulmonary Disease, Oral Health, Digestive Disorders, Musculoskeletal and Skin Disorders, Metabolic Changes, Sexual and Reproductive Issues, and Changes in Vision, Hearing, and Other Senses

Along with Data about Longevity and Causes of Death, Information on Acute and Chronic Pain, Descriptions of Mental Concerns, a Glossary of Terms, and Resource Listings for Additional Help

Edited by Jenifer Swanson. 660 pages. 1999. 978-0-7808-0233-9.

"This is a treasure of health information for the layperson." — *Choice Health Sciences Supplement, Association of College & Research Libraries, May '00*

"Recommended for public libraries."
— *American Reference Books Annual, 2000*

"Recommended reference source."
— *Booklist, American Library Association, Oct '99*

SEE ALSO *Healthy Aging Sourcebook*

■

Podiatry Sourcebook, 2nd Edition

Basic Consumer Health Information about Disorders, Diseases, Deformities, and Injuries that Affect the Foot and Ankle, Including Sprains, Corns, Calluses, Bunions, Plantar Warts, Plantar Fasciitis, Neuromas, Clubfoot, Flat Feet, Achilles Tendonitis, and Much More

Along with Information about Selecting a Foot Care Specialist, Foot Fitness, Shoes and Socks, Diagnostic Tests and Corrective Procedures, Financial Assistance for Corrective Devices, a Glossary of Related Terms, and a Directory of Resources for Additional Help and Information

Edited by Ivy L. Alexander. 543 pages. 2007. 978-0-7808-0944-4.

"**Recommended reference source.**"
— *Booklist, American Library Association, Feb '02*

"**There is a lot of information presented here on a topic that is usually only covered sparingly in most larger comprehensive medical encyclopedias.**"
— *American Reference Books Annual, 2002*

∎

Pregnancy & Birth Sourcebook, 2nd Edition

Basic Consumer Health Information about Conception and Pregnancy, Including Facts about Fertility, Infertility, Pregnancy Symptoms and Complications, Fetal Growth and Development, Labor, Delivery, and the Postpartum Period, as Well as Information about Maintaining Health and Wellness during Pregnancy and Caring for a Newborn

Along with Information about Public Health Assistance for Low-Income Pregnant Women, a Glossary, and Directories of Agencies and Organizations Providing Help and Support

Edited by Amy L. Sutton. 626 pages. 2004. 978-0-7808-0672-6.

"**Will appeal to public and school reference collections strong in medicine and women's health. . . . Deserves a spot on any medical reference shelf.**"
— *The Bookwatch, Jul '04*

"**A well-organized handbook. Recommended.**"
— *Choice, Association of College & Research Libraries, Apr '98*

"**Recommended reference source.**"
— *Booklist, American Library Association, Mar '98*

"**Recommended for public libraries.**"
— *American Reference Books Annual, 1998*

SEE ALSO *Breastfeeding Sourcebook, Congenital Disorders Sourcebook, Family Planning Sourcebook*

∎

Prostate & Urological Disorders Sourcebook

Basic Consumer Health Information about Urogenital and Sexual Disorders in Men, Including Prostate and Other Andrological Cancers, Prostatitis, Benign Prostatic Hyperplasia, Testicular and Penile Trauma, Cryptorchidism, Peyronie Disease, Erectile Dysfunction, and Male Factor Infertility, and Facts about Commonly Used Tests and Procedures, Such as Prostatectomy, Vasectomy, Vasectomy Reversal, Penile Implants, and Semen Analysis

Along with a Glossary of Andrological Terms and a Directory of Resources for Additional Information

Edited by Karen Bellenir. 631 pages. 2005. 978-0-7808-0797-6.

Prostate Cancer Sourcebook

Basic Consumer Health Information about Prostate Cancer, Including Information about the Associated Risk Factors, Detection, Diagnosis, and Treatment of Prostate Cancer

Along with Information on Non-Malignant Prostate Conditions, and Featuring a Section Listing Support and Treatment Centers and a Glossary of Related Terms

Edited by Dawn D. Matthews. 358 pages. 2001. 978-0-7808-0324-4.

"**Recommended reference source.**"
— *Booklist, American Library Association, Jan '02*

"**A valuable resource for health care consumers seeking information on the subject. . . . All text is written in a clear, easy-to-understand language that avoids technical jargon. Any library that collects consumer health resources would strengthen their collection with the addition of the** *Prostate Cancer Sourcebook.*"
— *American Reference Books Annual, 2002*

SEE ALSO *Men's Health Concerns Sourcebook*

∎

Reconstructive & Cosmetic Surgery Sourcebook

Basic Consumer Health Information on Cosmetic and Reconstructive Plastic Surgery, Including Statistical Information about Different Surgical Procedures, Things to Consider Prior to Surgery, Plastic Surgery Techniques and Tools, Emotional and Psychological Considerations, and Procedure-Specific Information

Along with a Glossary of Terms and a Listing of Resources for Additional Help and Information

Edited by M. Lisa Weatherford. 374 pages. 2001. 978-0-7808-0214-8.

"**An excellent reference that addresses cosmetic and medically necessary reconstructive surgeries. . . . The style of the prose is calm and reassuring, discussing the many positive outcomes now available due to advances in surgical techniques.**"
— *American Reference Books Annual, 2002*

"**Recommended for health science libraries that are open to the public, as well as hospital libraries that are open to the patients. This book is a good resource for the consumer interested in plastic surgery.**"
— *E-Streams, Dec '01*

"**Recommended reference source.**"
— *Booklist, American Library Association, Jul '01*

∎

Rehabilitation Sourcebook

Basic Consumer Health Information about Rehabilitation for People Recovering from Heart Surgery, Spinal Cord Injury, Stroke, Orthopedic Impairments, Amputation, Pulmonary Impairments, Traumatic Injury, and More, Including Physical Therapy, Occupational Therapy, Speech/Language Therapy, Massage Therapy, Dance Therapy, Art Therapy, and Recreational Therapy

Along with Information on Assistive and Adaptive Devices, a Glossary, and Resources for Additional Help and Information

Edited by Dawn D. Matthews. 531 pages. 1999. 978-0-7808-0236-0.

"This is an excellent resource for public library reference and health collections."
— *American Reference Books Annual, 2001*

"Recommended reference source."
— *Booklist, American Library Association, May '00*

■

Respiratory Diseases & Disorders Sourcebook

Basic Information about Respiratory Diseases and Disorders, Including Asthma, Cystic Fibrosis, Pneumonia, the Common Cold, Influenza, and Others, Featuring Facts about the Respiratory System, Statistical and Demographic Data, Treatments, Self-Help Management Suggestions, and Current Research Initiatives

Edited by Allan R. Cook and Peter D. Dresser. 771 pages. 1995. 978-0-7808-0037-3.

"Designed for the layperson and for patients and their families coping with respiratory illness. . . . an extensive array of information on diagnosis, treatment, management, and prevention of respiratory illnesses for the general reader." — *Choice, Association of College & Research Libraries, Jun '96*

"A highly recommended text for all collections. It is a comforting reminder of the power of knowledge that good books carry between their covers."
— *Academic Library Book Review, Spring '96*

"A comprehensive collection of authoritative information presented in a nontechnical, humanitarian style for patients, families, and caregivers."
— *Association of Operating Room Nurses, Sep/Oct '95*

SEE ALSO *Lung Disorders Sourcebook*

■

Sexually Transmitted Diseases Sourcebook, 3rd Edition

Basic Consumer Health Information about Chlamydial Infections, Gonorrhea, Hepatitis, Herpes, HIV/AIDS, Human Papillomavirus, Pubic Lice, Scabies, Syphilis, Trichomoniasis, Vaginal Infections, and Other Sexually Transmitted Diseases, Including Facts about Risk Factors, Symptoms, Diagnosis, Treatment, and the Prevention of Sexually Transmitted Infections

Along with Updates on Current Research Initiatives, a Glossary of Related Terms, and Resources for Additional Help and Information

Edited by Amy L. Sutton. 629 pages. 2006. 978-0-7808-0824-9.

"Recommended for consumer health collections in public libraries, and secondary school and community college libraries."
— *American Reference Books Annual, 2002*

"Every school and public library should have a copy of this comprehensive and user-friendly reference book."
— *Choice, Association of College & Research Libraries, Sep '01*

"This is a highly recommended book. This is an especially important book for all school and public libraries."
— *AIDS Book Review Journal, Jul-Aug '01*

"Recommended reference source."
— *Booklist, American Library Association, Apr '01*

■

Sleep Disorders Sourcebook, 2nd Edition

Basic Consumer Health Information about Sleep and Sleep Disorders, Including Insomnia, Sleep Apnea, Restless Legs Syndrome, Narcolepsy, Parasomnias, and Other Health Problems That Affect Sleep, Plus Facts about Diagnostic Procedures, Treatment Strategies, Sleep Medications, and Tips for Improving Sleep Quality

Along with a Glossary of Related Terms and Resources for Additional Help and Information

Edited by Amy L. Sutton. 567 pages. 2005. 978-0-7808-0743-3.

"This book will be useful for just about everybody, especially the 40 million Americans with sleep disorders."
— *American Reference Books Annual, 2006*

"Recommended for public libraries and libraries supporting health care professionals." — *E-Streams, Sep '05*

". . . key medical library acquisition."
— *The Bookwatch, Jun '05*

■

Smoking Concerns Sourcebook

Basic Consumer Health Information about Nicotine Addiction and Smoking Cessation, Featuring Facts about the Health Effects of Tobacco Use, Including Lung and Other Cancers, Heart Disease, Stroke, and Respiratory Disorders, Such as Emphysema and Chronic Bronchitis

Along with Information about Smoking Prevention Programs, Suggestions for Achieving and Maintaining a Smoke-Free Lifestyle, Statistics about Tobacco Use, Reports on Current Research Initiatives, a Glossary of Related Terms, and Directories of Resources for Additional Help and Information

Edited by Karen Bellenir. 621 pages. 2004. 978-0-7808-0323-7.

"Provides everything needed for the student or general reader seeking practical details on the effects of tobacco use." — *The Bookwatch, Mar '05*

"Public libraries and consumer health care libraries will find this work useful."
— *American Reference Books Annual, 2005*

Sports Injuries Sourcebook, 3rd Edition

Basic Consumer Health Information about Sprains and Strains, Fractures, Growth Plate Injuries, Overtraining Injuries, and Injuries to the Head, Face, Shoulders, Elbows, Hands, Spinal Column, Knees, Ankles, and Feet, and with Facts about Heat-Related Illness, Steroids and Sport Supplements, Protective Equipment, Diagnostic Procedures, Treatment Options, and Rehabilitation

Along with a Glossary of Related Terms and a Directory of Resources for Additional Help and Information

Edited by Sandra J. Judd. 651 pages. 2007. 978-0-7808-0949-9.

"This is an excellent reference for consumers and it is recommended for public, community college, and undergraduate libraries."
— *American Reference Books Annual, 2003*

"Recommended reference source."
— *Booklist, American Library Association, Feb '03*

∎

Stress-Related Disorders Sourcebook

Basic Consumer Health Information about Stress and Stress-Related Disorders, Including Stress Origins and Signals, Environmental Stress at Work and Home, Mental and Emotional Stress Associated with Depression, Post-Traumatic Stress Disorder, Panic Disorder, Suicide, and the Physical Effects of Stress on the Cardiovascular, Immune, and Nervous Systems

Along with Stress Management Techniques, a Glossary, and a Listing of Additional Resources

Edited by Joyce Brennfleck Shannon. 610 pages. 2002. 978-0-7808-0560-6.

"Well written for a general readership, the *Stress-Related Disorders Sourcebook* is a useful addition to the health reference literature."
— *American Reference Books Annual, 2003*

"I am impressed by the amount of information. It offers a thorough overview of the causes and consequences of stress for the layperson. . . . A well-done and thorough reference guide for professionals and nonprofessionals alike."
— *Doody's Review Service, Dec '02*

∎

Stroke Sourcebook

Basic Consumer Health Information about Stroke, Including Ischemic, Hemorrhagic, Transient Ischemic Attack (TIA), and Pediatric Stroke, Stroke Triggers and Risks, Diagnostic Tests, Treatments, and Rehabilitation Information

Along with Stroke Prevention Guidelines, Legal and Financial Information, a Glossary, and a Directory of Additional Resources

Edited by Joyce Brennfleck Shannon. 606 pages. 2003. 978-0-7808-0630-6.

"This volume is highly recommended and should be in every medical, hospital, and public library."
— *American Reference Books Annual, 2004*

"Highly recommended for the amount and variety of topics and information covered." — *Choice, Nov '03*

∎

Surgery Sourcebook

Basic Consumer Health Information about Inpatient and Outpatient Surgeries, Including Cardiac, Vascular, Orthopedic, Ocular, Reconstructive, Cosmetic, Gynecologic, and Ear, Nose, and Throat Procedures and More

Along with Information about Operating Room Policies and Instruments, Laser Surgery Techniques, Hospital Errors, Statistical Data, a Glossary, and Listings of Sources for Further Help and Information

Edited by Annemarie S. Muth and Karen Bellenir. 596 pages. 2002. 978-0-7808-0380-0.

"Large public libraries and medical libraries would benefit from this material in their reference collections."
— *American Reference Books Annual, 2004*

"Invaluable reference for public and school library collections alike." — *Library Bookwatch, Apr '03*

∎

Thyroid Disorders Sourcebook

Basic Consumer Health Information about Disorders of the Thyroid and Parathyroid Glands, Including Hypothyroidism, Hyperthyroidism, Graves Disease, Hashimoto Thyroiditis, Thyroid Cancer, and Parathyroid Disorders, Featuring Facts about Symptoms, Risk Factors, Tests, and Treatments

Along with Information about the Effects of Thyroid Imbalance on Other Body Systems, Environmental Factors That Affect the Thyroid Gland, a Glossary, and a Directory of Additional Resources

Edited by Joyce Brennfleck Shannon. 599 pages. 2005. 978-0-7808-0745-7.

"Recommended for consumer health collections."
— *American Reference Books Annual, 2006*

"Highly recommended pick for basic consumer health reference holdings at all levels."
— *The Bookwatch, Aug '05*

∎

Transplantation Sourcebook

Basic Consumer Health Information about Organ and Tissue Transplantation, Including Physical and Financial Preparations, Procedures and Issues Relating to Specific Solid Organ and Tissue Transplants, Rehabilitation, Pediatric Transplant Information, the Future of Transplantation, and Organ and Tissue Donation

Along with a Glossary and Listings of Additional Resources

Edited by Joyce Brennfleck Shannon. 628 pages. 2002. 978-0-7808-0322-0.

"Along with these advances [in transplantation technology] have come a number of daunting questions for potential transplant patients, their families, and their health care providers. This reference text is the best single tool to address many of these questions. . . . It will be a much-needed addition to the reference collections in health care, academic, and large public libraries."
— *American Reference Books Annual, 2003*

"Recommended for libraries with an interest in offering consumer health information." — *E-Streams, Jul '02*

"This is a unique and valuable resource for patients facing transplantation and their families."
— *Doody's Review Service, Jun '02*

■

Traveler's Health Sourcebook

Basic Consumer Health Information for Travelers, Including Physical and Medical Preparations, Transportation Health and Safety, Essential Information about Food and Water, Sun Exposure, Insect and Snake Bites, Camping and Wilderness Medicine, and Travel with Physical or Medical Disabilities

Along with International Travel Tips, Vaccination Recommendations, Geographical Health Issues, Disease Risks, a Glossary, and a Listing of Additional Resources

Edited by Joyce Brennfleck Shannon. 613 pages. 2000. 978-0-7808-0384-8.

"Recommended reference source."
— *Booklist, American Library Association, Feb '01*

"This book is recommended for any public library, any travel collection, and especially any collection for the physically disabled."
— *American Reference Books Annual, 2001*

SEE ALSO *Worldwide Health Sourcebook*

■

Urinary Tract & Kidney Diseases & Disorders Sourcebook, 2nd Edition

Basic Consumer Health Information about the Urinary System, Including the Bladder, Urethra, Ureters, and Kidneys, with Facts about Urinary Tract Infections, Incontinence, Congenital Disorders, Kidney Stones, Cancers of the Urinary Tract and Kidneys, Kidney Failure, Dialysis, and Kidney Transplantation

Along with Statistical and Demographic Information, Reports on Current Research in Kidney and Urologic Health, a Summary of Commonly Used Diagnostic Tests, a Glossary of Related Terms, and a Directory of Resources for Additional Help and Information

Edited by Ivy L. Alexander. 649 pages. 2005. 978-0-7808-0750-1.

"A good choice for a consumer health information library or for a medical library needing information to refer to their patients."
— *American Reference Books Annual, 2006*

Vegetarian Sourcebook

Basic Consumer Health Information about Vegetarian Diets, Lifestyle, and Philosophy, Including Definitions of Vegetarianism and Veganism, Tips about Adopting Vegetarianism, Creating a Vegetarian Pantry, and Meeting Nutritional Needs of Vegetarians, with Facts Regarding Vegetarianism's Effect on Pregnant and Lactating Women, Children, Athletes, and Senior Citizens

Along with a Glossary of Commonly Used Vegetarian Terms and Resources for Additional Help and Information

Edited by Chad T. Kimball. 360 pages. 2002. 978-0-7808-0439-5.

"Organizes into one concise volume the answers to the most common questions concerning vegetarian diets and lifestyles. This title is recommended for public and secondary school libraries." — *E-Streams, Apr '03*

"Invaluable reference for public and school library collections alike." — *Library Bookwatch, Apr '03*

"The articles in this volume are easy to read and come from authoritative sources. The book does not necessarily support the vegetarian diet but instead provides the pros and cons of this important decision. The **Vegetarian Sourcebook** is recommended for public libraries and consumer health libraries."
— *American Reference Books Annual, 2003*

SEE ALSO *Diet & Nutrition Sourcebook*

■

Women's Health Concerns Sourcebook, 2nd Edition

Basic Consumer Health Information about the Medical and Mental Concerns of Women, Including Maintaining Health and Wellness, Gynecological Concerns, Breast Health, Sexuality and Reproductive Issues, Menopause, Cancer in Women, Leading Causes of Death and Disability among Women, Physical Concerns of Special Significance to Women, and Women's Mental and Emotional Health

Along with a Glossary of Related Terms and Directories of Resources for Additional Help and Information

Edited by Amy L. Sutton. 746 pages. 2004. 978-0-7808-0673-3.

"This is a useful reference book, which makes the reader knowledgeable about several issues that concern women's health. It is recommended for public libraries and home library collections." — *E-Streams, May '05*

"A useful addition to public and consumer health library collections."
— *American Reference Books Annual, 2005*

"A highly recommended title."
— *The Bookwatch, May '04*

"Handy compilation. There is an impressive range of diseases, devices, disorders, procedures, and other physical and emotional issues covered . . . well organized, illustrated, and indexed." — *Choice, Association of College & Research Libraries, Jan '98*

SEE ALSO *Breast Cancer Sourcebook, Cancer Sourcebook for Women, Healthy Heart Sourcebook for Women, Osteoporosis Sourcebook*

Workplace Health & Safety Sourcebook

Basic Consumer Health Information about Workplace Health and Safety, Including the Effect of Workplace Hazards on the Lungs, Skin, Heart, Ears, Eyes, Brain, Reproductive Organs, Musculoskeletal System, and Other Organs and Body Parts

Along with Information about Occupational Cancer, Personal Protective Equipment, Toxic and Hazardous Chemicals, Child Labor, Stress, and Workplace Violence

Edited by Chad T. Kimball. 626 pages. 2000. 978-0-7808-0231-5.

"As a reference for the general public, this would be useful in any library."
— *E-Streams, Jun '01*

"Provides helpful information for primary care physicians and other caregivers interested in occupational medicine.... General readers; professionals."
— *Choice, Association of College & Research Libraries, May '01*

"Recommended reference source."
— *Booklist, American Library Association, Feb '01*

"Highly recommended."   — *The Bookwatch, Jan '01*

Worldwide Health Sourcebook

Basic Information about Global Health Issues, Including Malnutrition, Reproductive Health, Disease Dispersion and Prevention, Emerging Diseases, Risky Health Behaviors, and the Leading Causes of Death

Along with Global Health Concerns for Children, Women, and the Elderly, Mental Health Issues, Research and Technology Advancements, and Economic, Environmental, and Political Health Implications, a Glossary, and a Resource Listing for Additional Help and Information

Edited by Joyce Brennfleck Shannon. 614 pages. 2001. 978-0-7808-0330-5.

"Named an Outstanding Academic Title."
— *Choice, Association of College & Research Libraries, Jan '02*

"Yet another handy but also unique compilation in the extensive *Health Reference Series*, this is a useful work because many of the international publications reprinted or excerpted are not readily available. Highly recommended."   — *Choice, Association of College & Research Libraries, Nov '01*

"Recommended reference source."
— *Booklist, American Library Association, Oct '01*

SEE ALSO *Traveler's Health Sourcebook*

Teen Health Series

Helping Young Adults Understand, Manage,
and Avoid Serious Illness

List price $65 per volume. **School and library price $58 per volume.**

Alcohol Information for Teens
Health Tips about Alcohol and Alcoholism
Including Facts about Underage Drinking, Preventing Teen Alcohol Use, Alcohol's Effects on the Brain and the Body, Alcohol Abuse Treatment, Help for Children of Alcoholics, and More

Edited by Joyce Brennfleck Shannon. 370 pages. 2005. 978-0-7808-0741-9.

"Boxed facts and tips add visual interest to the well-researched and clearly written text."
— *Curriculum Connection, Apr '06*

Allergy Information for Teens
Health Tips about Allergic Reactions Such as Anaphylaxis, Respiratory Problems, and Rashes
Including Facts about Identifying and Managing Allergies to Food, Pollen, Mold, Animals, Chemicals, Drugs, and Other Substances

Edited by Karen Bellenir. 410 pages. 2006. 978-0-7808-0799-0.

Asthma Information for Teens
Health Tips about Managing Asthma and Related Concerns
Including Facts about Asthma Causes, Triggers, Symptoms, Diagnosis, and Treatment

Edited by Karen Bellenir. 386 pages. 2005. 978-0-7808-0770-9.

"Highly recommended for medical libraries, public school libraries, and public libraries."
— *American Reference Books Annual, 2006*

"It is so clearly written and well organized that even hesitant readers will be able to find the facts they need, whether for reports or personal information. . . . A succinct but complete resource."
— *School Library Journal, Sep '05*

Body Information for Teens
Health Tips about Maintaining Well-Being for a Lifetime
Including Facts about the Development and Functioning of the Body's Systems, Organs, and Structures and the Health Impact of Lifestyle Choices

Edited by Sandra Augustyn Lawton. 458 pages. 2007. 978-0-7808-0443-2.

Cancer Information for Teens
Health Tips about Cancer Awareness, Prevention, Diagnosis, and Treatment
Including Facts about Frequently Occurring Cancers, Cancer Risk Factors, and Coping Strategies for Teens Fighting Cancer or Dealing with Cancer in Friends or Family Members

Edited by Wilma R. Caldwell. 428 pages. 2004. 978-0-7808-0678-8.

"Recommended for school libraries, or consumer libraries that see a lot of use by teens."
— *E-Streams, May '05*

"A valuable educational tool."
— *American Reference Books Annual, 2005*

"Young adults and their parents alike will find this new addition to the *Teen Health Series* an important reference to cancer in teens."
— *Children's Bookwatch, Feb '05*

Complementary and Alternative Medicine Information for Teens
Health Tips about Non-Traditional and Non-Western Medical Practices
Including Information about Acupuncture, Chiropractic Medicine, Dietary and Herbal Supplements, Hypnosis, Massage Therapy, Prayer and Spirituality, Reflexology, Yoga, and More

Edited by Sandra Augustyn Lawton. 405 pages. 2006. 978-0-7808-0966-6.

Diabetes Information for Teens
Health Tips about Managing Diabetes and Preventing Related Complications
Including Information about Insulin, Glucose Control, Healthy Eating, Physical Activity, and Learning to Live with Diabetes

Edited by Sandra Augustyn Lawton. 410 pages. 2006. 978-0-7808-0811-9.

Diet Information for Teens, 2nd Edition

Health Tips about Diet and Nutrition

Including Facts about Dietary Guidelines, Food Groups, Nutrients, Healthy Meals, Snacks, Weight Control, Medical Concerns Related to Diet, and More

Edited by Karen Bellenir. 432 pages. 2006. 978-0-7808-0820-1.

"Full of helpful insights and facts throughout the book. . . . An excellent resource to be placed in public libraries or even in personal collections."
— *American Reference Books Annual, 2002*

"Recommended for middle and high school libraries and media centers as well as academic libraries that educate future teachers of teenagers. It is also a suitable addition to health science libraries that serve patrons who are interested in teen health promotion and education."
— *E-Streams, Oct '01*

"This comprehensive book would be beneficial to collections that need information about nutrition, dietary guidelines, meal planning, and weight control. . . . This reference is so easy to use that its purchase is recommended."
— *The Book Report, Sep-Oct '01*

"This book is written in an easy to understand format describing issues that many teens face every day, and then provides thoughtful explanations so that teens can make informed decisions. This is an interesting book that provides important facts and information for today's teens."
— *Doody's Health Sciences Book Review Journal, Jul-Aug '01*

"A comprehensive compendium of diet and nutrition. The information is presented in a straightforward, plain-spoken manner. This title will be useful to those working on reports on a variety of topics, as well as to general readers concerned about their dietary health."
— *School Library Journal, Jun '01*

Drug Information for Teens, 2nd Edition

Health Tips about the Physical and Mental Effects of Substance Abuse

Including Information about Marijuana, Inhalants, Club Drugs, Stimulants, Hallucinogens, Opiates, Prescription and Over-the-Counter Drugs, Herbal Products, Tobacco, Alcohol, and More

Edited by Sandra Augustyn Lawton. 468 pages. 2006. 978-0-7808-0862-1.

"A clearly written resource for general readers and researchers alike."
— *School Library Journal*

"This book is well-balanced. . . . a must for public and school libraries."
— *VOYA: Voice of Youth Advocates, Dec '03*

"The chapters are quick to make a connection to their teenage reading audience. The prose is straightforward and the book lends itself to spot reading. It should be useful both for practical information and for research, and it is suitable for public and school libraries."
— *American Reference Books Annual, 2003*

"Recommended reference source."
— *Booklist, American Library Association, Feb '03*

"This is an excellent resource for teens and their parents. Education about drugs and substances is key to discouraging teen drug abuse and this book provides this much needed information in a way that is interesting and factual."
— *Doody's Review Service, Dec '02*

Eating Disorders Information for Teens

Health Tips about Anorexia, Bulimia, Binge Eating, and Other Eating Disorders

Including Information on the Causes, Prevention, and Treatment of Eating Disorders, and Such Other Issues as Maintaining Healthy Eating and Exercise Habits

Edited by Sandra Augustyn Lawton. 337 pages. 2005. 978-0-7808-0783-9.

"An excellent resource for teens and those who work with them."
— *VOYA: Voice of Youth Advocates, Apr '06*

"A welcome addition to high school and undergraduate libraries." — *American Reference Books Annual, 2006*

"This book covers the topic in a lucid manner but delves deeper into every aspect of an eating disorder. A solid addition for any nonfiction or reference collection."
— *School Library Journal, Dec '05*

Fitness Information for Teens

Health Tips about Exercise, Physical Well-Being, and Health Maintenance

Including Facts about Aerobic and Anaerobic Conditioning, Stretching, Body Shape and Body Image, Sports Training, Nutrition, and Activities for Non-Athletes

Edited by Karen Bellenir. 425 pages. 2004. 978-0-7808-0679-5.

"Another excellent offering from Omnigraphics in their *Teen Health Series*. . . . This book will be a great addition to any public, junior high, senior high, or secondary school library."
— *American Reference Books Annual, 2005*

Learning Disabilities Information for Teens

Health Tips about Academic Skills Disorders and Other Disabilities That Affect Learning

Including Information about Common Signs of Learning Disabilities, School Issues, Learning to Live with a Learning Disability, and Other Related Issues

Edited by Sandra Augustyn Lawton. 337 pages. 2005. 978-0-7808-0796-9.

"This book provides a wealth of information for any reader interested in the signs, causes, and consequences

of learning disabilities, as well as related legal rights and educational interventions. . . . Public and academic libraries should want this title for both students and general readers."
— *American Reference Books Annual, 2006*

■

Mental Health Information for Teens, 2nd Edition

Health Tips about Mental Wellness and Mental Illness

Including Facts about Mental and Emotional Health, Depression and Other Mood Disorders, Anxiety Disorders, Behavior Disorders, Self-Injury, Psychosis, Schizophrenia, and More

Edited by Karen Bellenir. 400 pages. 2006. 978-0-7808-0863-8.

"In both language and approach, this user-friendly entry in the *Teen Health Series* is on target for teens needing information on mental health concerns."
— *Booklist, American Library Association, Jan '02*

"Readers will find the material accessible and informative, with the shaded notes, facts, and embedded glossary insets adding appropriately to the already interesting and succinct presentation."
— *School Library Journal, Jan '02*

"This title is highly recommended for any library that serves adolescents and parents/caregivers of adolescents."
— *E-Streams, Jan '02*

"Recommended for high school libraries and young adult collections in public libraries. Both health professionals and teenagers will find this book useful."
— *American Reference Books Annual, 2002*

"This is a nice book written to enlighten the society, primarily teenagers, about common teen mental health issues. It is highly recommended to teachers and parents as well as adolescents."
— *Doody's Review Service, Dec '01*

■

Sexual Health Information for Teens

Health Tips about Sexual Development, Human Reproduction, and Sexually Transmitted Diseases

Including Facts about Puberty, Reproductive Health, Chlamydia, Human Papillomavirus, Pelvic Inflammatory Disease, Herpes, AIDS, Contraception, Pregnancy, and More

Edited by Deborah A. Stanley. 391 pages. 2003. 978-0-7808-0445-6.

"This work should be included in all high school libraries and many larger public libraries. . . . highly recommended."
— *American Reference Books Annual, 2004*

"*Sexual Health* approaches its subject with appropriate seriousness and offers easily accessible advice and information."
— *School Library Journal, Feb '04*

Skin Health Information for Teens

Health Tips about Dermatological Concerns and Skin Cancer Risks

Including Facts about Acne, Warts, Hives, and Other Conditions and Lifestyle Choices, Such as Tanning, Tattooing, and Piercing, That Affect the Skin, Nails, Scalp, and Hair

Edited by Robert Aquinas McNally. 429 pages. 2003. 978-0-7808-0446-3.

"This volume, as with others in the series, will be a useful addition to school and public library collections."
— *American Reference Books Annual, 2004*

"There is no doubt that this reference tool is valuable."
— *VOYA: Voice of Youth Advocates, Feb '04*

"This volume serves as a one-stop source and should be a necessity for any health collection."
— *Library Media Connection*

■

Sports Injuries Information for Teens

Health Tips about Sports Injuries and Injury Protection

Including Facts about Specific Injuries, Emergency Treatment, Rehabilitation, Sports Safety, Competition Stress, Fitness, Sports Nutrition, Steroid Risks, and More

Edited by Joyce Brennfleck Shannon. 405 pages. 2003. 978-0-7808-0447-0.

"This work will be useful in the young adult collections of public libraries as well as high school libraries."
— *American Reference Books Annual, 2004*

■

Suicide Information for Teens

Health Tips about Suicide Causes and Prevention

Including Facts about Depression, Risk Factors, Getting Help, Survivor Support, and More

Edited by Joyce Brennfleck Shannon. 368 pages. 2005. 978-0-7808-0737-2.

■

Tobacco Information for Teens

Health Tips about the Hazards of Using Cigarettes, Smokeless Tobacco, and Other Nicotine Products

Including Facts about Nicotine Addiction, Immediate and Long-Term Health Effects of Tobacco Use, Related Cancers, Smoking Cessation, Tobacco Use Prevention, and Tobacco Use Statistics

Edited by Karen Bellenir. 440 pages. 2007. 978-0-7808-0976-5.

Health Reference Series